Orthomolecular Nutrition for Everyone

Megavitamins and Your Best Health Ever

HELEN SAUL CASE

AND 30 EXPERTS IN THE FIELD OF NUTRITIONAL MEDICINE

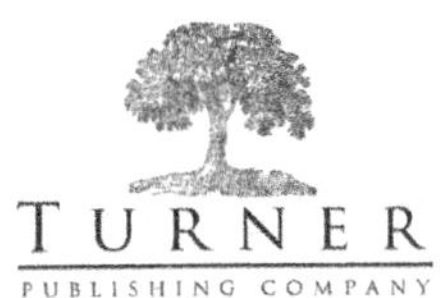

TURNER

PUBLISHING COMPANY

Turner Publishing Company
Nashville, Tennessee
New York, New York
www.turnerpublishing.com

Orthomolecular Nutrition for Everyone

The information contained in this book is based upon the research and personal and professional experiences of the author. It is not intended as a substitute for consulting with your physician or other healthcare provider. Any attempt to diagnose and treat an illness should be done under the direction of a healthcare professional.

The publisher does not advocate the use of any particular healthcare protocol but believes the information in this book should be available to the public. The publisher and author are not responsible for any adverse effects or consequences resulting from the use of the suggestions, preparations, or procedures discussed in this book. Should the reader have any questions concerning the appropriateness of any procedures or preparation mentioned, the author and the publisher strongly suggest consulting a professional healthcare advisor.

Library of Congress Cataloging-in-Publication Data
Names: Case, Helen Saul.
Title: Orthomolecular nutrition for everyone : megavitamins and your best health ever / Helen Saul Case.
Description: Nashville, Tennessee : Turner Publishing Company, [2017] | Includes bibliographical references.
Identifiers: LCCN 2016049160 | ISBN 9781681626574 (pbk. : alk. paper)
Subjects: LCSH: Orthomolecular therapy. | Vitamin therapy.
Classification: LCC RM217 .C38 2017 | DDC 615.3/28--dc23
LC record available at https://lccn.loc.gov/2016049160

Cover design: Maddie Cothren
Book design: Gary A. Rosenberg

Printed in the United States of America
10 9 8 7 6 5 4 3 2 1

Contents

Acknowledgments

Many thanks to Steven Carter, director of the International Society for Orthomolecular Medicine, for permission to include papers from the *Journal of Orthomolecular Medicine* (JOM). Thank you also to Jonathan E. Prousky, editor of JOM.

Thanks to the editorial board and contributors to the *Orthomolecular Medicine News Service.*

Special thanks are due to Thomas E. Levy, Ralph K. Campbell, and Jack Challem, "The Nutrition Reporter."

Thank you to all of the doctors and experts whose papers are included in this book, including Damien Downing, Nick Fortino, Harold D. Foster, Alan R. Gaby, Michael J. Gonzalez, William B. Grant, Claus Hancke, Rolf Hefti, Steve Hickey, James A. Jackson, Bo H. Jonsson, Christopher Lam, Stephen Lawson, Stuart Lindsey, Travis V. Meyer, Jorge R. Miranda-Massari, W. Todd Penberthy, Chris Revard, Hilary Roberts, Robert Sarver, Gert Schuitemaker, Robert G. Smith, Jerry Tiemeyer, Eddie Vos, Bradford S. Weeks, and Atsuo Yanagisawa.

Thank you to all the fathers and mothers of orthomolecular medicine, past and present, including Robert F. Cathcart, Adelle Davis, Ruth Flinn Harrell, Abram Hoffer, Frederick R. Klenner, and Hugh D. Riordan.

Thank you to my father, Andrew W. Saul, in particular. I am grateful to be your daughter and honored to be your colleague.

And thank you to my husband and both of my children for their constant love and support.

Foreword

Even today, orthomolecular medicine remains almost completely unknown to mainstream, traditional medical practitioners. Yet, in spite of this general unawareness, a small but steadily increasing number of such medical practitioners are beginning to realize that judicious vitamin, mineral, and nutrient supplementation does have a role to play in the wellness of their patients. However, the fact that proper supplementation can literally ***replace*** most prescription medicines is not even remotely appreciated. While it should not be stunning that the body responds better to the restoration of natural substances and nutrients when it is sick, most doctors still feel that the only truly effective therapies they have to offer their patients must be prescribed.

Helen Saul Case introduces the reader to orthomolecular medicine and its superior role in both reversing disease and maintaining good health. Quite literally, as initially put forth by Dr. Linus Pauling, the word "orthomolecular" means that the right molecules need to be given in the right amounts. Furthermore, it has now been well established that the right molecules to be given are those natural molecules that are depleted in the diseased tissues. In other words, orthomolecular medicine strives to restore a normal state in the body by reconstituting the levels of normal molecules both inside and outside the cells. Many cumulative years of clinical experience with this approach have now clearly demonstrated that when this can be achieved, the body heals itself very effectively. And prescription medications are only really indicated when this reconstitution of normalcy cannot be achieved and ongoing symptoms need to be suppressed in order to make the patient feel better.

In a very articulate and scientific manner, Mrs. Case demonstrates that an orthomolecular approach to daily living is the only consistently effective way to either regain or maintain good health. She asserts, quite accurately, that orthomolecular medicine is really just nutritional medicine. However, she quickly adds that there is simply not enough quality nutrition any longer available to singularly maintain good health. Quality supplementation of vitamins, minerals, and any of a wide array of other nutrient substances is absolutely essential to assist a quality diet in keeping the individual healthy.

Mrs. Case also points out that illness is literally the body's cry for vitamins, and that illness is the body's clearest sign that it is in need of nutrients. This is an incredibly elegant and simple way to summarize chronic illness and what it takes to restore health.

As the daughter of Andrew W. Saul, PhD, a renowned author and quite literally a founding father of orthomolecular medicine, it is not surprising to see how capably Mrs. Case is able to expound upon the science of orthomolecular medicine. She combines many of her personal and family experiences with her strong orthomolecular background to convey a large body of information in a straightforward and compelling manner. She offers many points of intuition and philosophy as well, some quite humorous, that very effectively draw the reader into an appreciation of everything orthomolecular medicine has to offer.

For anyone who is looking to understand the best and simplest ways to maintain good health, I highly recommend this wonderful book.

Thomas E. Levy, MD, JD

Preface

Orthomolecular (nutritional) medicine prevents and treats disease. This fact has been largely ignored by our current health care system, the media, and the medical literature. Why doesn't your doctor use nutritional therapy? Is it for lack of safety? Because it's not effective? Because it is expensive? It happens to be none of these. Nutritional medicine is safe, effective, and remarkably inexpensive, especially when compared to drug medicine.

Most vitamin research you hear about focuses on low, and therefore, inadequate doses of vitamins. Low doses do not get clinical results. High-dose vitamin therapy does; it has for decades. Anyone who has heard otherwise has heard wrong. The evidence from nearly 80 years of research by orthomolecular physicians proves it: nutritional therapy works.

As evidence, in this book are important papers from the *Journal of Orthomolecular Medicine.* This book intends to share a few of these remarkable papers with you. To access, for free, over 40 years of the *Journal of Orthomolecular Medicine,* please visit Orthomolecular.org.

Many articles from the *Orthomolecular Medicine News Service* are also included in this book. You can subscribe, free of charge, to the *Orthomolecular Medicine News Service* at http://orthomolecular.org/subscribe.html and you can access the article archive at http://orthomolecular.org/resources/omns/index.shtml. This noncommercial, peer-reviewed publication contains research, clinical experiences, and analyses by twenty-five natural-healing physicians and experts. For others who think this provides too much information, thank you for the compliment.

You will notice that I draw a great deal from my father, Andrew W. Saul. This is intentional. I think that if you are going to quote someone, you may as well pick the person who you think can say it best. After all, my father has been teaching others (that includes me) about vitamins, nutrition, and natural healing for forty years, and I happen to like his delivery. We are a father–daughter orthomolecular team. It seems only natural to me to quote the most influential person of my professional career.

PART ONE

What Is Orthomolecular Medicine (and Why Should We Care?)

"What you may first have to overcome is an old assumption that anything that is cheap and safe cannot possibly be effective. Freed of that assumption, health awaits you."

—ABRAM HOFFER, MD, PhD

Orthomolecular medicine is nutritional medicine. It uses vitamin, minerals, and nutritional supplements to prevent and cure real diseases. These are the very things you have been told not to take. This is the therapeutic approach you have been told does not work. This is the approach you have been told not to do. It is time for a change.

Life is hard, and sickness makes it harder. Doing what it takes to live healthfully is no walk in the park either. It takes effort and a whole lot of it. This can feel downright overwhelming.

Speaking of overwhelming, I worked myself up again the other day prowling the Internet for safe clothing fabrics, chemical-free feminine hygiene products, sustainable paper goods, and organic baby diapers. After what seemed like hours of reading, cost comparing, deciphering what was really meant when something was labeled "pure" or "natural," and weighing the benefits of cleaner living against inferior performance and poor reviews, I figured I'd be better off if instead I just wore nothing but an organic sheet, ditched the baby diapers altogether, and permitted my youngest child to answer nature's call outside in nature itself.

I'm not giving up, not yet, but it can drive a sane person crazy if you really start to dig into what chemical evils could be lurking in everyday household items, let alone your air, food, and water. Those who market sanitizers have folks believing they'll be healthier if they annihilate bacteria on every touchable surface, as if somehow the impossible task of making one's home sterile is supposedly "safer." When I think of this, I always remember when my babies' favorite pastime was to find my shoes, suck on the soles, and chew on the tread.

Simple and natural has its advantages. There is also better living through science and innovation. But maybe things are going a bit too far.

There are two sides to everything. The "natural" industry has instilled as much fear in the customer as the chemical industry. There are lists of possible associations to every cancer and disease imaginable, all linked to products we use. Are they wrong? Maybe they aren't. But in the meantime, even those of us who buy organic food, avoid pharmaceuticals, wear gloves when using cleaning products, sidestep freshly fertilized lawns, filter our drinking water, and wash our hands with plain old soap, we are becoming overwhelmed by the sheer number of hazards we feel we must avoid.

This is not to say there isn't room for improvement. It is satisfying indeed to see companies taking steps to "go green," to skip genetically modified ingredients, to harvest sustainable forests, to reduce waste in production, and to create recyclable packaging. It's nice being able to go to my local grocery store or local farmer and buy any number of organic products. But trying to make everything we touch clean, green, and pure is practically impossible, at least for now. All we can do is move forward and take steps in the right direction. Tackle the big stuff. Integrate healthy living. But don't let it run you over.

My dad always says, "You can't go wrong with the basics." In a world where we are constantly going to be exposed to chemicals, poisons, synthetic hormones, carcinogens, pathogens, and stress, doesn't it make a whole lot of sense to eat right, exercise, and take our vitamins? We simply cannot avoid some exposure to any number of things deemed harmful. But we have an opportunity to take small steps and make gradual changes that bring us closer to living healthfully. And for the moment, I'm going to wear the clothing I already own, and I may even let the baby continue to wear diapers.

This is why I love orthomolecular medicine: it focuses on the basics. Nothing could be more basic than the very building blocks of life. Every single cell in your body is made out of nutrients.

Orthomolecular medicine is nutritional medicine: it is the practice of using nutrients that are normal and familiar to the body to prevent and cure disease. This may sound difficult, but it doesn't have to be. It means we should eat right and take our vitamins.

Orthomolecular pioneer Abram Hoffer, MD, PhD, said, "Anyone who wishes to become familiar with orthomolecular medicine may do so by simply beginning with a whole-foods, sugar-free diet, and a few vitamins."[1]

This is something we can all do.

BUT WHY "ORTHOMOLECULAR"?

People get sick. It happens. The goal is to be less sick, less often. We may suffer through a cold, but we most assuredly do not want to suffer through cancer. And while an occasional cold is not overly problematic, chronic colds certainly would be.

Neither vaccination nor medication provides sufficient protection from disease. In many cases, medication also does not provide a sufficient cure. "Management" of disease using dangerous drugs is not a cure. For those people who take prescriptions for chronic or recurrent illness, this is not new information.

We have a choice. Sickness is inconvenient, uncomfortable, and expensive. Orthomolecular medicine provides a way out of the disease–drug–disease spin cycle. We do not have to limit ourselves to only one approach. We can do more than turn to medicines and surgery. There is another way, and in the opinion of orthomolecular doctors and specialists, a far better one.

Our body is designed to be well. "Orthomolecular" describes a way of living that promotes health and discourages disease. It encompasses a way of feeding the body with the very substances it requires to live. We depend on nutrients to survive. We depend on optimal levels of these nutrients to be healthy. Adopting an orthomolecular lifestyle can help you be healthy now, help you get better if you are not, and keep you healthy in the future. "Orthomolecular" is a fancy term but we do not need to use it. Rather the key is to *do* it.

Folks who are much smarter than us have come up with all sorts of complex ways to label the contents and biological processes of the body. We do not need to understand the chemical makeup of food to know we must eat. Understanding how water or exercise or sleep impacts our brain is not as important as simply making sure we drink water, exercise, and sleep. In the same way, knowing how to define nutritional therapy is not nearly as important as doing it.

The body is dependent on nutrients. Too few impact health, as do too many. Different circumstances, such as exercise, age, pregnancy, or diet, may impact the amount of nutrients a person needs at any given time. The body always requires nutrients, but amounts will vary based on one's biochemical individuality or one's life circumstances. The same person could need more of certain nutrients on certain days, and less on others. For example, a human body needs more vitamins when sick. This is not conjecture. This is established nutritional fact. More vitamin C is required for wound healing. Fever increases the need for thiamine. Aging increases the need for many nutrients; older people need more and absorb less. Children need proportionally more nutrients than adults do because they are growing. More nutrients are also required for women during pregnancy.

Orthomolecular Origins

By definition, *ortho-* means "right." Two-time Nobel Prize winner and molecular biologist Linus Pauling came up with the name "orthomolecular" to describe using the right molecules to heal the body and to keep it healthy in the first place. Now there was a word to describe the therapy physicians were successfully employing in their practice over three decades before there was even a name for what they were doing.[2]

In the late 1960s, Linus Pauling first used the word in an article titled "Orthomolecular Psychiatry" written for the journal *Science.* As explained in his book

How to Live Longer and Feel Better, an orthomolecular approach promotes and maintains good health by using optimal levels of substances that are normally present in the body and required for life.[3] The goal, Linus Pauling says, is to "establish and maintain optimum concentrations of essential molecules."[4] You have got to consistently feed the body nutrients it needs. This is what is necessary to be well. To be free of sickness or to heal from what currently ails you, you may require very large amounts of nutrients indeed. Time and time again, this fact was being confirmed in practice.

In the late 1940s and for the next several decades, Drs. Wilfrid and Evan Shute used large doses of vitamin E (up to 1,600 IU per day) to successfully treat some 30,000 patients for conditions including "acute coronary thrombosis, acute rheumatic fever, chronic rheumatic heart disease, hypertensive heart disease, diabetes mellitus, acute and chronic nephritis, and even burns, plastic surgery and mazoplasia."[5] Frederick R. Klenner was curing viral pneumonia and every case of polio he had the opportunity to treat and a "striking variety" of many other illnesses with high doses of vitamin C—to the tune of tens of thousands of milligrams per day.[6] These, and other, doctors were successfully treating real diseases with high-dose vitamins and doing so safely.

"High doses of vitamins were advocated shortly after they were first isolated. Claus Jungeblut, MD, prevented and treated polio in the mid-1930s using a vitamin. Chest specialist Frederick Klenner, MD, was curing multiple sclerosis and polio back in the 1940s using vitamins. William Kaufman, MD, cured arthritis similarly back in the 1940s. In the 1950s, Drs. Wilfrid and Evan Shute were curing various forms of cardiovascular disease with a vitamin. At the same time, psychiatrist Abram Hoffer, MD, PhD, was using niacin to cure schizophrenia, psychosis, and depression. In the late 1960s, Robert F. Cathcart, MD, cured influenza, pneumonia, and hepatitis. In the 1970s, Hugh D. Riordan, MD, was obtaining cures of cancer with intravenous vitamin C. Dr. Harold Foster and colleagues arrested and reversed full-blown AIDS with nutrient therapy, and, in just the last few years, Atsuo Yanagisawa, MD, PhD, has shown that vitamin therapy can prevent and reverse sickness caused by exposure to nuclear radiation. All of these doctors used very high doses, and consistently reported striking success rates. And all of these doctors reported great patient safety."[7]

You'll note that their protocols did not involve "massive drugging of patients." These physicians were getting success with vitamins at doses far above what the government declares "adequate."

THE RECOMMENDED DIETARY ALLOWANCE (RDA)

"RDA = Ridiculously Deficient Amount"

—STEVEN F. HOTZE, MD

Good health requires optimal doses of nutrients. You cannot drive to Vegas on a gallon of gas, nor can you expect insufficient nutrition to keep you well. A half cup of water may help you survive, but much more is considered necessary to thrive. Similarly, "If you give every homeless person you meet on the street twenty cents, you could easily prove that money will not help poverty," says Andrew W. Saul, PhD. "If you give RDA levels of vitamins, do not expect therapeutic results."

There are times when the RDA may be sufficient for a healthy individual, but there are *far more* people who would benefit from an increased intake of essential nutrients, not merely the amounts suggested to prevent deficiency. "Most vitamin research has used inadequate, low doses. Low doses do not get clinical results," says Dr. Saul. "Decades of physicians' reports and laboratory and clinical studies support the therapeutic use of large doses of vitamins and other nutrients. Effective doses are high doses, often tens or hundreds of times higher than the US Recommended Dietary Allowance (RDA) or Dietary Reference Intakes (DRI)."[8] Unfortunately, many of us do not even manage to obtain the low recommended amounts of vitamins every day, let alone the amounts required for the prevention and treatment of illness.

The RDA vs. Nature

"A 15-pound wild monkey takes in about 600 milligrams (mg) of vitamin C a day from its food.[9] An average human being weighs 180 pounds. That is the weight of twelve monkeys; twelve monkeys would get 7,200 mg. But the US RDA for vitamin C for a human is 90 mg per day for adult males; only 75 mg per day for adult females. That means that your vitamin C RDA is just over 1 percent that of a monkey. Who do you suppose made the mistake?"

—ANDREW W. SAUL, *The Orthomolecular Treatment of Chronic Disease*

People may be deterred from taking larger doses of vitamins due to the alleged "tolerable upper intake levels" arbitrarily set by our government. These intake levels are presented as "safety" limits. However, such "safety" limits are believed by many nutritionists to be too conservative and largely theoretical. In his paper "'Safe Upper Levels' for Nutritional Supplements: One Giant Step Backward" (see introduction to Part Two), Alan R. Gaby, MD, who also has a degree in biochemistry and is an expert in nutritional medicine, says that these limits are inappropriately restrictive.[10]

Research that *could* show just how effective large-dose vitamin supplementation can be is stifled by such "safety" limits. Saying, for example, that a dose of vitamin C over 2,000 milligrams (mg) per day is the "tolerable upper intake" could make any study aiming to use higher doses to treat disease unethical.

This is wrong.

People are understandably concerned about taking amounts in excess of the supposed "upper intakes." But they need not be. There's 80 years of research to support safety and efficacy of doses far greater than those indicated in the RDA or tolerable upper intake levels.

SAY NO TO DRUGS

"[E]ven after the billions of dollars of pharmaceutical-based research conducted over decades, there is little to show for it. In my opinion, no toximolecular substance will ever be a cure for anything."

—ABRAM HOFFER, MD

You will notice that "drug" is not part of any definition of "orthomolecular." Orthomolecular physicians consider drugs to be "toximolecular," that is, toxic to cells. And this makes sense. There isn't a single cell in the human body made out of a drug. "Restoring health must be done nutritionally, not pharmacologically," says Dr. Saul. "All cells in all persons are made exclusively from what we drink and eat."

Drugs are not normally present in the body. Nutrients are. More and more people agree that illness is not *really* due to a lack of pharmaceuticals. "Headaches are not caused by aspirin deficiency, nor are digestive problems due to insufficient intake of antacids," says Dr. Saul. Drugs may suppress symptoms of sickness, but they do not address the underlying cause of illness. What is worse, drugs come with a laundry list of harmful side effects. They are risky, if not downright dangerous. Vitamins, on the other hand, have an extraordinary safety record.[11] The "safety record" of pharmaceuticals, if you can call it that, is spectacularly awful.

The facts are scary. Over 100,000 people die each and every year from pharmaceutical drugs, taken as directed, as prescribed.[12] Rates of injury are mind numbing. Every year, over 1.5 million Americans will be injured due to drug errors at the doctor's office, nursing home, and hospital.[13] Count on errors to increase as prescriptions and prescription drug use increase. Seventy percent (70 percent) of Americans take at least one prescription medication—the majority of which are maintenance medications for long-term, chronic illnesses.[14] A third of us take two or more pharmaceuticals. And one in ten of us takes five *or more* prescription drugs. And sadly, one in five children is taking prescription medication.[15] Are children even allowed to say "no"?

We are inundated with drug advertisements on TV, in magazines, and online. At the same time, vitamin supplements are accused of being worthless or harmful, neither of which they are. Instead of being encouraged to take safe and essential nutrients, we are warned off the very thing that would help us get better, and would do so safely. "A drug in either low or high doses cannot act as a vitamin," says Dr. Saul. "However, vitamins in large doses can act as drugs, and with far greater safety."[16]

It should be clear to everyone that drugs are dangerous. But that doesn't stop us from taking them. In fact, we are taking more now than ever.[17]

The results? Lower rates of chronic disease? People getting better? Just the opposite is true. "It turns out that we are seeing increases in the number of patients with stroke, cardiovascular diseases, cancer, allergic diseases, psychiatric diseases, and various other health issues," says Atsuo Yanagisawa, MD, president of the International Society for Orthomolecular Medicine.[18] And you can be sure that the pharmaceutical industry is rising to meet the demand with a plethora of costly prescriptions, many of which are intended for lifelong use. As Dr. Hoffer said:

> "[E]ven after the billions of dollars of pharmaceutical-based research conducted over decades, there is little to show for it. In my opinion, no toximolecular substance will ever be a cure for anything. Natural means have been almost totally ignored. The body is composed of innumerable molecules developed over the past billions of years by the toughest test of all, survival. We are finely tuned organisms, with so many different compounds and reac-

tions and inter-reactions. Even after over 50 years of medical practice, it still surprises me that everything functions so well. So to think that one can insert a strange molecule that has never been there before, and hope to correct some malfunction, is the height of folly."[19]

"Thirty years ago, Henry Gadsden, the head of Merck, one of the world's largest drug companies, told Fortune *magazine that he wanted Merck to be more like chewing gum maker Wrigley's. It had long been his dream to make drugs for healthy people so that Merck could 'sell to everyone.'"*

—*SELLING SICKNESS*, 2006

If you think your doctor will prescribe a safer, cheaper, more effective, natural, orthomolecular alternative to drugs, think again. Seventy to 80 percent of the time, doctor's office and hospital visits involve prescription drug therapy.[20] We cannot count on our doctors to recommend vitamins instead of medicines. We must look into this for ourselves. "Many people have heard their doctors say, 'I have never seen any evidence that nutrient therapy cures disease,'" says Dr. Saul. "Those doctors are telling the truth: no, they personally have never seen the evidence. But that is not because it doesn't exist. It does."

It bears repeating: drugs are not really the answer. Good health does not come from medication. People who take medicines and do not get better are starting to catch on. People who suffer drug-induced side effects (which lead to more drug prescriptions to manage drug side effects) are catching on, too. A drug that you are instructed to take for the rest of your life is not a "cure." It is a sentence. And it is expensive.

Our perception is changing. We are getting smarter. We are learning that pharmaceuticals do not always work, and we are turning to alternatives. We do not have to rely on drugs, but we must (and do) rely on nutrients to be well.

VITAMINS PREVENT AND CURE DISEASE

"Facts do not cease to exist because they are ignored."

—ALDOUS HUXLEY

So what if we could use nutrition instead of drugs? We can. This is what nutritional therapy does. This is what orthomolecular medicine does. "The only compounds that have been used successfully in chronic ailments are the nutrients, vitamins, minerals, amino acids, essential fatty acids, and hormones," said Dr. Hoffer. "And when one tries to replace natural substances with compounds that are slightly different in order to have patent protection, the results are dismal."[21]

Orthomolecular medicine is twofold: prevention and treatment. A strong immune system fends off disease. Maintain a strong immune system, and it will work to keep you healthy. "A strong immune system is key to recovering from an infection, neutralizing and eliminating a toxin, and bringing diseased cells back to a state of good health," says Thomas Levy, MD. This requires that you give your immune system the tools it needs to do its job. "Good nutrition does not directly cure disease; the body does," says Dr. Saul. "You provide the raw materials and the inborn wisdom of your body makes the repairs. You provide the bricks and mortar and the mason builds the wall. Without supplies, the most skilled workman on earth can build nothing. Without plenty of nutrients, the body can't, either."

For those of us entrenched in a medical perspective, it may still be hard to believe: nutritional treatment is effective, cheap, and free of side effects.[22] Some may think, "Anything safe and cheap can't possibly be effective, right? And aren't those vitamins expensive?" Not compared to medical treatment of disease, that's for sure. The evidence shows that vitamins have been safely preventing and curing disease for decades. Just because your doctor hasn't done it, does not mean it hasn't been done. When it comes right down to it, if you do not spend your money on prevention and taking care of your health, you will most assuredly spend it on disease. Funerals aren't cheap either.

VITAMINS ARE SAFE

"Nobody dies of poisoning by an overdose of vitamins."

—LINUS PAULING, PHD, CHEMIST AND DOUBLE NOBEL LAUREATE

Could you hurt yourself with vitamins? You could try, but you would certainly have a hard time doing so. Of course, there is a right way and a wrong way to do anything. However, "The number one side effect of vitamins is failure to take enough of them," says Dr. Saul. "Vitamins are extraordinarily safe substances."

Just because it is possible that you could hurt yourself with an overdose of vitamins does not make it likely that you will. Dr. Hoffer said, "Any discussion of side effects or of toxic reactions without specifying the doses is meaningless, for at zero levels nothing is toxic and at sufficiently high levels everything is toxic, including oxygen and water." Just like with oxygen and water, you require vitamins to live. Nutrients are essential. The only question, then, is dose.[23]

Pay attention. This is important: injury from vitamin insufficiency and deficiency is far more likely than injury from vitamin overdose. Tens of billions of doses of vitamins are taken each year and there is not even *one* vitamin death per year.[24]

Nutrients are good for you. Go ahead and get plenty. Abundance is a good thing. It is deficiency that is a problem.

Vitamins have a very large margin for error, and, therefore, for safety. Drugs do not. Vitamins are infinitely safer than drugs. Minerals are also remarkably safe, though not quite as safe as vitamins. Still, both vitamins and minerals are safer than any pharmaceutical or over-the-counter drug. Period.

Even the word *overdose* needs to be evaluated when it comes to vitamins. Are you "overdosing" because you took more than the measly RDA of vitamin C? Is 1,000 mg of vitamin C a megadose? If you are chuckling, then you too know that 1,000 mg of vitamin C a day is certainly not overdoing it. Those who choose to take orthomolecular doses of vitamin C know that sometimes the body may require 100,000 mg per day or more in times of severe illness.

As long as people have this idea that any amount over government recommendations is an overdose, we will suffer the consequences of failing to obtain what the body truly needs to keep healthy. Consider this: almost all animals make their own vitamin C. Adjusted for weight, pound for pound, animals make the human equivalent of between 1,500 and 15,000 mg per day or so of vitamin C right inside their bodies. They make even more vitamin C when they are sick or under stress. The RDA would have us believe that just 75 mg per day of vitamin C is sufficient for women, and a paltry 90 mg per day is enough for men.[25] Oh, *please.* Is all of Mother Nature wrong or, just maybe, did our government make a teensy tiny mistake?

Just because we have this preconceived notion of what is "a little" of a vitamin and what is "a lot" does not make it true. A small dose is often an ineffective dose, and doses much greater than our government recommendations can be safe and beneficial.

We should always be mindful of the supplements we take. We should still go to the doctor and discuss our health concerns. But we don't always have to do what the doctor says. And unless you see an orthomolecular doctor, you can expect that "orthomolecular" will not be heard in any answer to a question posed in the exam room.

THE BALANCED DIET MYTH

"Man is a food-dependent creature. If you don't feed him, he will die. If you feed him improperly, part of him will die."

—EMANUEL CHERASKIN, MD, DMD

Prevention of disease is by far the best approach to health. But any glance at a meal on the average American dinner table will illustrate that most people are not really thinking about their health. We may simply prefer what our parents fed us, what we are used to, or what tastes good to us. I think most folks know by now that eating lots of vegetables and fruits is healthy. *We just don't want to do it.* Advertisements, sensationalist media, false information, biased research, inadequate government recommendations, food pyramids, the financial interests of drug companies, and fad diets certainly cloud the judgment of well-meaning eaters everywhere. On top of it all, we go to doctors who promptly prescribe medication for our health issues and address problems with medication with more medicines. We have come to believe this is right and normal. But no matter what we are told, no matter what we hear or what we read, we have to do what is right for us and our bodies. And a "balanced diet" just is not going to cut it.

"Eat a balanced diet and you will obtain all the vitamins and minerals you need." Yeah, right. How many times have you heard *that* one? Frankly, "balanced" is one thing our diets should not be. The scale should be tipping full over in favor of all of the vegetables and fruits we are eating. Everything else goes on the other side. In addition to that great diet, we should also take vitamins. Even if we eat right, we still won't achieve optimal levels of certain vitamins and minerals, including vitamin C and vitamin E. Vegetables and fruits are not as nutritious as they used to be, nor are they as tasty. (Have you eaten a store-bought tomato lately?) Thanks to mineral-depleted soils and our desire for bigger, more attractive, pest- and weather-resistant produce, the vitamin and mineral content has gone down.[26] (Speaking of tomatoes, you may taste a delicious tomato again if you buy local and organic or grow your own.) Let's fill in any nutritional gaps with proper supplementation. This is orthomolecular nutrition.

Some people require more nutrients than others.[27] While the Recommended Dietary Allowances would have you think otherwise, requirements often vary. Age, pregnancy, illness, stress, and environment all affect the quantity of nutrients a body needs. There is no dose that works for everyone, every time. Supplements should supplement a healthy diet, and if you are not eating healthy food, you need supplements all the more. If you are suffering from illness, your need is even greater. The RDA simply will not do.

A little of a vitamin may be enough to prevent deficiency. More often, dosages of vitamins in amounts much higher than government recommended dietary allowances are required for good health. It depends on the individual. It depends on the need. A dry sponge holds more liquid. Similarly, a sick or stressed body requires more vitamins. The very idea that we can obtain all the nutrients we need through our food is substantially untrue. It's a nice legend. Even if you eat a predominantly organic, plant-based diet, it is hard to do, let alone if you eat like most Americans.[28]

We cannot possibly still believe that the "well-balanced" diet advice is working. Look at what is actually in the take-out bag. There are lots of crappy restaurants, but we can still call out the giant: McDonald's. I couldn't tell you the last time I grabbed a "meal" there, but 1 percent of the world's population could tell you. That's a huge number of people frequenting a restaurant notorious for non-nutritious food. Two billion dollars a year in advertising makes for colossal sales, and business owners have no intention of letting that stock go down.[29] We certainly do not have to eat there. I imagine most folks reading a book with the word "orthomolecular" in the title aren't anyway. But I say we put these hardworking fast-food employees out of business. And before you shame me for applauding job losses, I am no more apologetic about canning fast-food restaurant workers due to lowered demand for inferior, highly processed, notoriously unhealthy food than I would be if we needed to lay off doctors or hospital staff or gravediggers because folks were living longer, dying older, and spending many more years alive and healthier. What a treat it would be if such jobs began to disappear. Imagine what other jobs might take their place.

Can Supplements Take the Place of a Bad Diet?

by Andrew W. Saul, PhD

Excerpted from *J Orthomolecular Med.* 2003; 18 (3 & 4): 213–216.

Can supplements take the place of a bad diet? They'd better. In spite of decades of intense and well-funded mass education, the great majority of adults and children in the United States still do not consume the government's recommended daily quantities of fruits and vegetables.

Vitamins Provide for Special Concerns

Traditional dieticians have set themselves the heroic but probably unattainable goal of getting every person to eat well every day. Even if obtained, such vitamin intake as good diet provides is inadequate to maintain optimum health for everyday people in real-life situations. Tens of millions of women have a special concern. Oral contraceptives lower serum levels of B vitamins, especially B_6, plus niacin (B_3), thiamin (B_1), riboflavin (B_2), folic acid, vitamin C, and B_{12}.[1] It is uncommon, even rare, for a physician to instruct a woman to be sure to take supplemental vitamin C and B-complex vitamins as long as she is on the Pill.

Vitamins Fill in Nutritional Gaps

It is widely appreciated that at least 100 IU of vitamin E (and probably 400 IU or more) daily is required to prevent most cardiovascular and other disease. Yet it is literally impossible to obtain 100 IU of vitamin E from even the most perfectly planned diet. To demonstrate this, I've challenged my nutrition students to create a few days of "balanced" meals, using the food composition tables in any nutrition textbook, to achieve 100 IU of vitamin E per day. They could attempt their objective with any combination of foods and any plausible number of portions of each food. The only limitation was that they had to design meals that a person would actually be willing to eat.

As this ruled out prescribing whole grains by the pound and vegetable oils by the cup, they could not do it. Nor can the general public.

"Supplements" by definition are designed to fill nutritional gaps in a bad diet. They fill in what may be surprisingly large gaps in a good diet as well. In the case of vitamin E, doing so is likely to save millions of lives. A 1996 double-blind, placebo-controlled study of 2,002 patients with clogged arteries demonstrated a 77 percent decreased risk of heart attack in those taking 400 to 800 IU of vitamin E.[2] Again, such effective quantities of vitamin E positively cannot be obtained from diet alone.

To illustrate how extraordinarily important supplements are to persons with a questionable diet, consider this: children who eat hot dogs once a week double their risk of a brain tumor. Kids eating more than twelve hot dogs a month (that's barely three hot dogs a week) have nearly ten times the risk of leukemia as children who eat none.[3] However, hot-dog-eating children taking supplemental vitamins were shown to have a reduced risk of cancer.[4] It is curious that, while theorizing many "potential" dangers of vitamins, the media often choose to ignore the very real cancer-prevention benefits of supplementation.

Vitamins Supply Nutrients Easily and Cheaply

Critics also fail to point out that supplements are economical. For low-income households, taking a three-cent vitamin C tablet and a five-cent multivitamin, readily obtainable from any discount store, is vastly cheaper than getting those vitamins by eating right. The uncomfortable truth is that it is often less expensive to supplement than to buy nutritious food, especially out-of-season fresh produce. Milligram per milligram, vitamin supplementation is vastly cheaper than trying to get vitamins from food.

Few people can afford to eat several dozen oranges a day. A single large orange costs at least 50 cents and may easily cost one dollar. It provides less than 100 milligrams (mg) of vitamin C. A bottle of 100 tablets of ascorbic acid vitamin C, 500 mg each, costs about five dollars. The supplement gives you 10,000 mg per dollar. In terms of vitamin C, the supplement is 50 to 100 times cheaper, costing about one or two cents for the amount of vitamin C in an orange. Those who wish to follow Linus Pauling's perennially wise recommendation to take daily multigram doses of vitamin C can do so easily and cheaply.

Vitamins Supply Nutrients Essential to Health

Since the time of the ancient Egyptians, through the time of Hippocrates, and right up to the present, poor diet has been described and decried by physicians. Little has changed for the better, and much has changed for the worse. Though nutritionists place a nearly puritanical emphasis on food selection as our vitamin source, everyone else eats because they are hungry, because it makes them feel better, and because it gives pleasure. No one likes the "food police." Telling people what they should do is rarely an unqualified success, and with something as intensely personal as food, well, good luck. We could, of course, legislate Good Food Laws and make it against the law to make, sell, or eat junk. That is as likely to work as Prohibition.

Our somewhat less draconian choice of "noble experiment" has been to educate, to implore, and to exhort the citizenry to be "choosy chewers," to "eat a balanced diet" and to follow the food groups charts. The result? Obesity is more prevalent and cancer is no less prevalent. Cardiovascular disease is still the number-one killer of men and women. "Health is the fastest growing failing business in western civilization," writes Emanuel Cheraskin, MD, in *Human Health and Homeostasis*.[5] "We can say with reasonable certainty that only about 6 percent of the adult population can qualify as 'clinically' healthy." We can try to sort out each of the many negative behavior variables (such as smoking), which certainly must be factored in. When we have done so, we are left with the completely unavoidable conclusion that our dinner tables are killing us.

Decide for Yourself

The good diet vs. supplement controversy may be reduced to four logical choices:

1. Shall we eat right and take supplements and be healthy?
2. Or, shall we eat right and take no supplements, be vitamin E and C deficient for our entire life span, and greatly increase our risk of sickness and death at any age?
3. Or, shall we eat wrong and take no supplements, and be even worse off?
4. Or, shall we eat wrong, but take daily vitamin supplements, and be a lot less sickly than if we did not take supplements?

While each of these four options constitutes a popular choice, there is one best health-promoting conclusion:

Supplements make any dietary lifestyle, whether good or bad, significantly better. Media supplement scare-stories notwithstanding, taking supplements is not the problem; it is a solution. Malnutrition is the problem. As it has for thousands of years of human history, so the malnutrition problem remains with us today. The biggest difference is that we are now malnourished even though overeating. Only in the last century have supplements even been available. Their continued use represents a true public health breakthrough on a par with clean drinking water and sanitary sewers, and can be expected to save as many lives.

REFERENCES FOR "CAN SUPPLEMENTS TAKE THE PLACE OF A BAD DIET?"

1. Wynn V. Vitamins and oral contraceptive use. *Lancet* 1975 Mar 8;1(7906):561–564.

2. Stephens NG, et al. Randomized controlled trial of vitamin E in patients with coronary artery disease: Cambridge Heart Antioxidant Study (CHAOS). *Lancet* 1996; 347:781–786.

3. Peters JM, et al. Processed meats and risk of childhood leukemia (California, USA). *Cancer Causes Control* 1994;5(2):195–202.

4. Sarasua S, Savitz DA: Cured and broiled meat consumption in relation to childhood cancer: Denver, Colorado (United States). *Cancer Causes Control* 1994;5(2):141–148.

5. Cheraskin E. *Human Health and Homeostasis*. Birmingham, AL: Natural Reader Press, 1999.

Vitamin Censorship

"Withholding information from public search is wrong. Censorship at a public library is very wrong."

—ANDREW W. SAUL, PhD

The *Journal of Orthomolecular Medicine* (JOM) is still not adequately indexed by Medline, a public, taxpayer-funded online library. PubMed indexes three articles from JOM. Yep, just three. If you would like to circumvent the censorship and read the rest, you can access over 40 years of the *Journal of Orthomolecular Medicine* at Orthomolecular.org.

ORTHOMOLECULAR IS AN INDIVIDUALIZED APPROACH

"Each person must take an individualized program, which they can discover if they are lucky to have a competent orthomolecular doctor. If they do not, they can read the literature and work out for themselves what is best for them. I believe the public is hungry for information. As more and more drugs drop by the wayside, the professions are going to become more and more dependent on safe ways of healing people, and using drugs is not the way to do that. Using nutrients is."

—ABRAM HOFFER, MD

The concept of "biochemical individuality" is that each of us has unique nutritional needs. We all require "water" and we all require "food." How much we each require at any given time will vary. The same is true with nutrients. This is the rule rather than the exception. *Orthomolecular medicine recognizes this, and can be safely tailored to fit the needs of an individual.*

Good health is not one-size-fits-all. The flippant punchline of the old patient-doctor joke is: "Take two aspirin and call me in the morning." This isn't really amusing anymore. Until recently, many people were being told, and without jest, to take aspirin for its blood "thinning" effect. How many of their doctors recommended high-dose vitamin E to prevent clotting and heart attacks?[30] Based on the relentless poor press vitamin E gets, probably none of them.

"Take this and let me know how it works for you" is not a bad concept, but it is a bad idea when you are talking about the administration of drugs that inherently carry serious side effects. (That includes aspirin.) Patients become test subjects, and only they and their loved ones suffer the consequences if things do not go right. To think that a drug in a one-size-fits-all pill somehow addresses the needs of all folks across gender, weight, race, age, and health history is unwise and unsafe. This is no way to operate, especially when there is another way, one that is vastly safer and often more effective.

We all have to take responsibility for our own health. We cannot, and should not, rely on others to do it for us. We can choose to live a lifestyle that supports good health. We have to work at it every single day. We cannot believe, even for a second, that some pill at our doctor's office has all the answers. It simply isn't true. We need not and should not rely on our current disease-care system to provide us with the answers for wellness. We must look into nutritional medicine for ourselves. "There is a lifestyle change that prevents, arrests, and reverses serious chronic disease," says Dr. Saul. You can be well. Ultimately, it is you, not your doctor, who must do it. Fortunately, vitamins can help.

Vitamin Pill Popper

"The easiest way to cure any disease is never to get it."

—ANTON W. OELGOETZ, MD

An orthomolecular lifestyle can appear a bit strange. We take handfuls of vitamin pills every day. We will swallow a dozen or so at restaurants or pop tabs in the car. We take them before family gatherings, stressful events, or long drives. We swallow them down at breakfast, lunch, dinner, bedtime, and in-between. Vitamins are in my purse, our gym duffels, and our cars. We carry vitamins for the kids in the diaper bag. We often have a few in our pockets. They are in our fridge, basement, and bathroom. We have a three-tier kitchen cabinet stock full of vitamin bottles and a larger stash in the cellar. We travel with huge bottles of vitamin C in our suitcases. If we forget to pack any, we will make a special trip to grab what we need when we arrive. We will even ship them in advance to the homes of relatives when we intend to stay for an extended visit. Vitamins are our constant companions.

When you take as many vitamins as we do, good prices are important. We literally buy ten pounds of C powder at a time. My dad will buy twenty. In fact, I just purchased nearly a year's supply of vitamin C capsules this morning while I was waiting at the doctor's office. (It was a really good sale.) There I was, waiting in the exam room for my annual gynecological checkup, and I was ordering vitamin C, via a website app on my phone. Saving money on something our family uses all the time just makes sense. I'm the only person I know who took advantage of Black Friday to buy vitamins.

This may seem a bit crazy to some folks—all the pill popping, that is. To me it is crazy *not* to take vitamins. We like investing in a healthy present and future. And it is working. Every day. We believe in "nutritional insurance," a phrase coined by biochemist Roger J. Williams, discoverer of pantothenic acid (B_5), and we happily pay for it. Each time my husband fills up his week's supply of vitamin pill boxes, he says, "I like taking vitamins."

I do too.

Steps to Better Health: Are You Sick of Sickness?

by Helen Saul Case

From the *Orthomolecular Medicine News Service,* October 19, 2013.

Better health? It takes effort. You have got to want it, and then you have got to work for it. There is no one-step solution. We need to eat right *and* drink plenty of water *and* take our vitamins *and* drink fresh, raw, vegetable juice *and* exercise *and* reduce stress. All of these things make your immune system stronger and your body inhospitable to sickness. This isn't easy. But isn't suffering from illness harder?

Know Your Options

I was raised in a household where instead of drugs we used vitamins. They are far safer and often more effective. When I went off to college, I thought I'd give mainstream medicine a try. Not only did drugs not cure my own "feminine ailments," they actually made things worse. I went back to what I knew: vitamins and nutrition work. I'm not a doctor, but I believe you don't have to be a doctor to help yourself. My father, orthomolecular educator Andrew W. Saul, explained that medical doctors are trained to practice medicine and prescribe medications. Natural, vitamin alternatives just aren't visible in the medical tool bag. I sought out nutritional cures because I needed to. I go to my doctor, but I don't always get the drugs she recommends. Using vitamins and nutrition to prevent and cure illness works better for me. Sure, we can always go to our doctors with our health problems. But wouldn't it be nice to not *need* to go?

Ditch the Drugs

Adding a chemical to your body doesn't address the underlying cause of illness. No cell in the human body is made out of a drug. You have a real choice: medication or nutrition. One of these two choices is remarkably safer, cheaper, and, in many cases, more effective than the other. Guess which one that is? People put their faith in pharmaceuticals because they are sick and they want to get well. But when drugs don't work, which is surprisingly often, we have to make a decision. We can choose to keep returning to the disease-medicate-disease-medicate spin cycle, or we can choose to get onto excellent nutrition and a healthy lifestyle. You may find that your doctor agrees but simply needs some education about the benefits of vitamin supplements.

Take Your Vitamins

I sure do. There is no single magic bullet in the list of essential nutrients. They are all important. The right dose is crucial. High doses help the body get adequate amounts of essential nutrients when it needs them. Many people do know the value of great nutrition, but knowing how to use high doses of vitamins to treat our health issues is another story. Which vitamins should we take? How much? (Really, *that* much?) Do they work? Yes. Vitamins do work, and you don't have to take my word for it. Experienced physicians Abram Hoffer, MD, Thomas Levy, MD, Carolyn Dean, MD, Ian Brighthope, MD, Ralph Campbell, MD, Michael Janson, MD, and many others have shown time and time again the safety and efficacy of nutritional therapy. Clinical evidence is strong. Vitamins and nutrition can prevent and arrest chronic disease.

Know That You Can Do This

Learn about your options, especially those you aren't likely to hear about in the doctor's office. Read studies on effective vitamin therapy, and then check the references. If you don't have time for all of that, orthomolecular books can help. You don't need to be reliant on a drug-based medical system.

OUR HEALTH, OUR RESPONSIBILITY

Perhaps all this is not for everybody. Taking responsibility for our own health is no easy task. But it is worth it. As you keep reading, you will find out why.

PART ONE REFERENCES

1. Hoffer, A., A. W. Saul. *Orthomolecular Medicine for Everyone: Megavitamin Therapeutics for Families and Physicians.* Laguna Beach, CA: Basic Health Publications, 2008.

2. Saul, A. W. "A Timeline of Vitamin Medicine." *Orthomolecular Med News Service* (Feb 15, 2014): http://orthomolecular.org/resources/omns/v10n08.shtml (accessed May 2016).

3. Pauling, L. *How to Live Longer and Feel Better.* Corvallis, OR: Oregon State University Press, 2006.

4. Ibid.

5. Hoffer, A. "The True Cost of Cynicism." *J Orthomolecular Med* 7(4): (1992): http://www.doctoryourself.com/hoffer_shute.html (accessed May 2016). Saul, A. W. "Vitamin E: Safe, Effective, and Heart-Healthy." *Orthomolecular Med News Service* (Mar 23, 2005): http://orthomolecular.org/resources/omns/v01n01.shtml (accessed May 2016). Saul, A. W. "Shute Vitamin E Treatment Protocol." http://www.doctoryourself .com/shute_protocol.html (accessed May 2016).

6. Saul, A. W. "Hidden in Plain Sight: The Pioneering Work of Frederick Robert Klenner, M.D." *J Orthomolecular Med* 22(1) (2007): 31–38.

7. Saul, A.W., ed. *The Orthomolecular Treatment of Chronic Disease: 65 Experts on Therapeutic and Preventive Nutrition.* Laguna Beach, CA: Basic Health Publications, 2014.

8. Ibid.

9. Milton, K. "Nutritional Characteristics of Wild Primate Foods: Do the Diets of Our Closest Living Relatives Have Lessons for Us?" *Nutrition* 15(6) (Jun 1999): 488–498. http://www.2ndchance.info/wildprimatediets.pdf (accessed May 2016).

10. Gaby, A.R. "'Safe Upper Limits' for Nutritional Supplements: One Giant Step Backward." *J Orthomolecular Med* 18(3–4) (2003): 126–130.

11. Saul, A.W., J.N. Vaman. "No Deaths from Vitamins—None at All in 27 Years." *Orthomolecular Medicine News Service* (Jun 14, 2011): http://orthomolecular.org/resources/omns/v07n05.shtml (accessed May 2016).

12. Starfield, B. "Is US Health Really the Best in the World?" *JAMA* 284(4) (Jul 26, 2000): 483–5.

13. Associated Press. "Drug Errors Injure More Than 1.5 Million A Year: Report Calls for All Prescriptions to be Electronic by 2010." (Jul 20, 2006): http://www.msnbc.msn.com/id/13954142 (accessed May 2016). Saul, A.W. "How to Make People Believe Any Anti-Vitamin Scare: It Just Takes Lots of Pharmaceutical Industry Cash." *Orthomolecular Med News Service* (Oct 20, 2011): http://orthomolecular.org/resources/omns/v07n12.shtml (accessed May 2016).

14. Mayo Clinic News Network. "Nearly 7 in 10 Americans Take Prescription Drugs, Mayo Clinic, Olmsted Medical Center Find." (Jun 19, 2013): http://newsnetwork.mayoclinic.org/discussion/nearly-7-in-10-americans-take-prescription-drugs-mayo-clinic-olmsted-medical-center-find/.

15. Gu, Q., C. F. Dillon, V. L. Burt. "Prescription Drug Use Continues to Increase: U.S. Prescription Drug Data for 2007–2008." *NCHS Data Brief* (42) (Sept 2010):1–8. http://www.cdc.gov/nchs/data/databriefs/db42.htm (accessed May 2016).

16. Saul, A.W., ed. *The Orthomolecular Treatment of Chronic Disease: 65 Experts on Therapeutic and Preventive Nutrition.* Laguna Beach, CA: Basic Health Publications, 2014.

17. Kantor, E. D., C. D. Rehm, J. S. Haas, et al. "Trends in Prescription Drug Use among Adults in the United States from 1999–2012." *JAMA* 314 (17) (Nov 3, 2015).

18. Saul, A.W., ed. *The Orthomolecular Treatment of Chronic Disease: 65 Experts on Therapeutic and Preventive Nutrition.* Laguna Beach, CA: Basic Health Publications, 2014.

19. Hoffer, A. Introduction to "Placebo Medicine" by A. W. Saul. http://www.doctoryourself.com/placebo.html (accessed May 2016).

20. Centers for Disease Control and Prevention. FastStats. Last updated April 27, 2016. "Therapeutic Drug Use." http://www.cdc.gov/nchs/fastats/drug-use-therapeutic.htm (accessed Nov 2015). Centers for Disease Control and Prevention. National Center for Health Statistics. "National Ambulatory Medical Care Survey: 2010 Summary Tables." http://www.cdc.gov/nchs/data/ahcd/namcs_summary/2010_namcs_web_tables.pdf (accessed Nov 2015).

21. Hoffer, A. Introduction to "Placebo Medicine" by A. W. Saul. http://www.doctoryourself.com/placebo.html (accessed May 2016).

22. Hoffer, A., A. W. Saul. *Orthomolecular Medicine for Everyone: Megavitamin Therapeutics for Families and Physicians.* Laguna Beach, CA: Basic Health Publications, 2008.

23. Hoffer, A. "Side Effects of Over-the-Counter Drugs." *J Orthomolecular Med* 18(3–4) (2003): 168–172.

24. Saul, A. W. "No Deaths from Vitamins. Absolutely None. 31 Years of Supplement Safety Once Again Confirmed by America's Largest Database." *Orthomolecular Med News Service* (Jan 14, 2015): http://orthomolecular.org/resources/omns/v11n01.shtml (accessed May 2016).

25. Office of Dietary Supplements. National Institutes of Health. "Vitamin C: Fact Sheet for Health Professionals." https://ods.od.nih.gov/factsheets/VitaminC-HealthProfessional/ (accessed April 2016).

26. Davis, D.R., M.D. Epp, H.D. Riordan. "Changes in USDA Food Composition Data for 43 Garden Crops, 1950 to 1999." *J Am Coll Nutr* 23(6) (Dec 2004): 669–82.

27. Hoffer, A., A. W. Saul. *Orthomolecular Medicine for Everyone: Megavitamin Therapeutics for Families and Physicians.* Laguna Beach, CA: Basic Health Publications, 2008.

28. Centers for Disease Control and Prevention. CDC Newsroom. "Majority of Americans Not Meeting Recommendations for Fruit and Vegetable Consumption." Press Release. (Sept 29, 2009): http://www.cdc.gov/media/pressrel/2009/r090929.htm (accessed May 2016). Casagrande, S. S., Y. Wang, C. Anderson, et al. "Have Americans Increased Their Fruit and Vegetable Intake? The Trends between 1988 and 2002." *Am J Prev Med* 32(4) (Apr 2007): 257–63.

29. O'Brien, K. "How McDonald's Came Back Bigger than Ever." *The New York Times Magazine* (May 4, 2012): http://www.nytimes.com/2012/05/06/magazine/how-mcdonalds-came-back-bigger-than-ever.html?_r=0 (accessed May 2016).

30. Saul, A.W. *Orthomolecular Medicine News Service.* "Vitamin E: Safe, Effective and Heart-Healthy." (Mar 23, 2005): http://orthomolecular.org/resources/omns/v01n01.shtml (accessed April 2016).

CHAPTER 1

Confessions of an Orthomolecular Lifer

"When in doubt, try nutrition first."

—ROGER WILLIAMS, PHD, IN *NUTRITION AGAINST DISEASE*

I've been doing this since I was born. I've been doing this since *before* I was born. Of course, I have my mother and father to thank for that. My father has been teaching others about orthomolecular medicine for over 40 years. My mom practiced orthomolecular principles when she was pregnant with me. I have lived my entire life with access to, and guidance about how to use, a massive amount of information about the power of vitamins to cure and prevent illness. This orthomolecular stuff comes naturally to me, and not because I have an MD after my name, which I most assuredly do not. I was just born lucky.

Being lucky, though, has very little to do with how healthy anyone is. Sure, I had a great start in life. Once I had to take care of my own health, things changed. When I went to college, I thought I knew better. My parents couldn't be right about everything, I suspected. I lived a college lifestyle that included eating and drinking unhealthy foods and staying up late, and generally ignoring all I had been taught by my parents. I went to the doctor with my health problems and took the medicines they prescribed. When another health problem surfaced, or the same ones returned, back I would go for more. I found, as many people do, that the drugs did not really help me get better. Often one illness would lead to another opportunistic infection, and one drug that did not work would lead to another, often more expensive, often stronger, more dangerous drug that also did not always work. I had to deal with the negative side effects of drug treatment, too. I was not achieving good health by taking pharmaceutical drugs.

They provided a bandage only, one that needed to be changed often. And for some reason, the wound underneath just would not heal. This was unacceptable, especially since I suspected that I knew better.

I did not like suffering. I did not like all the things sickness restricted me from doing. For example, I was not going to have a whole lot of sex if I had a yeast infection. I was not going to be able to go hang out with my friends if I was coughing up a lung. And I was not going to be able to do anything at all if I was on my back with a migraine headache for a week or more out of every month. Some folks feel that all the work one has to do to keep healthy is a pain in the rear. I think dealing with sickness is far harder than anything I have ever had to do to stay well.

After going off track during my college years, I decided to go back to what I knew worked: building and maintaining a strong immune system with vitamins and nutrition. I finally said yes to that juicer my dad wanted to get me for Christmas, and I started using it. All the time. I began paying more attention to what I ate, what I drank, and the vitamins I needed to take. I worked at it every day. I made a point to practice healthy habits, and in the process of doing all of this, I was able to treat myself effectively and safely and, better yet, to stay healthier in the first place. Not a single doctor I ever went to told me about how nutrition could help me get better and stay that way. I found myself limiting the advice I received from doctors to diagnosis only. Then I would place their recommended prescription in my pocket, go home and take vitamins instead. Why? Because they worked better. They always had.

I do not mean to disparage the medical community. They are an essential piece of the health puzzle. But unfortunately for most doctors and their patients, they have dropped a few puzzle pieces on the floor, and they do not even know it. They do the best job with what they have, but they are missing the whole picture. People who have been raised doing what I still do to this day know beyond a shadow of a doubt that those forgotten pieces are the most important, despite what they might have heard otherwise.

Getting orthomolecular doses of nutrients into one's body, often in much larger amounts than current government health recommendations, has allowed my family to be spared from needing to rely on expensive, often ineffective pharmaceutical and over-the-counter drugs. We have the wonderful freedom of choice. We have options. This is an awesome feeling, especially when it is a Sunday night, someone is sick, and the doctor's office is closed. No need to panic. Vitamins to the rescue.

My parents instilled in me a way of doing things that has allowed me to avoid taking antibiotics or other prescription medications for what ails me. This same teaching has allowed me to be less sick and to feel less awful and recover more quickly when I am. We all get sick. How we get better is where we differ.

I figured this out at a pretty young age. It only took a few years of health mistakes to get a grip on what really worked. My job writing orthomolecular books, I tell myself, is to help others do this too, so they can benefit from what I have been so lucky to have just been born with: the knowledge and understanding to practically apply the use of orthomolecular medicine for the best health possible. You don't have to be a doctor to do this yourself. (My dad has been saying this for four decades.) I'd like to share with you how.

My lack of amazement with our current health care system has been continually strengthened by the fact that I know a way out. No matter what the problem, nutrients help, and certainly do no harm. Time and time again I have watched orthomolecular medicine do what conventional medicine did not. And if they both work, I have seen orthomolecular medicine do it better.

Having utilized orthomolecular principles my entire life, I have a strong basis for comparison. I know this stuff works. So did my parents. Eventually, so will my children. Even at ages two and four, they had a sense for it. So too have dozens upon dozens of medical doctors who have come to see the value of nutrients to prevent and cure disease.

"Wow. That C. I got better quick!"

—OUR FOUR-YEAR-OLD DAUGHTER

Putting in the effort to live healthy is a remarkably positive experience. I reap the benefits of feeling good, being well, and the ability to share that with the next generation. Health care costs are not a burden in this house, and thank goodness. Instead, I can complain about the high cost of eating the best food possible. But I don't. Good health is worth it. People struggle to pay such high health care deductibles these days. I prefer to pay for great food and vitamin supplements instead.

Here's what that looks like:

We buy lots of whole foods, as local, as fresh, and as organic as possible.

We eat a plant-based diet.

We limit the amount of meat we eat, especially red meat. If we do eat it, it is grass fed and organic.

We take handfuls of vitamins.

We drink lots of (as clean as possible and filtered) water.

We stay active with regular exercise.

We get outside.

We play.

We make a point to limit screen time.

We make a point to rest, relax, and re-center.

We take care of our relationships between ourselves, our children, and our families.

We get out and see people, face-to-face.

We make time for ourselves.

Everyone is different. You must do what works for you, and what works for you is different than what may work for another. This is especially true when it comes to doses of nutrients. Some folks need more. Some need less. The amount varies from day to day, year to year, even moment to moment. The good news is:

Vitamins are very safe.

Vitamins are relatively cheap (especially compared to the alternative).

Vitamins are very effective.

You can do this. It takes time. Don't expect to learn everything overnight. I've been doing this my whole life and I'm still learning. We all are. As Will Rogers said, we are all ignorant, just on different subjects.

HEALTH FIRST, FAMILY SECOND, JOB THIRD

Growing up, it was our motto for living. It still is: health comes first, family second, our job and everything else are third. This is our hierarchy of priorities, the order of what is most important. It is not a rigid rule but rather a guideline that has the incredible power of putting focus where it belongs.

My brother and I heard it thousands of times while we were growing up, as my father heard it from his father. Health is first. You simply must take care of yourself. Then comes family, a close and important second. Your job and everything else are third. When we were little, "job" was replaced with "school."

There is great comfort in having defined priorities. Let's start with the first one: health. I don't feel guilty if I take a sick day from work, or take care of a child with a cold instead of doing other planned activities. I know that it is more important to get well and heal. "Health first" guides our family's entire way of living, from the food we eat to the exercise we plan into our week. Health is not just a priority in a decision-making moment, but always.

Family is second. While work and school are very important, family is more so. Do we have to check our e-mail on a Sunday? Whatever is in there will still be there Monday morning. The inbox can wait. Health comes before family. You must take care of yourself so you can take care of them. In the event of an emergency on an airplane, you must put on your oxygen mask first, then provide for your child.

"Take your vitamins."

"Yes, Mom. Yes, Dad."

It sounds so simple, really. But like the old advice to eat right and exercise, it may be far harder for some to put into practice. That's why it's handy to have a book like this.

Take your vitamins! *Orthomolecular Nutrition for Everyone* will confirm, Mom and Dad are still right.

We'll navigate the grocery store, delve into the importance of specific nutrients, and find out why nutrients, in doses probably much larger than expected, help us stay healthy and cure sickness. We'll talk about the good, the bad, and the ugly when it comes to fat, sugar, and carbohydrates and the popular diets that embrace them or shun them. We'll talk about a healthy lifestyle that will make it near impossible for disease to dominate you. Here you will learn how to be well, and how to stay well, and how to do it all yourself.

Third is our job. At the very least, work gives us the means by which we survive. If we are lucky, our job is also fulfilling, satisfying, and provides additional purpose and meaning. Yet health and family come before it. Approaching work in this manner has a way of providing life with some well-needed balance. Work is important, no doubt about it. It is not *all important.* Are those extra hours at the office, away from time with our children, really going to translate into something of importance in the end? Will there be a plaque for us on the wall? Would it matter if there were? There are times when work must be prioritized and families must make sacrifices, but *balance* is key.

I don't think about this much anymore. "Health first, family second, job third" has become my silent, internal mantra. It is just the way I do things, the way my family does things, automatically and willingly. It helps maintain perspective and keep what is most important, or what should be, at the forefront of our minds and reflected in our actions.

Now that we're introduced, let's get even more personal.

WHERE THE POOP GOES

I have never wished to be a kid again, but this may be the single exception. Kids don't have to worry about where the poop goes. Adults do. I know more about our property's septic system than I ever wanted to know. And now, if you choose to continue reading, so will you.

Our septic tank is very small. For those of you who have one, you'll know that a 300-gallon tank for a family of four is undersized. There's not a whole lot of room in there. It can get full of solid stuff relatively quickly, a lovely thought indeed. However, the possible risks associated with failure to keep up with yearly pump-outs hadn't really occurred to us. At least not until there was a problem.

One spring, an eye-catching shimmering pond developed over one end of our leach field. It was a fragrant pool of sludge that, when caught in a gentle southeasterly breeze, shared its foul smell generously with any folks who dared venture into our backyard. It was especially pungent on those hot summer days.

Luckily, it was actually an easy problem to fix, thanks to excellent advice from a reputable repair company. Water conservation helped, and so did staggering loads of laundry, showers, and dishwashing throughout the day to ease the load on the system at any one time. Still, the field was draining too much on one side, which was more water volume than the leach line could properly handle. I was truly impressed when the repair took a matter of a few seconds: turn a ring at the end of the pipe that worked with the water level to control the outflow to the field. I was also impressed that the fella sent to do the repair took his glove *off,* reached his bare hand down into our wastewater distribution box, scooped away some of the contents of our family's bowels from the tube's opening, made the adjustment to the ring, looked at it for a minute, then looked at his hand, casually wiped his fingers on his pants, and put his glove back *on.*

The glove came off again later.

"Sign, please," he said as he handed me a pen.

And then I washed my hands.

There would appear to be only two kinds of people in the world comfortable with handling other people's poop: those who work in the septic business and parents. (For that matter, "parents" should be extended to include any "caregiver." Nurses must have stomachs of steel. How could one survive otherwise?)

My husband could tell you distinctly of the day he "caught" a heaping handful of poop that had escaped the small child he was changing, before he could manage to get a diaper back on. Yes, he gagged. And washed his hands next to a dozen times. But every future encounter of the excrement kind no longer phased him, nor me for that matter. I have had my share of feces on my hands too. And I am still alive. (So is he.) The body's immune system is really tough. Thank heaven for that.

Turd Watch

My children will be mortified that I have recorded this, so I'll let them guess which it was. For one of our children, my husband designated bath time in our house as "Turd Watch." For several months, one of our little cuties just loved to let it go in the bath. The water was warm and relaxing and comfortable. Kind of like still being in mother's womb. Why not have a bowel movement? It must have seemed a logical moment. A few toots from a baby behind, and we were on alert. Invariably, the baby would not disappoint. My husband and I were so inoculated, we would deftly reach into the water with our bare hands, snatch the turd, and quickly toss it in the toilet before it started to break down into soup—or worse: pieces too small to grab but too big to go down the drain without manual intervention. Time was of the essence, as the small child who had just emitted the mess would, upon first sight as it floated by, scream bloody murder and try to crawl up the sides of the tub to escape the evil intruder. Then the bath was most certainly over, although the addition of feces to the water necessitated further bathing (and a new tub of water).

Lest we think handling turds is dangerously unsanitary, I would like to point out that *E. coli* is *everywhere.* Some people fear it. Others do not. We can argue that hand washing is in order. But panic is unnecessary.

No Need to Panic

Think of the beach, for example. There are times when the Great Lakes are so overloaded with *E. coli* (and who knows what else) that those in charge close the beach. It's not exactly sterile when reopened for swimming. Closures are due to "elevated levels" of *E. coli*. When reopened, those levels are simply normal. *E. coli* is still there. It's always there.

E. coli in the water comes from many sources. Shoreline sewage-treatment plants, runoff water from urban areas and from manure on farms, and, yes, seagulls poo in the water too. Just watch your children play. They will swallow *mouthfuls* of that water. They may even occasionally contribute to the *E. coli* levels. Somehow, amazingly, they survive. We all have.

How is this possible?

The Lake Huron Centre for Coastal Conservation tells their Canadian beach-goers, "Fortunately very few strains [of *E. coli*] are pathogenic. . . . The *E. coli* present in humans do not cause diseases in people." In fact, they say, it's the other stuff they worry about. "Although for the most part *E. coli* is not pathogenic, its presence in recreational water, especially at elevated levels, has been taken to indicate fecal contamination and the likelihood that pathogens such as Salmonella, Streptococci, Cryptosporidium, Giardia, Enterovirus, etc. could be present."[1]

Oh, what to do, what to do. For one, we should remember a quote attributed to Louis Pasteur: "The germ is nothing; the terrain is everything." A healthy body fights disease. A healthy body can avoid illness in the first place. Germs are everywhere. They are natural, normal, and always around. On every beach, on every surface, they cannot be avoided. But only some people will fall victim to illness.

Germs Are Everywhere

Sorry, germophobes. There is no way to be free of germs. We are swarming with them. Everything is. If you fear them, you will forever be afraid.

Sure, some pathogens are more dangerous than others, but let's consider, for example, that half of those untreated *survive* the bubonic plague. I realize that 50 percent is a dreadful mortality rate, but let's look at the glass half full of lake water just for a moment. The plague still exists. My dad told me about plague warning signs at a state park. The sweet little squirrels. Who knew? There were signs instructing you to keep away from the squirrels because they carry, yep, you guessed it: *plague*. The *Los Angeles Times* reported in their plague article that,

"In California, there have been 42 human cases of plague since 1970. Nine were fatal."[2] Apparently, there are plague-ridden squirrels in Yosemite Park, and Lake Tahoe and. . . . I can't go on. We're all gonna die!

Let me try again: half of us are gonna die!

Well, folks, if that's how we looked at these things, we would never leave the house. There is a pretty amazing system in place to keep you free of disease, to fight off infection that may try to get the best of you, and no, it's not the health care system. It's your immune system and it's brilliant. All you have to do is take care of it.

EBOLA, ENTEROVIRUS, DIRTY DISHES, AND PLAGUE

From the *Orthomolecular Medicine News Service,* September 13, 2014.

by Andrew W. Saul, PhD

If Abraham Lincoln were to describe the germ theory, I think he might have put it something like this:

"You can infect all of the people some of the time, and some of the people all of the time; but you cannot infect all of the people all of the time."

The question, of course, is, why? Why do some people have high resistance to illness? Why do some people seem to get sick looking at a picture of a germ? Certainly their level of nutrition, perhaps more than any other single factor, is reason number one. I think "germs" are a much smaller reason.

I first learned this in tenth grade, not from my biology teacher, but from the sickest kid in school: my lab partner, Mike. (If you haven't just finished eating, and if you have no immediate culinary plans, may I add that the whole disgustingly delightful story awaits you at http://www.doctoryourself.com/germs.html.)

Frantic media alarms over Ebola and other viruses fill the airwaves. All this cannot help but make you panic just a little. And personally, I think it's intended to. Some businesses, and a lot of people who invest in them, stand to make a pile of money if they can keep you frightened and on edge. Such a state makes you into an obedient follower, and most especially, a willing consumer.

Cantankerous Contagion Questions

Ebola and enterovirus cannot be any greater threat than was the Black Death. The highly contagious plague famously killed tens of millions of people. It did not vanish after the Middle Ages, either: there are deaths from plague every year, in the United States, today.

So have you had your plague shot? You haven't? Then why isn't your doctor urging you to get one? Do you know anyone who has had a plague vaccination? Then why is there no plague epidemic?

Now to ***really*** scare you. (This next bit is satire.) I have just discovered a life-threatening new epidemiological phenomenon, and I am announcing it right here, right now:

Saul, A. W. (October 2014). Soiled dishes syndrome (SDS): An overlooked public health disaster in the making. *J Overblown Med Anxiety 1* (1).

To summarize: A major epidemic is looming on the horizon, largely due to hurried housewives, careless bachelors, lazy teenagers, and slovenly college students. It is called Soiled Dishes Syndrome (SDS). SDS is caused by food particles, lipstick traces, grease, grime, milk rings, and other culinary crud left on cups and cutlery by sloppy dishwashers in a hurry. Suspected for decades by patrons of every Greasy Spoon restaurant on the planet, SDS is certain to spread an extraordinary variety of viruses and bacteria at a truly alarming rate. If you've ever shared a student-apartment kitchen sink with way too many others, you have been exposed to SDS. If you've ever eaten off plates and silverware that were not autoclaved for at least an hour, you are at risk of pushing up the daisies. If you've ever had your own kids do the dishes. . . well, words fail me.

What can be done? Absolutely, positively nothing. Even if you are a scrupulously careful dishwasher yourself, sooner or later you will eat off dishes that look clean but actually still have two or three (million) invisible bacteria on them. Then, over the lips, past the gums, look out stomach, here they come.

The situation is hopeless. Nasty microbes are simply everywhere. Dire problems are expected for babies who put their fingers in their mouths (Soiled Fingers Syndrome, or SFS), toddlers who put toys in their mouths (Toddler Toy Syndrome, or TTS), and adults who put anything but a brand-new toothbrush in their mouths (AWPABABNTBITM). Vaccinations for SFS, TTS, and especially AWPABABNTBITM are needed immediately. It is recommended that a million zillion tax dollars be granted to the pharmaceutical industry without delay.

Until a vaccine is developed, here are two ways to protect yourself:

1. Don't eat fresh food, because fresh food is not sterile (UFS, Unsterilized Food Syndrome).
2. Do not drink directly from a juice bottle, blow a whistle, or ever, EVER play a harmonica, trumpet, or clarinet (UEES, Unsterilized Everything Else Syndrome). We expect that summer camp counselors and philharmonic horn and woodwind sections will soon be dropping like flies.

I hope you know that I am kidding.

As Lincoln said, quoting what the girl said as she put her foot into her stocking, "It strikes me that there is something in it." Exposed to a limitless quantity of potential pathogens every day, it is nothing short of remarkable how nearly seven billion people manage to be alive at one time on this utterly unimaginably unsterile Earth.

Thank heaven for homeostasis, the body's active promotion of life.

I used to define homeostasis for my students by (badly) impersonating John Travolta's dancing in *Saturday Night Fever*. I'd do his famous one-hand-pointing-up-and-out, one-hand-pointing-down-and-away move, and smoothly say, "Stayin' alive."

Nobody missed the homeostasis question on the exam.

It is the preference of nature to keep you alive. Your anatomy was assembled and grown without regard for your opinion. Your physiology carries on immeasurably complicated biochemistry every second of your day, night, and life without ever asking you how. I maintain that a healthy body will fight, and beat, the vast majority of viral and bacterial invaders *if* nutrient intake dosages are sufficiently high for prevention, and, if need be, astronomically high for cure of serious illnesses. The prescription? It's the simplest imaginable: Follow a healthy lifestyle. Live right, exercise right, eat right, and get your rest. Take your vitamins every day, at every meal, especially lots of vitamin C, and don't let anyone tell you otherwise.

And while you're at it, wash those dishes. I mean, why push your luck?

Germs Are Good and Strong Immune Systems Are Better

"There is no dispute that a competent immune system is the best way to keep a disease from developing and taking hold in the first place."

—THOMAS LEVY, MD

Ever live on a farm? Hang out with kids who did? Well, you are all the healthier for it. Fewer allergies and less asthma are associated with kids who live on farms.[3]

Dirt is good. If you too have a toddler who puts everything in his or her mouth, you understand what is at work here. Children will invariably be exposed to all sorts of little microorganisms. We too. And yes, once in a while they or we will get a sniffle or get a fever or get sick. But that is okay. As long as it is not too serious, this is the body's normal, natural way of combating inevitable exposure to pathogens. It is all part of a system way smarter than us. But as long as we give our immune system the right tools to do its job, runny noses won't turn into hospital visits. And yes, this can be done. My kids are three and five and have yet to need an antibiotic. We use vitamins and nutrition instead. Because they work.

The body's immune system is strong. Orthomolecular medicine makes it stronger. Germs are everywhere. We need them, really. Think about gut bacteria, for example. These microorganisms are essential for keeping us healthy.

Keeping the Tank Clean

If you've never had a close friend who likes to talk about their most recent excretory event with you, I'm here to help make up for lost time.

In keeping with our subject matter, your colon is like a septic tank. You have got to get the poop out. So, for starters, staying regular is a great way to keep things moving along. This is not as self-evident as it may seem. Many folks are not going as often as they should. My father has seen hospital patients go two weeks without a bowel movement. Personally speaking, I don't let a day go by without one.

Detoxifying is something that seems to get a lot of attention these days. Overall, it's a good concept. Get rid of toxins. Sounds good to me. But you do not need a whole lot of expensive products to help you do that. First off, avoid toxins as much as you can, like in your food, for example. Second, eat lots of fiber-rich fruits and veggies to keep your bowels moving along, and the toxins too. Third, take C.

Vitamin C is your friend. Let's talk about incredibly toxic mercury. "Both acute and chronic exposures to mercury can be effectively treated with vitamin C," says Thomas Levy, MD, "and typically most of the damage from such poisoning can be prevented and/or promptly repaired." Additionally, "Pesticides are diverse in chemical structure but they are usually susceptible to neutralization by vitamin C," he says. "Vitamin C also tends to readily repair the damage done by many pesticides." Not bad. Especially considering that vitamin C is "arguably the safest of all nutrients that can be given."[4] If you are concerned about lead poisoning, high-dose vitamin C helps there too. To learn more, please see the article in this book entitled "How Doctors Use Vitamin C Against Lead Poisoning."

That's not all. According to niacin researcher W. Todd Penberthy, PhD, niacin (B_3) is also a powerful detoxifying agent.[5] And don't forget to drink plenty of water.

Feces and Fences

Our neighbor has a big heart. And many outdoor kitties that she has rescued and lovingly taken care of for years. She also adopted a dog, Lily, who, upon walking through my sludgy septic field heard me say, "That's right, Lily. Walk in my poop for a change!" Don't worry, we all get along. We actually don't have a fence between our yards. Our family is a sympathetic bunch too. Three rescued cats share our indoor space.

With pets naturally come pet by-products. If we took a moment to consider just how much time we dealt with poop on a day-to-day basis, we might be shocked. For goodness' sake, my mom has to schedule regular appointments with the veterinarian to give her poor cat enemas. Ugh.

Middle Schoolers

I had no idea I would have so many poop-related stories to tell you. Maybe it was all pent up (so to speak) and just looking for the proper venue in which to come out. That brings us to when I used to teach middle school.

Frankly, I think anyone who chooses to teach middle school should know full well that "messing with kids' heads" is part of the job assignment. Students are still ever so slightly gullible at this age, an adorable quality that fades dramatically once they enter high school. This penchant to still believe that what one's teacher is saying must be true allows for some good-natured fun in between assignments. I learned early on: if you don't keep class interesting, you lose their attention entirely. I was not the only teacher who operated with this understanding.

It was exam time and the students were settling in to take an end-of-the-year final. It was so quiet up and down the hall you could hear a pin drop. In the parking lot outside the classroom window next door, a septic-company truck pulled in to empty the port-a-potties that had been set up for the construction workers repairing the school roof. The children had to be quiet, facing forward to start their exam. But the very audible machine suction occurring right over their shoulders, right outside their window, right behind their backs was too obvious to ignore. Looking quietly forward as they were supposed to, all they could do was listen. Their teacher, however, did not spare them his commentary, and proceeded to give them a play-by-play. He described the large quantity of matter being sucked into the hose, details about how it must smell, and, of course, explained that the worker had finished with the hose and proceeded to open up and eat his sandwich, sucking his fingers as sandwich juice dripped onto them. Without washing his hands. I'm pretty sure that wasn't actually happening. But it didn't matter. In their heads it was. Ah, the power of suggestion. That's all you have to do to get a middle schooler. They were understandably appalled, but a few smiles flashed across the room and the students' pre-exam tension was eased just a bit. Next door and listening, I, however, was in hysterics.

We may as well face reality: we deal with doo-doo every day. Become a parent or become a dog owner. You know exactly what I am talking about. Feces is at the front of your mind. When did he go last? When will he need to go again? How did it look? Did he pass that penny he ate? I hope he goes soon! I'm pretty sure this level of concern is normal. Take care of yourself. Take care of your family. Pay attention to where the poop goes.

In the words of Monty Python, "And now for something completely different."

TURN OFF THE TV. AND PHONE. AND LAPTOP. AND TABLET. AND . . .

Part of the whole "do what's right for your body" thing means lifestyle examination. How we live can directly or indirectly impact our health. I'm keenly aware of this as I stare at my computer screen writing this very sentence.

Modern technology is addictive. Just look around. People are starting at screens. Ever try to ignore them for a while? Some of us would have nothing to do.

They say you never forget how to ride a bike. But perhaps we have forgotten to go get on one.

We Are All Doing It. And We Like It.

Tailor-made entertainment is effortless. It's fun. All we need is a screen and we're set for hours. But should we be? The worst part of healthy living is the "healthy" part. It involves "doing." And "doing" can be just about the hardest thing ever, especially when tantalizing, satisfying bubblegum for the mind can be yours for just a simple press of a button or swipe of a finger.

"Oh, I'm not supposed to sit on my rear, watch eight hours of television, and eat bonbons?"

Apparently, that sort of thing isn't good for us. But it sure *feels* good, right? Many of us could spend a very satisfactory day eating chocolate and knocking out half a season or more of *Game of Thrones.* I don't know about you, but I *like* doing nothing.

Fortunately for my health, I like doing *something* even more.

Wretched Excess

During the holiday season, my father rates Christmas light displays. The more ridiculous the display, the more "points" are given. Houses with modest, thoughtful, seasonally proper décor with matching lights in tasteful rows receive few if any points. No points at all are given to those classy New England homes with a clear candle in each front window and beautiful fresh greenery on the door. The more gaudy, overdone, obnoxious, or "hanky" an exhibit is, the better it scores. ("Hanky" was a term he coined to describe decorations that might only comprise of a half-working string of blinking lights flung over a branch and left to swing awkwardly in the wind, or perhaps a half-deflated air Santa near an out-of-season rotten pumpkin.)

However, the most points are reserved for people who have managed to decorate with wretched excess. No, these folks didn't stop with the house. They decorated the barn, the second garage, the mailbox, the doghouse, and the dog.

There is true joy in wretched excess. We want to go to Charlie's Chocolate Factory. We love our all-you-can-eat buffets. We are fascinated by the *Guinness Book of World Records*. More is better, right?

What's the Problem with Too Much?

Maybe there isn't one. Some folks will fuss and say there's no real reason they should turn off the screens. They enjoy being able to disconnect from their day by connecting to prefab entertainment. Screen time can be family time too.

Are memories made on the couch? I'm certain some are. I like curling up and watching movies with my husband. Content often leads to conversation. I also enjoy playing video games with my kids. They have to think, use strategy, and it's just plain fun. We like to Skype with Grandpa and Grandma. The kids like the drawing programs on the touch pads, and I like the portability and convenience of countless stain-free markers, crayons that don't break, pencils that need not be sharpened, and free "paper." Streaming Internet radio often accompanies the kids during bath time with countless kids' songs. And television these days is packed with fun-to-watch, addictive shows.

As always, the statistics may make us think twice about TV and everything else available via screens.

Children are spending on average seven hours every single day in front of screens. Seven hours. Because kids are so good at multitasking (for example, texting and watching TV at the same time), they actually pack ten hours and 45 minutes of media content into that seven hours.[6] Remember, that's an *average*. For every child who spends less time in front of illuminated panels, there is another spending far more.

As for adults, we are setting an example, good or bad. Adults are exposed to screens about eight hours a day, with TV accounting for just over five of those hours.[7] At work, many of us have to stare at a computer all day. Once we get home, we don't put our smartphones away. We check our e-mail, even if work ended hours ago. We turn on the TV. We may as well check the weather even if we aren't going outside. There are good shows to catch. The same is true on the weekends. If you are bored, get your phone out and look busy, right? It's kind of handy to have a GPS right in your pocket when you need directions. You don't have to interact with the locals.

How many people still use their phone during dinner, even though it is generally frowned upon? I have literally watched kids text each other from across the table, rather than simply look up and have a conversation. Standing in line? Grocery shopping? Make a call. Take a call. Browse the Web. Tweet. Send a selfie. People do it all the time. Maybe we shouldn't.

Still, screens can be therapeutic. When someone is tired or down, they turn on the television. It is easy. It is entertaining. There's often something interesting online. (Another funny cat video perhaps?) There's shopping, gossip, funny commercials, sports clips, you name it. It's all very alluring. It's all rather addictive. The question is, is it actually good for us?

It depends on what we watch (especially what kids watch), and it depends on what it is replacing. My husband and I went out the other night. We ate dinner, walked the pier, and watched the sunset from a gazebo. It was your classic date, and it was fantastic. While taking in the spectacular warm-red sunset, my husband nudged me, smiled, and said, "Look. They're on a date." He was referring to a young couple on a bench behind us. There they were, sitting together, each looking at his or her phone. I'm sure they were just Googling "best sunsets ever."

The Good Old Days

I remember a 90-year-old family friend of ours who used to wait by her mailbox for the delivery each day. Like many older folks, she really looked forward to getting an envelope to open. My folks would often mention this example when encouraging us to write to our grandparents.

It is not that different for us. It is still exciting to get mail. Except now our "mail" glows on a backlit screen and is delivered immediately, day or night, with the added expectation from the sender that we reply instantly. After you hear your phone chime, how long do you wait before you read a text message? Most of us probably do so directly.

Talk with Your Kids About TV

"All television is educational television.
The only question is: what is it teaching?"
—NICHOLAS JOHNSON

Can screens be part of a wholesome, productive, normal childhood? You bet. Screens are a fact of life. I sit here staring at a screen in order to make a living, as often does my husband. But when we think about how we want to spend our free time, we try to put screens last on the list. Our family spends oodles of time outside, talking, playing, traveling, and visiting with friends. We keep the TV off while we eat dinner as a family and avoid seats in restaurants near screens too.

Overall, when it comes to TV, our kids don't watch much, and when they do, it's "good" TV. We stick to educational programming, and we watch shows before they do if we have any question about wholesomeness (an acceptable level of violence and so forth). We often watch programs with them and talk about what we see. We mute commercials or change the channel during them. They get exposure to new and interesting subjects, new vocabulary, and are often inspired by what they see.

While what they watch may be more important than how much they watch, we still place limits on usage to encourage other activities. Being able to use an electronic device is a privilege in our house. The kids have to be well-behaved, or no TV and no iPad. When they do get screen time, we limit it to no more than one and a half hours, as my parents did when I was younger. We figure it is a good sign that our kids have no trouble finding something to do when the TV is off.

There is a way to do it right. There's also a way to do it wrong. I have seen people so hooked on their devices that they don't talk with their spouse, interact with their children, eat right, exercise, or go to sleep.

There is only so much time in a day. The hours you spend watching TV or playing video games means fewer hours doing something else, whatever that may be. One activity will naturally displace another. We often ask ourselves, when the TV is on: is this really the best way to spend our time?

It would seem, as with many things, that moderation is key. If you find yourself choosing to marinate in media on your own rather than play outside with your kids or watch an actual ball game with friends, or you Facebook family rather than visit them, maybe it is time to shut down the computer, silence the cell phone, go breathe some fresh air, and interact one on one in the same physical space with those you love.

Health Problems and Good Ol' TV

If you are wondering why I am bothering to talk about screen time in a book about nutrition, here's your answer: more screen time means more health problems.

Harvard knows their stuff. And they say, "Extensive research has confirmed the link between TV viewing and obesity in children and adults, in countries around the world."[8].

Carolyn Dean, MD, ND, describes such technology devices as "modern pills for people."[9] And it feels sooooo good. The excitement of looking forward to screens, actually getting the time to engage with them—it's the best. Except for the letdown after hours have gone by and your life has become no more interesting. And you find yourself with little to talk about. (I passed level 103?) Ever talk to a kid who does nothing but play video games? It's like talking to an alien. I have no idea what they are saying. This always makes me kind of sad. These kids spend so much time in an imaginary world, they fail to live in the real one.

The more time we spend sedentary in front of screens, the less time we spend exercising, eating right, and interacting with real, actual people. Failing to eat right and exercise means we put ourselves at increased risk for chronic disease.

A study published in the *Journal of the American College of Cardiology* about "recreational sitting," screen time, death, and heart disease, concluded that, yes, screen time means you are much more likely to die or suffer cardiovascular disease regardless of physical activity.[10]

The more time kids spend in front of the television, the fatter they are.[11] This goes for us adults too. It makes sense, really. We are sitting still, often with a snack, as more unhealthy food choices are advertised to us. It's incredible that we ever leave the house. I guess sometimes we run out of snacks.

One nice thing about eating healthy food is that you aren't eating junk. This may seem overly self-evident, but each time you eat something that is good for you, you're filling your stomach, curbing hunger, and not eating something bad.

"Turn off the TV and go outside!" We should take our parents' and grandparents' advice. Find a safe place to play and go take in a daily dose of nature.

My dad used to always mute the commercials when we were kids. I do the same. My kids don't need their little brains flooded with cartoons that advertise drugs or happy actors enjoying unhealthy food. It's a well-circulated little factoid that makes a big impact: parents only spend 38.5 minutes a week in meaningful conversation with their kids. Maybe we can chat while the TV is on mute.

TAKE CARE OF YOURSELF NOW AND LATER

It is far easier not to eat right and not to exercise. But if you don't take care of yourself now, you are bound to do it later. And managing sickness is much more difficult to do than just taking care of yourself in the first place.

Most of us want to do whatever the heck we want. Being told how we should eat, move, talk, live, sit, stand, and work: it all gets rather oppressive. We constantly rein in our desires. We shouldn't tell the boss to stick it. We shouldn't send our kids off in a traveling carnival. We shouldn't toss the dog feces found in our own yard back into the neighbor's yard where they belong. And we probably shouldn't watch too much TV.

Quiet your mind. Read a good book or get some fresh air. Being plugged in also means we are tuned out to the things that are happening around us in the now. Screens are easy. Real interaction with real people is harder and requires action and imagination to fill the time, rather than entertainment being provided to us on a platter. Fight the addiction. Anyone who plays Candy Crush knows it. A good friend of mine uninstalled all such games off of her phone. She said to me, "I don't like how unproductive they made me, so I deleted them." It is hard to turn away from media. The moment we have a break, we get all excited about interacting with devices. Let's get back to getting excited about interacting with each other.

Speaking of which . . .

HANGOVER RELIEF

"I read a book about the evils of drinking, so I gave up reading."
—HENNY YOUNGMAN

I am confident my folks would be mortified if I wrote this down. It certainly has no place in a health book, right?

Ah, what the heck.

For me, the utilization of orthomolecular medicine hasn't always been because of my desire for good health. Sometimes, I use it for the express purpose of recovery after indulging in bad habits. Hey, we are supposed to get out and socialize, face to face. And every once in a while it is healthy to let loose a little bit, right?

Thank goodness for vitamin C. Among its many powerful functions, which we will address in the chapter dedicated to the nutrient, vitamin C is a safe alternative and effective antibiotic, antiviral, antihistamine. It is also an excellent cure for hangovers. Vitamin C is an antitoxin, which sure comes in handy when we are intoxicated. We know it is not a good idea to drink too much, but knowing to do the right thing does not necessarily mean we always do it. If one suspects that too many drinks have gone down the hatch (and that a headache in the morning is likely to follow), drinking a boatload of water and taking a massive dose of C before bed can do wonders. I know this to be true because I've done it, and while I'm not proud to admit it, I know full well I'm not the first who has put down one too many cocktails at the "Best Wedding Party Ever!"

Vitamin C is awfully handy for accelerating the detox process. Practically speaking, this is what I do: After a night of a few too many adult beverages, right before I head to bed, I take about 10,000 to 15,000 milligrams (mg) of vitamin C, swallow a couple of pints of water, and then sleep it off. The next day, I'll be remarkably functional. I also take vitamin C the next morning if there is any lingering feeling of "ugh" left over. And if I don't take vitamin C at all the night before, I can still take large doses in the morning (in an attempt to get to saturation) to knock out a hangover. Once saturation is reached, the hangover is usually much better, or gone entirely. The only trouble here is if you are *really* sick and you can't hold anything down, don't count on the C to stay down either. You can only expect vitamin C to help counteract an average amount of poor judgment.

Using vitamin C to feel better should not justify the use of alcohol, or make you think you can drink more without consequence. Vitamin C is not a miracle cure for reckless overindulgence. But C can be a helpful bandage when needed. And if you find that you end up with a sore throat or just feel icky after drinking certain wines or liquors (what is in that blue stuff?!), vitamin C can help you feel better, too. Nutrients sure are useful when you don't have time to be sick.

We all need to let loose once in a while, I suppose, and I figured I'd pass along this tidbit of helpful info just in case you need a Sunday morning—or an entire *Sun-day*—after a wild night out to be little more manageable.

TAKE A MODERATE STANCE AND IRRITATE EVERYBODY

I have found that nothing quite irritates people like being a moderate. Unless you also tell them you take handfuls of vitamins. Then you're not only an extremist, but you're also nuts. But when it comes right down to it, taking the middle road seems to bother folks on both sides of the argument. Still, here is where I stand:

I have angered many a pediatrician because my children only get some vaccinations, namely those required by state law for school entry. We do not get them all. We do not get none. We have found few friends in the middle. (Additional information is provided later in this book in these articles: "Don't Vaccinate Without Vitamin C" and its companion, "Vaccinations, Vitamin C and 'Choice.'")

I am a stay-at-home mom. I believe in raising my own children. I am convinced I can do it best. I also have a career as an author, a speaker, and an educator.

I believe in moderate amounts of strenuous exercise (is that an oxymoron?), but you won't find me running an ultra-marathon. I'm not down on fitness. Quite the contrary. If pushing yourself toward a lofty goal keeps you fit, have at it. Certainly the problem with the American people is not that we get too much exercise.

I believe in health care, not disease care. Our family chooses to heal from illness and, better yet, work to prevent it entirely with vitamins and nutrition, not medication. It seems to really annoy others, especially physicians and the pharmaceutical industry, that nutritional therapy works so well for many. Still, many folks I know don't want in on it. Sure, they'll *ask,* but then they will quickly tune out the sentence that follows. Nothing quite ends a conversation like talking about taking large doses of vitamins. (Perhaps you are the exception.)

I believe in going to doctors, but not always doing what they say. Am I a moderate for keeping myself and my children off of medication? According to recent trends, I'm downright fanatical. We have a rare condition in our household called "good health." There may be some trying to come up with a drug for it, but until then, we just haven't needed to take pharmaceuticals.

I eat really good-for-me food. I also have a treat once in a while.

I eat meat, but not much. I was raised lacto-ovo vegetarian until the age of eight. From then on, I ate a little meat, mainly poultry. These days, I still choose to eat some meat. It's far less than most people: we have it about once weekly. (I really like tacos.) Many a vegetarian or vegan may rise up to point out the error of my ways. On the other hand, if I'm accused of being vegetarian, which oddly enough I often am, meat eaters will proclaim that one can simply not be nourished eating a nourishing plant-based diet. I can tell you, as many a veggie eater can, there are plenty of nonmeat foods that pack a punch of protein and vitamins.

Discussing religion or politics with a moderate viewpoint might just land you in one heck of a passionate argument. What defines "healthy living" appears to incite the same level of emotion.

It's okay. We don't all have to agree with one another. As the singer Ricky Nelson said, "You can't please everyone, so you've got to please yourself." Perhaps he should have said instead: You can't please *anyone.* You must, then, please yourself.

"Don't take chances. Take vitamins."

—ME

CHAPTER 1 REFERENCES

1. Crowe, A. "E. coli: A Permanent Resident of our Beaches?" The Lake Huron Centre for Coastal Conservation: http://laehuron.ca/index.php?page=e-coli (accessed May 2016).

2. Rocha, V. "Plague-Infected Squirrels Found at Yosemite National Park Campground." *Los Angeles Times* (Aug 14, 2015): http://www.latimes.com/local/lanow/la-me-ln-plague-infected-squirrels-20150814-story.html (accessed May 2016).

3. Schuijs, M. J., M. A. Willart, K. Vergote, et al. "Farm Dust and Endotoxin Protect Against Allergy Through A20 Induction in Lung Epithelial Cells." *Science* 349(6252) (Sept 4, 2015): 1106–1110. doi: 10.1126/science.aac6623.

4. Levy, T. E. *Vitamin C, Infectious Diseases, and Toxins: Curing the Incurable.* Philadelphia, PA: Xlibris Corporation, 2002.

5. Hoffer, A., A. W. Saul, H. D. Foster. *Niacin: The Real Story.* Laguna Beach, CA: Basic Health Publications, 2012.

6. Henry J. Kaiser Foundation. "Generation M2: Media in the Lives of 8- to 18-Year-Olds." (Jan, 20 2010): http://kff.org/other/event/generation-m2-media-in-the-lives-of/ (accessed May 2016).

7. Council for Research Excellence (CRE). "Ground-Breaking Study of Video Viewing Finds Younger Boomers Consume More Video Media than Any Other Group." (Mar 26, 2009): http://www.prnewswire.com/news-releases/ground-breaking-study-of-video-viewing-finds-younger-boomers-consume-more-video-media-than-any-other-group-61955592.html (accessed May 2016).

8. Harvard School of Public Health. "Television Watching and 'Sit Time'" http://www.hsph.harvard.edu/obesity-prevention-source/obesity-causes/television-and-sedentary-behavior-and-obesity/ (accessed May 2016).

9. Dean, C., with T. Tuck. *Death by Modern Medicine.* Belleville, ON: Matrix Vérité Media, 2005.

10. Stamatakis, E., M. Hamer, D. W. Dunstan. "Screen-Based Entertainment Time, All-Cause Mortality, and Cardiovascular Events." *J Am Coll Cardiol* 57(3): 292–299.

11. Cox, R., H. Skouteris, L. Rutherford, et al. "Television Viewing, Television Content, Food Intake, Physical Activity and Body Mass Index: A Cross-Sectional Study of Preschool Children Aged 2–6 Years." *Health Promot J Austr* 23(1) (Apr 2012): 58–62. Zimmerman, F. J., J. F. Bell. "Associations of Television Content Type and Obesity in Children." *Am J Public Health* 100(2) (Feb 2010): 334–340. Robinson, T. N. "Television Viewing and Childhood Obesity." *Pediatr Clin North Am* 48(4) (Aug 2001):1017–1025.

CHAPTER 2

Oh, What to Eat?

"A diet of minimally processed foods close to nature, predominantly plants, is decisively associated with health promotion and disease prevention. . . . The case that we should, indeed, eat true food, mostly plants, is all but incontrovertible."

—DAVID KATZ, MD

It's possible that we already know exactly what we need to eat. We just don't want to eat it. At a restaurant the other day, I asked a young waitress which salad on the menu was best. She took a moment to think, and then she finally admitted that she didn't eat lettuce. Her favorite menu item was deep fried meat—schnitzel. I suppose I was asking a bit much considering I had landed in a German restaurant that day. Schnitzel was their specialty. I imagine some folks at popular fast-food restaurants don't know which salad on their menu is best either.

Perhaps we actually want to eat right, and we just don't see to it that we do. Eating right can be a challenge. Every meal. If you are learning what to eat and what not to eat, you know full well how much time you spend reading and learning about food. If you believe in preparing your own meals from fresh ingredients, you know full well how much time and energy that takes too. Have a garden? That's work. Trying to avoid pesticides, genetically modified organisms (GMOs), preservatives, and additives? That's work too. Making sure you are actually chewing and swallowing the best food possible takes willpower. It takes dedication. It takes work. Every meal.

EAT YOUR VEGETABLES. I MEAN IT.

Raw veggies? Cooked veggies? Which should we eat? Eat them cooked. Eat them raw. Eat them juiced. Eat them all. (I'm a poet, and don't know it.)

What matters is the *veggie* part. With a nod to the brilliant Dr. Seuss, the hero in *Green Eggs and Ham* might have done better to eat green vegetables rather than green eggs and skip the ham entirely, unless he chose to eat the occasional serving of the organic, grass-fed, nitrate-free variety.

Vegetables are good. Period. Juiced. Raw. Dried. Cooked. Pureed. Canned. Candied. Okay, maybe not candied. But even so, would sugared veggies be better for you than a Twinkie? Probably. I imagine the *wrapper* is better for you than the Twinkie in it. (At least it has less sugar.) Some preparation methods will affect the nutrient content of vegetables. And of course, the less processed the better. But if you are eating vegetables in whatever form, *at least you are eating vegetables.* The more vegetables you eat, the less room you have to eat something else less healthy. Ideally they would all be fresh, raw, or lightly steamed, straight from your own organic garden. If you can't do that, get as close to that as you reasonably can. Just eat the vegetables. Often and in quantity.

So Processed Foods are Safer?

Folks sometimes get hung up on produce because they worry about pesticides. It can't be good for us if it is covered with chemicals, right? Certainly we should avoid ingesting pesticides when possible. But skipping the vegetable entirely is the wrong way to do it.

I have actually heard people say that they would rather eat factory foods over fresh produce because at least they know it will be "safer." That's hardly the case. Processed foods come from pesticide-coated ingredients too, but lack the abundant nutrients found in fresh, whole food. Processed foods are boiled, fried, baked, irradiated, pasteurized, preserved, colored, and then fortified with a sorry amount of nutrients in an attempt to add back what is lost during production or in order to introduce additional vitamins into our diet that we don't get nearly enough of because we are eating too many processed foods in the first place. In fact, processed foods are so depleted of nutrients that fortification is legally required to make sure that some nutrition is present. This tactic doesn't create healthy food. It's just less bad, but only barely.

Oh, the things we will do for shelf life, a consistent product, and our extreme fear of pathogens! Processed food may look healthy, and the box probably tells you it is, but it is never as healthy as the whole food from whence it came. And even there is some question. How "good" were those foods when they arrived at the factory doors?

The benefits of eating veggies far outweigh the risks of exposure to small quantities of pesticides. That being said, to reduce your exposure to chemicals, you can buy organic (better for the environment too), and you can wash your produce with soap and water to remove as much toxic residue as possible. Adding a little vinegar helps too.

Vegetable-Juicing Wars

Health magazines and health advocates often argue about which kind of vegetable is best. For example, an article in *Natural Health* magazine did not support juice cleanses. Instead of patting folks on the back for at least attempting to get more veggies in their diet, the author of the article spent a great deal of time putting down juice fasts, arguing that store-bought "kale-and-whatever" juices are too sugary, provide inadequate calories, lack protein, fat and fiber, and folks are likely to go back to their old habits afterward anyway.[1] She may have a point, but just barely. I say, if it is a vegetable, eat it. Juice it. Drink it. Mix it with something tasty, like an apple, so you can get it down. If juice fasting appeals to you, go for it. It is never a bad idea to consume lots of vegetables. If the structure and rigidity of a seven-day juice cleanse will make that happen, do it. It's better than not juicing at all.

"Juice" that you achieve by mixing some sort of powder into water is not going to be the same as the kind you get from your own juicer in your kitchen. And yes, it's true: store-bought beverages are not superior to fresh, homemade vegetable juice. But perhaps bottled greens are the gateway drug to better health. One healthy habit often leads to others. Making a conscious effort to obtain more vegetables in one's diet would hopefully extend beyond premade smoothies and right into one's own kitchen, where fresh vegetables are being prepared and eaten in abundance.

To the author's credit, the last paragraph of the article in *Natural Health* promotes grabbing a juice beverage now and then, especially if one's diet has been suboptimal that day, and forgoing sugary varieties in favor of vegetable-based homemade concoctions. Good idea.

Perhaps folks reading *Natural Health* magazine are ready for the next push. I mean, they are already reading *Natural Health* magazine, right? They are health-nut-school graduates looking to make their diets even better. Hats off to them.

But for the average gal who picked up a copy of the magazine off the table at her massage appointment, let's encourage *her.* Ideally, we would all eat an organic, plant-based diet, consume healthy fats, drink plenty of water, exercise regularly, and juice too. Until then, I feel we must encourage eating of *all* vegetables.

Sugar in Vegetables?

Eat them anyway. Eat lots. Strive to get a variety of vegetables in your diet, but don't stress about the sugar in carrots. In the hierarchy of food, vegetables win hands down every time.

TIME TO GET JUDGMENTAL

I suppose it is high time I share with you what we have been eating. The best way I can do that is to tell you what our average shopping cart is filled with each week. And yes, there are tons of vegetables in it.

Groceries in Our Shopping Cart

I'm sure we aren't the only ones doing it. I can see the casual glances of other folks in line scanning the contents of our shopping cart. I'm glancing right back at theirs. Perhaps our quick looks at each other aren't really that casual. They are making judgments or assumptions about the items I have selected, as I am about theirs.

My dad used to tell me that if you want to know how to eat right, look in the shopping carts of all the others folks and don't buy what they are buying. (He was in fact quoting nutritionist Dr. Carlton Fredericks.) Unfortunately, in all the years I have been scanning the contents of carts, they are still right.

I make a point to select the best food possible. I read labels. I put stuff back on the shelf if I need to.

How Putting Back Food Got Me in Trouble

When we were first dating, this did not please my husband one bit. Everything he put in the grocery cart I took out. I simply couldn't buy foods loaded with sugar, or containing preservatives, artificial flavors, artificial colors, or chemicals. I would not buy altered, processed food donning "low fat" or "low sugar" labels that invariably contained fillers that were much worse. Tensions rose on one particular day until, at last, he wheeled around on his heels and stopped dead in the middle of the aisle and declared, "I *hate* shopping with you."

My reshelving the Oreos might have been the final straw. But there we were, having one of our first "conversations" about what good food was made of. It sure is awfully hard to say good-bye to things you have always eaten and enjoyed.

Sometimes being right also means being lonely. Thankfully, in my case, my husband stuck by my side. Over time, and it didn't take long, he realized like so many folks do, that there really is a food hierarchy. Some things we simply should not eat. Others, like fruits and vegetables, we should always eat and do so in quantity. The only way to ensure one over the other is to not buy any junk in the first place.

It's Not So Taboo to Be a Health Nut These Days

There are lots of folks making adjustments to what they buy at the grocery store. Many folks are reading labels. Carefully.

Unfortunately, many of the adjustments Americans made to their grocery lists over the years have harmed rather than helped their health. For example, people took the advice to eat less saturated fat, and (often unknowingly) ate more sugar instead. The ol' food pyramid that suggested people eat more grains than greens was a problem all along. Americans had no problem doing it, however. The grains people ate were not the filling, more nutritious whole grains. Folks went straight to the refined products. Ever eat a homemade whole-wheat-crust pizza? You are full after one slice. Not like the enormous pie you get from your local pizza joint, of which you could probably eat half.

Our government's current advice is simple: make your plate half fruits and vegetables at every meal. Hopefully we will. Based on my nonscientific shopping-cart snooping, it would seem we still have some work to do.

OUR FAVORITE FOODS

So what does our family put in our grocery cart? Some vegetables, like carrots, we buy all year long, regardless of season. Others, like tomatoes, we don't buy until they are in season and we can obtain locally grown varieties. We buy organic food whenever possible. If it looks fresh and healthy and doesn't cost a fortune, into the cart it goes. Quality is important. So too is quantity, especially in the summertime when there is an abundance of affordable produce. However, when buying up the bulk summer harvest, "organic" is a bonus, but not necessarily a requirement for us. We can afford to eat more vegetables when they cost less. When we buy locally grown produce at roadside stands, talking with the farmer about their use or avoidance of certain pesticides can further drive our purchasing decisions. Washing and peeling also helps reduce some pesticide exposure.

For health reasons and for the sake of the environment, we avoid buying genetically modified (GMO) foods and meat from animals that have been fed a diet that contains genetically modified organisms. If something new ends up on the GMO list (like zucchini), we make a point to avoid it and buy organic instead. Unless an item is clearly labeled indicating no GMO contents, eating organic is the only way to ensure that what we eat is not genetically modified.

You also won't find any sugar-laden beverages on our shopping list. If you want something to drink at our house, there is water or milk, and occasionally fruit juice. We are not perfect. We also have beer. But it usually has time to gather dust before anyone gets into it.

Our Shopping List:

Every item here is organic if possible.

- ❑ Bulk greens, spinach, lettuce, cabbage, romaine, and kale
- ❑ Mushrooms, red and yellow onions, bell peppers, avocados, bananas, eggplant, olives, scallions, celery, sweet potatoes, white/red potatoes, carrots, cucumbers, radishes, apples, oranges, grapes, green beans, tomatoes, and (less frequently) cauliflower, broccoli, Brussels sprouts, and asparagus; sweet corn (when in-season)
- ❑ Fresh fruit (in season when possible) such as peaches, plums, blueberries, strawberries, cherries, pomegranates, watermelon, kiwi, pears, apples, and pears
- ❑ Fresh cilantro, parsley, rosemary, and thyme
- ❑ Lemons and limes
- ❑ Fresh garlic and ginger
- ❑ Cheeses, sour cream, cottage cheese, and grass-fed butter
- ❑ Eggs (when we can't get them locally), milk, and cream
- ❑ Fresh or frozen berries
- ❑ Whole-milk yogurt
- ❑ Dry and canned beans and legumes
- ❑ Pumpkin, flax, and sunflower seeds

- ❑ Pureed baby food
- ❑ Applesauce
- ❑ Seaweed, roasted red peppers, pickles, hummus
- ❑ Grass-fed meat (pork, poultry, beef, bacon) or wild-caught fish (to avoid GMO feed and antibiotics)
- ❑ Fresh bread

Foods We Like but Buy Less Often:

Every item here is organic if possible.

- ❑ Olive and coconut oils; organic canola oil; vinegars (red, balsamic, apple cider, and rice)
- ❑ Brown rice, quinoa, oatmeal, whole-wheat flour, and white flour
- ❑ Ice cream
- ❑ Croutons (or I make my own)
- ❑ Tofu
- ❑ Wild-caught tuna, canned
- ❑ Hot sauce, dried spices, hot peppers, and mayonnaise
- ❑ Snack crackers for the kids
- ❑ Peanut butter and jelly
- ❑ Local raw or organic honey
- ❑ Nuts (pecans, peanuts, cashews), dried cranberries, sunflower seeds
- ❑ Prepared soups for quick meals; organic chicken stock/broth
- ❑ Raisins and prunes
- ❑ Ketchup and mustards
- ❑ Sprouted-grain organic bread or waffles (to freeze)
- ❑ Corn chips and shells
- ❑ Boxed macaroni and cheese
- ❑ Tea and coffee
- ❑ Pasta and ingredients for sauce
- ❑ Granola or oat O's
- ❑ Snack bars made of nuts
- ❑ Juice (for taking vitamin C)

Our Rare Purchases:

Every item here is organic if possible.

- ❑ Baking supplies, including: cocoa, sugar, dark chocolate, molasses, shortening, and extracts (like vanilla and peppermint)
- ❑ Sauces for ethnic cuisine (hoisin, soy, chili, coconut milk)
- ❑ Hot dogs (for summer cookouts) and pepperoni (for homemade pizzas)

Perhaps the inside of our fridge looks kind of boring, at least to anyone wanting a quick-fix blast of sugar. It is loaded with vegetables, some dairy, and just about everything—save fruits, veggies, nuts, and cheese for snacking—involves work to make into a meal. Many of our menu items involve planning and preparation. Absolutely none of them have instructions like, "Remove foil to expose tater tots." Want bread? You'll probably have to make it. Want soup? You'll probably have to cook it. While we do buy some prepared foods, most food preparing is done by us.

We went grocery shopping yesterday. I just looked in the fridge and all of our cabinets. What you see here is pretty much what we have in the house—or forgot to buy. Sure, the list will probably change here and there as the years go by and we learn about new foods.

As you may have noticed from our list, we have great local grocery stores that carry a wide selection of organic foods. We go there weekly. That's about how long it takes to eat up the fresh food from the previous shopping trip. Some folks may feel that fresh food is expensive. It can be. However, I find that the "gourmet" animal proteins like organic cheese and meat are far pricier. Therefore, we see to it that we eat plenty of the less expensive legumes and cheaper animal products such as eggs and yogurt.

OUR MEALS

"Health comes from the kitchen. Your first hobby is to discover the fun of cooking."

—ADELLE DAVIS, *Let's Eat Right to Keep Fit*

There are lots of whole foods on our plates. For example, last night my hubby and I cooked and ate our once-monthly (if that) steak dinner. We don't actually plan it that way, but that's about the frequency at which steak shows up on our table. Organic steak is expensive. It is an occasional treat. Next to our moderate cut of meat was a huge pile of green beans, and next to those, sliced tomatoes with garlic and basil. Processed food occasionally makes it to the table, but not nearly as often as whole foods. What is processed is mainly organic, such as boxed macaroni and cheese for the kids, and canned soup. You won't find TV dinners, boxed lasagna, pot pies, or pocket pizzas in our freezer. We still order a pizza once in a while, and by "once in a while" I mean every three months or so. Better yet, we make our own.

My husband loves to cook; I do too. Most of our meals are made at home, but we still eat out in restaurants. We especially like to eat breakfast out with the kids about once a week, and usually after we've all had a glass of homemade veggie juice. We don't turn up our noses at family barbecues or evening meals. We just eat *really clean* whenever we are in control of what ingredients go on our plates. This doesn't always involve cooking. Many times, "meals" are simply collections of good foods, but not in the form of a prepared dish. For example, the kids love variety plates for lunch. I'll put carrots and celery with blue cheese, chips with hummus or homemade guacamole, prunes, cheese with mustard, apple slices with or without peanut butter, cut fruit, and so on, all on one plate. They love to select what they eat next, and we have found the good food goes down better when they have many choices.

The following list includes some of our main menu items. All of our meals are served with piles of vegetables or fruit in them, on them, and/or on the side.

Our Menu Ideas:

- ❑ Pinto burgers (whole wheat, shredded carrots, eggs, sage, salt, and pinto beans)
- ❑ Salads (three times a week for dinner), loaded with whatever we have veggie-wise as well as hard-boiled eggs, avocados, nuts, and seeds
- ❑ Wild-caught fish (once a week, if affordable)
- ❑ Tacos, enchiladas, or nachos with beans, or ground beef, or shredded chili-powder potatoes

- ❑ Soup: mushroom, lentil, or other bean or pea soups
- ❑ Eggplant omelet
- ❑ Oatmeal
- ❑ Chili: turkey, beef, or bean based
- ❑ Tofu stir-fry
- ❑ Portobello burgers with roasted red peppers, onions, and garlic aioli
- ❑ Meatloaf or lentil loaf
- ❑ Broccoli or spinach quiche
- ❑ Rice (or quinoa) with mixed vegetables and mozzarella cheese (hot sauce and butter served on top)
- ❑ The occasional (monthly) steak dinner
- ❑ Homemade half-whole-wheat pancakes or French toast (with fruit)
- ❑ Baked dark-meat chicken and vegetables
- ❑ Pasta with homemade sauce
- ❑ Crockpot stews
- ❑ Homemade pizza
- ❑ Guacamole (yes, sometimes it is a meal)

If you have found yourself judgmental of my shopping cart or my dinner table, that's okay. You don't have to like, cook, eat, or buy what we do. I want to share with you what we like to do, at least for now, and it works for us. It works because we are happy, healthy, and fit.

The more my family learns about food, the more variety we have in the house and the more varied a diet we eat. We are often adjusting and changing our list and incorporating new ingredients into our menu. We spend most of our budget on fresh fruits and vegetables and work meals around them to prevent spoilage. Breakfast and lunch are generally simple meals in our house, and dinner more elaborate (as we have more time to cook when one parent entertains the little ones).

"Everything in Moderation"

It's a silly phrase, really. The word *everything* means to some folks exactly that: everything. It allows the justification of bad behavior: "I'll just have *some* soda every day . . . every meal." But that doesn't really work, does it? We can't have everything in moderation, or at least we shouldn't. There are many substances you could put into your body that you simply have to say no to. Heroin, for instance. If there are foods you can't control yourself around (and those foods aren't fruits and vegetables) you may have to avoid them completely.

We could find a way to demonize all foods. We can say olive oil is good for you, but if you drink down a quart a day, it's not so good anymore. We'll eat spinach, but then the next media-driven *E. coli* scare will have folks sidestepping fresh greens in stores. Some will fuss about the natural sugar in fresh fruit even when eating fruit is a much better choice than not eating fruit.

The goal is to move up the food continuum. To adopt a food hierarchy, as it were. Eat the best food you can for the money you have to spend.

You notice there are plenty of items conspicuously absent from our family's shopping list and meals. There are entire aisles in the grocery store we never go down. They include the soda aisle, the factory-made cookies and candy aisle, and the sugary cereal section. We don't buy sugary baked goods either. We eat few snack foods (occasionally organic crackers), precious few frozen entrees (we've bought perogies here and there), a small number of convenience foods (organic mac and cheese for the kids and the occasional can of organic soup), and no mixes (except for organic dressing spice mixes). We avoid processed meat, except for the occasional addition of organic pepperoni on our homemade pizza. Artificial and "imitation" anything are missing. This also means, for the most part, that all these things are missing from our diet.

Could we eat even better? Sure we could. Probably everyone can. It is a process. Much of our health success can be attributed to lack of temptation. When we go to our cabinets for food, that is exactly what we get: real food. Not having junk in the house means we are far less likely to eat junk. We can't always eat organic food when we eat out, nor can we expect all of our friends and family to cook like we do. We just do the best we can, when we can. At parties, you'll see me load up on items from the veggie tray and salad bowl first. Then, if there is room, I'll enjoy some of the standard American fare.

For those "I can't take any more of this healthy stuff" days, yes, we have a tub of dark chocolate chip chocolate ice cream in the freezer. Just to make us feel better, it's organic. There is also a single bag of potato chips in the bread box. And therein lies the other rule about eating well: you can't. Not all the time, that is. Do your very best to eat right most every day, most every meal. If you eat wrong, recognize it; see yourself doing it, and work to make a change. It's not easy. It never is. There may be foods you can't keep in the house at all. For example, you won't find thin mint cookies or chocolate brownies on our countertops. If they are in our vicinity, they get eaten instantly and in quantity. We know we simply can't have them around. Treats we can control our intake of, like that tub of ice cream in the freezer, are easy to keep around. We have the self-control needed to keep from eating too much too often. A little bit of ice cream now and again keeps us from throwing our hands up and racing to the corner store to eat something much worse.

SECRET ICE CREAM

Everyone has their secrets. For years, my husband kept one from me. Eventually, I figured it out.

One evening long ago in years BC (before children), I was on the couch with a migraine. It was the worst ever. It was the migraine that changed my life, literally. Afterward, I changed careers. I adopted regular, healthy stress-reduction activities. I focused on getting optimal doses of the vitamins and nutrients my body needed. But this particular headache was before all that, and there I lay comatose, unable to do anything because of the pain. I couldn't take it anymore. I wanted drugs.

My dear husband headed to the store to buy some caffeine-laden migraine pain-relief pills, but it took a while. He finally came home after what seemed like forever, bottle in hand.

"What took so long?" I strained. He paused. He looked guilty. I *knew* he was up to something.

"Well?" I squawked.

He admitted he had stopped for frozen custard after the supermarket.

"Really?!" I shot back, instantly furious. I couldn't *believe* him. Here I was, suffering with unimaginable pain, and he took his sweet time eating sweets. Shameful.

"I ate it in the car on the way home?" he asked rather than stated. "I went through the drive through!" he added, as if somehow that made it better.

It didn't. I wanted to relate to him just how much my head hurt. But I didn't even want to talk. I just couldn't believe it. The idea that I had to suffer with a crippling headache even one minute longer than I needed to because he had to order his chocolate custard on a sugar cone made me ferociously indignant. I was in no mood for excuses. I flatly accused him of eating "secret ice cream" and demanded he tell me how many other times he had eaten frozen treats without my knowledge.

And so it was revealed. For the next few weeks, anytime we drove by an ice cream stand I'd point and question him accusingly. "Ever have any *secret* ice cream there?!"

"Um . . . yes."

It turns out there had been several times when he had surreptitiously slipped out to get himself a frozen dessert. It wasn't always when he was supposed to be doing something else. Sometimes he would go during his lunch break or maybe when he was on his way to hang out with a buddy.

With my headache now gone, his failure to promptly get pain reliever to me no longer concerned me. It was the fact that I had no idea he was eating secret ice cream in the first place. Even worse, I was being left out.

Once in a while I'll ask my husband if he's had any secret ice cream lately. Occasionally, he will confess on his own. He will tell me about a time he was thinking of having some secret ice cream, or a new place we should try because he knows it's . . . um . . . good. To this day we joke about it. My kids now have secret ice cream too. Our daughter will announce to Daddy when he gets home, "We had secret ice cream today!"

Like I said, everybody has their secrets.

(If you are interested in learning more about how to treat, prevent, and lessen the duration of migraine headaches so you don't have to resort to drugs, you may wish to consult my books *The Vitamin Cure for Women's Health Problems* and *Vitamins & Pregnancy: The Real Story*. Among other things, they discuss the detailed rationale for using niacin, magnesium, and vitamin C. Migraines are truly awful, and knowing how to successfully use nutritional therapy has been extremely helpful for me.)

EATING MEAT

Since our family only eats meat once a week or so, I feel I can afford to get the more expensive grass-fed and organic kind. Nonorganic meat is still pretty pricey too. (I'm pretty sure that's the reason I was raised vegetarian.)

The American Heart Association would like you to keep your meat (preferably lean) consumption to no more than 6 ounces a day.[2] We are eating nearly twice that.[3] Most of it is red, and nearly a quarter of it is processed.[4] According to an article in *Public Health and Nutrition* (2011), "Red meat still represents the largest proportion of meat consumed in the U.S. (58%). Twenty-two percent of the meat consumed in the U.S. is processed."[5] The Heart Association encourages us to eat more chicken, fish, and beans.[6] I imagine beans don't have quite the curb appeal as does a nice juicy steak.

According to the Food and Agriculture Organization of the United Nations in their 2009 publication *The State of Food and Agriculture,* Americans are eating about 279 pounds of meat, on average, per person each year.[7] If you divide that by 365 days in a year, that's an average of about 12 ounces a day of meat per person. In actuality, the amount is even higher. Vegetarians and vegans are eating none; someone else is eating their 12 ounces per day. Unless we are getting that all down in one sitting, it would be safe to say at least two out of three of most Americans' meals used to be able to stare right back. Are we all eating organic grass-fed animals? At that rate, who could afford to?

Meat costs plenty. It is no surprise that current forecasts project that our daily intake is heading down,[8] and some of us don't eat any at all. Some of us want to eat less meat and to make the meat we do eat the best possible for us and our environment. If we were attempting to buy and eat organic grass-fed meat to the tune of 12 ounces a day, it would be downright extravagant. Fish isn't cheap either. But beans sure are.

We all need protein. How we get it can change. For some of us, it already is changing. For more of us, it should.

According to the movie *Fast Food Nation* (2006), 25 percent of the country eats fast food every day. I imagine precious few of these meals are meat-free.

A Vegetarian Eats a Hot Dog

At the age of eight, when I was in third grade, I was finally allowed to select and eat meat. I had been waiting for this. I knew *exactly* what I would pick. Since forever I longed to be a normal child and eat an actual grilled hot dog (instead of a tofu "not" dog). Finally, when I came of age, my dad said he would buy some franks if that's what I really wanted. My excitement peaked. We headed off to the grocery store. It went downhill from there.

Instead of buying one package of hot dogs like most normal parents would do, my father bought somewhere around ten packs of weenies, maybe more. (Yes, they were, in fact, on sale.) He hefted them onto the store's conveyor belt, lugged the bulging bag back to our car, dumped the slippery packages onto the kitchen counter, and then unceremoniously stuffed them into the bottom of our refrigerator. I'm not exactly sure why, but the sheer quantity of tubed meat being manhandled that day wasn't particularly appealing. Still, I was determined to have my hot dog.

I'm not sure if there is any scientific evidence showing that kids who are caught smoking and then, as punishment, are forced to smoke a whole pack of cigarettes ever resolve to be nonsmokers. I imagine such conditioning just jump-starts a bad habit. At the very least, it raises ethical questions about such parenting. I can tell you, however, from my personal experience with hot dogs, that after voluntarily consuming my fill of the bulk-pack cheap red weenies, I have not been enticed to eat any more of them.

It's probably better that way. Hot dogs are terrible for you. That hasn't slowed most Americans down any. According to The National Hot Dog and Sausage Council (yes, there is one) Americans eat, on average, 70 hot dogs per person every year.[9] Only a few years ago, they estimated the hot dog intake at 60 per person. I don't think we should be proud.

Pass the Mustard, or Just Pass on the Hot Dog?

by Andrew W. Saul, PhD

From the *Orthomolecular Medicine News Service,* July 2, 2010.

More hot dogs are eaten at the Fourth of July holiday than at any other time of the year. The National Hot Dog and Sausage Council says that "during the Independence Day weekend, 155 million will be gobbled up" and that Americans will consume more than seven billion hot dogs over the summer. "Every year," they proudly proclaim, "Americans eat an average of 60 hot dogs each."[1]

That looks to be a modest average of just over one hot dog per week per American. But there are at least seven million vegetarians in the U.S., and another 20 million who would be inclined to avoid meat.[2]

This means that even if you do not eat any hot dogs at all, someone else is eating your share.

But a hot dog or two a week? Big deal!

Maybe it is. Children who eat one hot dog a week double their risk of a brain tumor; two per week triples the risk. Kids eating more than twelve hot dogs a month (three a week) have nearly ten times the risk of leukemia as children who eat none.[3]

And it is not just about kids. Of 190,000 adults studied for seven years, those eating the most processed meat, such as deli meats and hot dogs, had a 68 percent greater risk of pancreatic cancer than those who ate the least.[4] Pancreatic cancer is especially difficult to treat.

Think twice before you serve up your next tube steak. If your family is going to eat hot dogs, at least take your vitamins. Hot dog eating children taking supplemental vitamins were shown to have a reduced risk of cancer.[5] Vitamins C and E prevent the formation of nitrosamines.[6–8]

It is curious that, while busy theorizing about the many "potential" dangers of vitamins, the news media have largely ignored this clear-cut cancer-prevention benefit from supplementation.

May I also suggest that you have your kids chew their hot dogs extra thoroughly. In landfills, "Whole hot dogs have been found, some of them in strata suggesting an age upwards of several decades."[9]

Bon appétit.

REFERENCES FOR "PASS THE MUSTARD"

1. http://www.hot-dog.org.

2. *Vegetarian Times*. Vegetarianism in America. http://www.vegetariantimes.com/features/archive_of_editorial/667 (accessed May 2016).

3. Peters JM, Preston-Martin S, London SJ, et al. Processed meats and risk of childhood leukemia. *Cancer Causes Control* 1994; 5(2):195–202.

4. Nothlings U, Wilkens LR, Murphy SP, et al. Meat and fat intake as risk factors for pancreatic cancer: the multiethnic cohort study. *J Nat Cancer Inst* 2005;97:1458–1465.

5. Sarasua S, Savitz DA. Cured and broiled meat consumption in relation to childhood cancer: Denver, Colorado (United States). *Cancer Causes Control* 1994;5(2):141–148. 6. Tannenbaum SR. Preventive action of vitamin C on nitrosamine formation. *Int J Vitam Nutr Res Suppl* 1989;30:109–113.

7. Lathia D, Blum A. Role of vitamin E as nitrite scavenger and N-nitrosamine inhibitor: a review. *Int J Vitam Nutr Res* 1989;59(4):430–8.

8. Cass H, English J. *User's guide to vitamin C*. North Bergen, NJ: Basic Health Publications, 2002.

9. *Smithsonian*, July 1992, p 5.

Our family's transition into meat eaters meant that now we would enjoy a bit of poultry: a turkey at Thanksgiving and an occasional summer "chicky" barbecue. Red meat almost never made it through the door, save the hog dogs that did. I'm pretty sure my mom would eat a hamburger now and again, but I never saw her do it. What was once "vegetarian" became "plant-based," a way of eating that my husband, children, and I have adopted. My husband really likes preparing and cooking meat. He will spend all day on a smoked something-or-other. But he also enjoys plenty of nonmeat meals each week with me. He used to eat more meat. He now eats less. He's happy with the transition. He likes how he feels. As my dad says, "By moving towards a vegetarian diet, you automatically reduce your too-high intake of protein, fat, and sugar. It is just that simple. There is no diet plan to buy."

I am no longer vegetarian. I eat a plant-based diet, which isn't really a "diet" at all. I just eat that way.

EATING FAT

Fats don't make us fat, but this is news for a lot of people. Many foods, including dairy products, have been demonized for their fat content, and over time, the fats have been steadily removed from milk products until ingesting the drain-water-flavored skim milk became commonplace and folks entirely forgot what actual milk tastes like. Those fortunate enough to get it straight from the cow will argue that whole milk at the store is a far cry indeed from real milk. Raw milk is loaded with beneficial bacteria, digestive enzymes, vitamins, and more. Pasteurized milk, unfortunately, kills off beneficial bacteria, destroys enzymes, and lowers milk's vitamin content.[10]

I eat dairy. I enjoy some milk, but mostly I eat cultured dairy like yogurt and cheese. I also adore sour cream and butter. When we were younger, dairy was a source of fat and protein for us growing kids who ate a lacto-ovo vegetarian diet. My father would bring home raw goat and cow's milk from the farm where he worked milking cows. We ate a lot of cheese. It made many a vegetarian dish taste better. Just like dressing made a salad better. Cheese is often given a hard time. I get it. It's not for everybody. Can it really be part of a healthy diet?

Cheese Is Making Us Fat

Is it? Or is it everything else we are also eating? And everything else we aren't?

Back in the early 2000s, the United States Department of Agriculture

(USDA) worked with their creation, the Dairy Management Incorporation, to get more cheese into fast-food menus. People just weren't eating enough cheese, I guess. A focus on low-fat dairy options meant too much whole milk and fat were left over.[11] What could be done? Cheese in Pizza Hut pizza crust? Brilliant! In 2010, 40 percent more cheese was added to Domino's pizzas.[12] People were buying cheesier pizzas and loving them. Business boomed. Scratch that. Business booms. You won't see me ordering a whole-wheat crust with half the cheese, no sir. If I'm having a pizza, I'm having a PIZZA. Who's with me? Cheese is the best part. And the Parmesan cheese-sprinkled sauce, and the garlic-cheese crust . . .

Then there is talk about fat and how too much is a bad idea. Believe it or not, eating fat does not make you fat. Whole milk is not really the problem. In my opinion, neither is cheese. Hold on, I'll explain.

"Most of us realize by now that fats don't make you fat," says Hyla Cass, MD. "In fact, fats are essential in keeping your body healthy."[13] Of course, what kind of fat you eat does matter. The healthiest fats are polyunsaturated fats, the omega-3 and omega-6 fats, such as those found in fish oil.[14] They are essential. Your body requires these fats but cannot make them. You have to eat them. We are actually doing all right with our consumption of omega-6 fatty acids, found in milk, meat, seeds, nuts, and veggie oil.[15] It is the other one, omega-3 fatty acids, we really have to pay attention to. As with many things, our ratio is off. Many Americans consume too many omega-6 fatty acids and not nearly enough omega-3s. Omega-3 fatty acids are found in foods like flaxseed, fatty fish, and eggs. Many folks also choose to take a supplement in order to get a mercury-free dose of omega-3s. Monounsaturated fats are also good for you. This type of fat is found in foods like avocados and olive oil. You'll notice, however, that cheese does not fit into either of these categories.

The moral of the story is we should limit the saturated animal fats found in meat, and, yes, cheese. This is no time to go on the cheese diet. If you do eat meat and cheese, buy organic grass-fed to limit your exposure to antibiotics, hormones, and pesticide residue.[16] And as far as cheeses go, aged cheese is better for you. Select ones, like cheddar, Gouda, and Swiss, that have aged for months. They digest more easily.

It is no secret that many eat what is not good for them. But adding extra cheese to a pizza isn't really the deeper issue here. I happen to agree with the Agriculture Department on this one. I think cheese can fit into a healthy diet. It's the other thousand meals eaten each year that are void of fresh, raw produce that are the problem. It is a matter of portion and proportion. Americans eat way too much of the wrong things and nowhere near enough of the right things.

"Agriculture Department data show that cheese is a major reason the average American diet contains too much saturated fat," says the *New York Times* in an article entitled "While Warning about Fat, U.S. Pushes Cheese Sales."[17] Cheese may not be the only problem. "Research has found that the cardiovascular benefits in cutting saturated fat may depend on *what replaces it* [emphasis added]. Refined starches and sugar might be just as bad or even worse, while switching to unsaturated fats has been shown to reduce the risk of heart disease."[18]

What replaces it, eh? "Low fat" often comes loaded with fillers and additives. Fat tastes good. Without it, normally fat-based products tend to taste poor. If you don't believe me, go read the ingredients on a container of diet yogurt, often given a catchy, seemingly healthy-sounding label like "Light and Fit," which describes nothing about the product or the real health consequences for the consumer buying it. If you can get past all the indigestible fillers like modified food starch and the paint they use to color it to make it look like food, you can still "enjoy" cancer-causing, good bacteria–killing fake sweeteners, and nasty preservatives. Ick. You'd be better off eating a whole-milk yogurt, cream and all, without the added bad ingredients. Really. And if you aren't eating a low-fat version of the same food, what are you eating instead? Are you selecting foods loaded with refined starches and sugar that are just as bad as or even worse than that excess saturated fat? "According to the Center for Health Statistics, the American obesity epidemic started in the early 1980s—not coincidentally at the same time the market was flooded with low-fat products," said Dr. Hyla Cass.[19] "Suddenly, the rate of overweight adults went through the roof."

I see. Tack on all that cheese to a pizza crust made of refined white flour, processed meat loaded with nitrates (preservatives), and top it off with sugary sauce (sweet sauce is popular 'round these parts) and a sugary drink (fake or real sugar, it doesn't matter; both are bad, folks), and you've got a recipe for disaster.

Hmm. Sugar's no good. And skip the refined starch? Dang. Nix the cheese and suddenly there's no pizza on the table anymore. Perhaps that's for the better.

But I am unwilling to live a pizza-free life. And I have an astonishing amount of company.

Maybe an occasional pizza is not the problem. Maybe the extra cheese on it is not a problem either. But eating nothing but processed food with few to no vegetables is a problem. Must we say it again? Cheese alone is not the issue. It's all the other junk food folks are eating and all the good stuff we aren't.

When I was growing up, I couldn't stand it when my parents would ruin a perfectly good pizza night by making us drink a glass of fresh, homemade vegetable juice first. I just wanted to eat the pizza, for goodness' sake, like a normal child. But as we watch "normal" children, now turned adults, suffering with health problems, it may be no surprise that I do *exactly* the same with my children as my parents did with us. Nothing quite gets that glass (or sippy cup) of veggie juice down like a hot, bubbly slice of cheesy goodness waiting on a child's plate right in front of them.

Even better, we ensure quality ingredients by making our own pizza pies. It's fun, too. The kids love to help. You may want to get yourself a pizza stone. They rock. (Pun intended.) We make our pies with homemade dough and sauce, and top with nitrate-free pepperoni. Oh yes, and lots of organic cheese.

Do It with Veggies

Take everything with a grain of salt, or a cube of cheese, as it were. Avoid the hype, don't eat bad things, and go back to the least publicized stuff out there: good ol' veggies.

I have an idea. Let's do it with veggies. Let's get the veggie farmers rich beyond their wildest dreams. Let's get *excessive.* Instead of cheese, let's grind veggies into pizza crust and stuff the crust with peppers and take the toddler approach: don't tell anyone.

Of course, the toddler approach in our household is different. We tell them exactly what they are eating. There is no prejudice. Nobody in our kids' presence is allowed to turn up their nose at any good food our kids choose to eat. Don't like prunes? Cabbage? Spinach? Fine. Keep it to yourself. My kids like 'em. Our kids are aware of what goes into their bodies. Might we puree some greens and add it to tomato sauce? Sure. But we will also tell them it's in there.

Americans are tricky. Many have not been raised with an appreciation or taste for a plant-based diet. Is more cheese on a pizza a problem for them? Probably. And so is every other unhealthy, commercially processed, high-calorie, high-sugar, low-nutrition meal they eat. Would they eat a veggie-er processed pizza if they knew about it? Who knows? Nobody's tried it yet.

"YOU ARE WHAT YOU EAT"

I've never liked that phrase. I don't want to be a floret of broccoli. Neither does any kid. They all make fun of the phrase. It's just no good. It doesn't really bolster the health food community any, and yet it seems to be the best slogan they've got.

At some point we have to stop blaming the folks who make commercials and advertisements and start taking personal responsibility for what we put into our mouths. Nobody is forcing anyone to eat junk food. We buy it, we ingest it, and we will suffer the consequences if we choose to continually ignore what has been known for, like, ever. If we eat junk, we will feel like junk eventually. If we eat well, we will feel well. So yes, whether I like the phrase or not, we are what we eat.

Or maybe, as said by biochemist Adelle Davis, author of *Let's Get Well,* "We are indeed much more than what we eat, but what we eat can nevertheless help us to be much more than what we are."[20]

A Calorie Is a Calorie, or Is It?

There are those who will argue that a candy calorie is the same as a lettuce calorie.[21] I have literally watched nutrition guests on TV talk shows compare a spinach, tomato, and grilled-chicken salad to the calorie equivalent of three Klondike bars.

Scientifically speaking, yes, a calorie is a calorie. It is the energy required to raise the temperature of one gram of water by one degree Celsius.

Reasonably speaking, no. To simply call a calorie a calorie, no matter where it originates, sends an unfortunate message that only calories count. To equate a candy or dessert calorie with that of a healthy vegetable distracts from the truth. It is unconstructive. It clouds our judgment from what is really important. To focus on calorie intake alone is never enough. Calories are not created equal.

Eating 1,000 calories in the form of candy is very different from eating 1,000 calories in the form of vegetables. One is good for the body; the other is not. For example, Dr. Mark Hyman said, "Coke will spike blood sugar and insulin and disrupt neurotransmitters, leading to increased hunger and fat storage, while the thousand calories of broccoli will balance blood sugar and make you feel full, cut your appetite and increase fat burning. Same calories—profoundly different effects on your body."[22]

Furthermore, for 1,000 calories you could eat *100* cups of Romaine lettuce (at 10 calories a cup) or about one and a half cups of little jelly beans (at 4 calories *per bean).* One is nutritious. The other is not. Eat all the lettuce you can hold. Believe me, you'll quit well before you reach 100 cups. Do not eat jelly beans. (Then you needn't bother counting jelly bean calories.) Speaking in more reasonable terms, a large, low-calorie salad packed with an array of vegetables will fill you and nourish you. The calorie-equivalent few bites of jelly beans will do neither. This would seem so obvious. Why isn't the media catching on?

Don't get hung up on good calories. Over time, you may find, as I have, that I don't get caught up on calories *at all.* Still, there will be folks out there who measure how much lettuce they eat for fear of too many lettuce calories. Obsessing over vegetable calories is counterproductive. Calories from lettuce and all other vegetables are always and forever something we can and should eat plenty of.

Eat all the fresh fruits and vegetables you want. Period. Eat both. Eat plenty. Do not get out your scale or your calculator. It is liberating indeed to ignore the numbers and commit yourself to eating the best food possible. Eating the best food possible means you can ignore the numbers, and you can ignore the numbers if you eat the best food possible. Most of the produce our family buys doesn't even have a nutrition label on it.

There are lots of other foods that have to be monitored and, ideally, avoided: items packed with processed ingredients, namely sugar, and those boasting "low calorie" on the label as they are often packed with other unhealthy ingredients. Vegetables are not one of them. Fruits are not one of them. For anyone that's about to argue about the sugar content of fruits and vegetables, your case is about as strong as the one about lettuce calories. By volume, there is far less sugar in fruits and vegetables then in processed candy or desserts and far more nutrients. The sugar in our fresh fruits and vegetables is not what makes Americans fat. Conversely, Americans are not fat because we eat too many fruits and vegetables. Eat lettuce. Eat carrots. Eat apples and (gasp!) bananas. Have the occasional ear of corn. Eat *organic.* Don't fight the calorie battle so hard that you forget you are trying to win the calorie war.

This is the truth: vegetables and fruits, whole and fresh especially, are good for you. Do not fuss about the quantity. Quantity is good. Fret about all the other nutritionally void foods you are eating. Fret about soda, fret about processed foods, and fret about candy and fried food and fast food. Do not fret over the calorie content of carrots.

And for the folks who are certain it was all that dressing on the spinach salad that made it as calorie dense as a pile of Klondikes, they would still be missing the whole point. Vegetables are almost always the better food choice. Yes, even if you have to put dressing on them. I say, "If the dressing gets the salad down, eat the dressing." Skip unnatural store-bought dressings that are loaded with sugar or artificial sweeteners, preservatives, artificial color, GMO ingredients, additives like monosodium glutamate (MSG), or that are labeled "low fat" or "low calorie" (they instead just increase the content of unhealthy fillers and/or sugar to make them taste better). But if your favorite calorie-packed blue cheese dressing is the only way you are going to get those vegetables down, then get it on the salad. Fresh vegetables with dressing are always better than no vegetables. And since most Americans are in the "way too few vegetables" category,[23] it's time to eat some dressing. Want a healthier salad topper? Make your own dressing and use your own spices. Switch to olive oil and vinegar (like a high-quality balsamic), or get creative. Sometimes, I just shake a bunch of hot sauce (some prefer salsa) over my salad. Tastes like a taco. Over time, you may find you need less dressing or even none at all.

When you know what calories you should eat, and which ones you shouldn't, the only barrier left is free will. Some will argue that folks don't have access to good food. That is largely untrue. Some will say cost is a factor, but I'd like those folks to compare the cost of a fast-food meal or a pack of name-brand cookies to a pile of fresh vegetables. They may be surprised to see that a switch to the good stuff isn't that noticeable in the wallet. For others, even if good food does end up costing more (see section on the cost of good food), the money saved avoiding health problems and doctor visits and pharmacy bills makes up for it.

There are so many ways to do this right, and there are so many ways to do this wrong. Just see that you are on the right side of the equation.

"You cannot mistreat your body for 20, 50, or 70 years and then expect a doctor to give you a wonder drug to cure your ills. You cannot expect that any more than you could drive your car recklessly, miss stoplights, and break speed limits for years and expect the judge to let you off with a clean license. There is only one basic cause of disease, and that is unhealthful living. Unhealthful living leads to unhealth; this is simple enough to be easily overlooked. Healthful living leads to health; this is nature's law for all living beings. If this seems self-evident to you, that's good. You then realize that we can't fool Mother Nature, at least not forever."

—ANDREW W. SAUL, PhD

Organic: Is It Worth It?

I'm one of "those people" who buys organic whenever reasonably possible. I'll pay a little more for delicious sweet-cream butter from cows raised on grass. The taste alone is worth it. I'll pay more for the organic veggies I juice (organic carrots taste better), and I'll even swing for the pricey organic meat.

For the most part, I'm willing to pay about 25 percent more for organic food, and I can be convinced to pay even a tad more if the food is undeniably superior in taste and quality. We buy massive quantities of produce; it takes up about 75 percent of our shopping cart.

And then there are apples. Last winter, our grocery store was selling organic apples for a buck. Each. Ouch. Keeping a bounty of healthy goodies in our house was mighty expensive. I imagine when the typical shopper sees such prices, they think the same, and walk right on by the apple display.

On the other hand, the local farmer's market will sell us sixteen enormous apples for four dollars. No, they aren't organic. While they are "homegrown" in the summer, they may or may not be local in the wintertime. But the sheer *quantity* of fresh produce we manage to pile high in our countertop baskets for a quarter of the cost, is reason enough to use soap when we washed them, peel them if desired, and eat and juice them anyway.

Some purists just gasped. In fact, I can hardly believe myself.

Over the years, organic produce has infiltrated and nearly, but not quite, taken over our countertops, cabinets, and refrigerator shelves. This winter, organic apples became more reasonably priced at our local grocery store. (They are now sold by the bag, bringing down the per unit price a bit.) I have to admit, the more I learn about nonorganic food, the guiltier I feel about the food I feed my children. Why would I expose their little, developing bodies to conventionally raised apples, especially when apples are such a big part of their diet?

Good question. I bet you know my answer. We eat as much organic food as possible. We also eat (far less) conventionally farmed foods when the quality and prices dictates it be so. And we take lots of vitamin C to help us neutralize our inevitable exposure to toxins.

We are constantly working on our good health. Anybody who does it knows it is a daily task. Choices are exercised meal to meal, moment to moment. There is always a way to improve, to avoid more chemicals, to eat more cleanly, to increase the ratio of fruits and vegetables to other foods in every meal. When we can, we do it. But when eating better means that we can afford to eat better, we just get the produce in the cart. I would argue that eating some nonorganic produce is still a far better choice than other not-so-healthy foods that could displace them. Eating one food replaces the need to eat another. Our stomachs are only so big.

You will notice that when you start eating clean and taking your vitamins, when you don't, you *feel* it. My husband and I were both rather uncomfortable after a Christmas dinner party. I am pretty sure nothing served could be labeled "organic." We came home, took our vitamins, and marveled that folks could eat that food every day and not feel awful. Or, maybe they do.

Can't afford organic? Grow a garden. The next best thing: make friends with someone who does. You will find yourself inundated with pound after pound of produce that will simply go bad if it isn't shared. And one more tip: compost your fruit and veggies scraps. When I was a little girl, an apple core tossed into our compost heap turned into our very own organic apple tree. We moved a long time ago, but the tree is still there.

Protective Vitamins for Toxin Exposure

No matter how you live your life, you will be exposed to some toxins. It is inevitable. We can reduce our exposure, and we should, by choosing to eat whole, organic foods, and drink clean filtered water. But no matter how hard we try, they are there. All we can do is stack the deck in our favor.

This is a very compelling reason for folks to always take their vitamins, and that means everybody: children (including those unborn), adults, and the elderly. Vitamin C is especially important. In large doses, vitamin C is an effective antitoxin. Please see the chapter on vitamin C for more.

Buy Directly from the Farmer

Community Supported Agriculture (CSA) was a good idea for our family for one very particular reason: we got used to eating large quantities of greens. Not all farm shares are made equal, but the particular one we joined provided us with pounds of fresh organic greens every week, including arugula, spinach, bok choy, purslane (that one even grows by our driveway), dandelion greens (ditto), chicory, mustard greens, kale, and several varieties of lettuce. What they grew is what we ate. We couldn't let it go to waste, so we learned to eat it all, every week, all summer long.

Creativity was inevitable. Besides eating the greens fresh and raw in numerous salads, we'd throw them in a sauté pan with some garlic or a stir fry or into soup. Cooking them had the added advantage of using greens that were soon to wilt or go bad. Juicing took care of the rest. However, as a note of caution, do not juice a pound of (only) mustard greens in order to "use them up." About four excruciatingly spicy sips (and one tummy ache later), the rest of the offensive liquid will likely be discarded and thus wasted.

We were practically overwhelmed with greens, and we got used to it. We always ate quite well, but the sheer magnitude of good, fresh food provided by the CSA nearly tripled the number of vegetables we consumed. When the CSA ended for the season, we were so used to abundance that it was carried over to the way we shop and reflected in the choices that went into our grocery cart every week. Many items the CSA provided we wouldn't have necessarily bought in quantity on a regular basis. Kale, for example. I wasn't familiar with its flavor or its multiple uses, so I generally avoided it. For many folks, food items that are unfamiliar are often left untouched. Since kale had become part of our diet, it remained there, as did several other greens we learned to eat.

And this wasn't all. We were exposed to new varieties of root vegetables, fruits, herbs, and legumes. Oftentimes, the cost of fancy vegetables, like heirloom tomatoes, kept them from ever making it to our home. The CSA gave us the opportunity to eat these foods without the financial burden of the three-dollar grocery store tomato. It also works for those who don't have a vegetable garden.

Of course, exposure and abundance aren't the only advantages of a farm share. Participating in a CSA connects you with the food you eat and with where it was grown. You and your family learn what is in season, and when. You can support organic farming and sustainable farming practices. You support local business and local families. Your bounty rises and falls with how well the farmer's crops do that year: if the weather is spectacular, you all end up with a massive haul. If it is a tough growing season, you share that risk with the farmer. While your pocketbook may not like it, a lesson is learned for sure.

Supermarkets provide a false sense of security. We can get practically any food we want, in any quantity, any time of year (and sometimes pay dearly for it). In reality, the supply of fresh food is more unpredictable than our grocery store shelves would have us believe. There is much to be gained by the experience, whether you live in the country or the city. Give it a try and get used to eating real fresh food.

When in Doubt, Avoid Sugar

"Sugar is an addiction far stronger than what we see with heroin."
—ABRAM HOFFER, MD

We never like to be told no. Even when Mom said we couldn't have that cookie, kids would sneak into the kitchen, stealthily remove one from the cookie jar, and eat it anyway. It's human nature, I suppose. We like eating sugar.

Realizing that sugar addiction can be likened to heroin addiction should make anybody think twice before they consume it. There is no safe dose of heroin. You do, however, require a small amount of sugar. But not all sugar is made equal.

The advice to eat lots of vegetables may be just as important as the advice to avoid sugar. Not the kinds in fruits and vegetables, but refined sugars.

Sugar is not good for you. Just because something claims to contain "real sugar" does not make it a health food. Just because you may be better off with a little real sugar over artificial sweeteners or corn syrup, does not make it okay to sigh in relief that a product contains actual sugar. And sugar often comes from GMO sugar beets. Not that this makes cane sugar or organic sugar of any kind any healthier, for that matter. If you are suffering with yeast infections, urinary tract infections, (or any infection), weight gain, mood disturbances like anxiety or depression, to name just a few negative sugar-induced side effects, removing refined sugar from your diet is the right thing to do.

Should Sugar Be Regulated?

This next article by Robert G. Smith, PhD, Research Associate Professor in the Department of Neuroscience, University of Pennsylvania, discusses the dangers of sugar and will remind us to maintain our resolve to keep sugar out of our diets.

Toxic Sugar

by Robert G. Smith, PhD

From the *Orthomolecular Medicine News Service,* April 24, 2012.

An article in the prestigious journal *Nature* explains that sugar, especially fructose, widely available in soft drinks and other processed foods, is responsible for many serious noncommunicable diseases, such as heart disease, cancer, diabetes, obesity, and liver failure.[1,2] One of the contributing reasons is that fructose and other high-calorie substances such as alcohol cannot be directly utilized by the body's tissues so they must be metabolized by the liver, where they generate toxicity and set the body on a path to diabetes.[3] Further, fructose interferes with the body's sense of satiety, so that an excess of calories tend to be ingested. This overwhelms the liver, which then must convert the overdose of sugar into fat, which harms the liver and can lead to diabetes. Thus, sugar such as fructose, when added to processed foods, has been compared to alcohol in its toxic effect. Even nonobese people are susceptible to "metabolic syndrome," in which fructose induces hypertension, cardiovascular disease, insulin resistance, and damage to biological molecules such as proteins and lipids.[1–3]

Soft drinks that contain mainly sugar, such as sodas and filtered fruit juices, don't have enough nutrients to keep the body healthy and free from disease. They provide calories without essential nutrients that you would find in the whole fruit. These "empty" calories then replace other foods such as whole grains, fruits, and vegetables that are the main sources of essential nutrients. But added sugar is not limited to soft drinks. Added fructose, as in high-fructose corn syrup or just plain sugar (i.e., sucrose, which is 50 percent glucose and 50 percent fructose), is found in a wide variety of processed foods, such as breakfast cereal, juices, jellies and jams, candy, baked goods, sauces, desserts, and even ready-made dinners and processed meat. Fructose tastes sweet but does not satisfy hunger as well as more nutritious foods.

The high added-fructose content of processed foods is addictive in a similar way to alcohol, especially for young children. This has caused an epidemic of obesity in both children and adults. Further, the metabolism of fructose in the liver is similar to that of alcohol because it tends to perturb glucose metabolism, generating fat and causing insulin resistance, which leads to inflammation and degeneration of the liver and many other problems.[4] Overall, this dietary pattern caused by overloading our bodies with fructose is a vicious cycle that leads to widespread deficiencies of nutrients such as vitamins and essential minerals, along with damage and inflammation throughout the body. This vicious cycle of sugar addiction, consistent with the "metabolic syndrome," is in large part responsible for the high death rate from the modern diet.

If the modern diet could be adjusted to satisfy hunger without excess calories and to contain a larger proportion of essential nutrients, the epidemic of disease from added sugar might be averted. When ingested in the form of fruit, fructose is less harmful because it is absorbed slowly by the gut and importantly is accompanied by essential nutrients. Supplements of essential nutrients can help, but only if knowledge about the adequate doses and their benefits is made widely available. Examples are supplements of vitamin A, B vitamins, vitamin C, vitamin E, magnesium, omega-3 and -6 essential fats, which in the proper forms and doses can help prevent dietary deficiencies that cause heart disease, cancer, and diabetes.[5] Other lifestyle choices can help, for example, reducing total calories, increasing ingested fiber, and getting more exercise.[3] But the benefits of these healthy choices have not been convincing to the modern consumer. Ubiquitous high-pressure marketing of soft drinks contributes to the problem.

To correct the problem of sugar overconsumption, it has been suggested that sugar be regulated like alcohol and tobacco.[1] The goal would be to change habits to reduce consumption. Many schools have already banned the sale of sodas but have replaced them with juices or artificial drinks that contain added sugar. According to this suggestion, the sale of sweetened drinks and processed foods containing added sugar could be limited in school vending machines or elsewhere during school hours. Age limits on the sale of sugary foods in stores might also help. A limit or ban on television commercials advertising products containing added sugar might also be helpful. A tax on sugar, especially high-fructose corn syrup, could be used to fund research into essential nutrients and advertise their benefits. The idea behind such regulation would be to persuade the public, especially children, to consume less sugar and more nutritious foods.[1,2] This could greatly benefit public health.

It has been argued that similar regulation of alcohol is widely accepted because it has kept alcohol consumption under control.[1] For example, in other areas of our lives, changes in what is perceived as acceptable behavior have been successful, such as bans on smoking in public places, designated drivers who don't drink alcohol, and the inclusion of air bags in cars. To some, a similar type of governmental regulation of sugar would seem justified because at the cost of some loss of personal freedom it could improve health and cut short the epidemic of noninfectious disease.

On the other hand, many people see regulation of sugar by taxing foods containing added sugar as abhorrent and draconian. After all, although it is addictive,[4] sugar doesn't cause the danger of being drunk on the highway, and it doesn't present an imminent danger to health comparable to smoking. It's more insidious than that. And sugar has long been part of the dietary habits of many cultures. Thus, any governmental regulation of food will have many critics who explain that regulation would be ineffective, and further, we should be able to purchase and eat any food according to our preference.

The underlying issue in this debate is public access to knowledge about nutrition. If the harm that added fructose causes to our health could be widely publicized, along with information about inexpensive and readily available healthy alternatives, this could lead to better health for millions of people. It would cause shoppers to consider other choices, such as vegetable juice or a glass of water, along with unprocessed nutritious foods and vitamin supplements in adequate doses. What is needed is a campaign that provides practical information about diet: what nutrients we need, how to determine the proper doses, and the dangers of a processed-food diet. This could include televised advertisements and health programming, as well as curricula taught at levels from grade school to medical school. It might also include more informative labeling about the nutrient content of food, as well as more healthy and tasty food served at restaurants and dining rooms. Marketplace pressure might then convince food companies to sell more healthy food with a minimum of added sugar and an adequate content of essential nutrients. Orthomolecular medicine, the practice of treating illness by providing sufficient doses of essential nutrients to prevent deficiencies, can help to provide this information.[5–8] We can all become healthier by forgoing added sugar and other processed foods that lack essential nutrients. And when this is impossible, we can supplement with these essential nutrients to prevent the epidemic of obesity, cardiovascular disease, diabetes, and cancer.

REFERENCES FOR "TOXIC SUGAR"

1. Lustig RH, Schmidt LA, Brindis CD. The toxic truth about sugar. *Nature* 2012;482:27–29.

2. Jacobson MF. Liquid candy: how soft drinks are harming Americans' health. Center for Science in the Public Interest, 2005. Available at: http://www.cspinet.org/new/pdf/liquid_candy_final_w_new_supplement.pdf.

3. Bremer AA, Mietus-Snyder M, Lustig RH. Toward a unifying hypothesis of metabolic syndrome. *Pediatrics* 2012;129:557–570.

4. Lustig RH. Fructose: metabolic, hedonic, and societal parallels with ethanol. *J Am Diet Assoc* 2010;110:1307–1321.

5. Brighthope IE. *The Vitamin Cure for Diabetes.* Laguna Beach, CA: Basic Health Publications, 2012.

6. Roberts H, Hickey S. *The Vitamin Cure for Heart Disease.* Laguna Beach, CA: Basic Health Publications, 2011.

7. Hoffer A, Saul AW. *Orthomolecular Medicine for Everyone.* Laguna Beach, CA: Basic Health Publications, 2008.

8. Hoffer A, Saul AW, Foster HD. *Niacin: The Real Story.* Laguna Beach, CA: Basic Health Publications, 2012.

LEARNING LABELS

The more you know, the less you may want to know, and it would seem many Americans are content to be in the dark. But for those who have suspected there's more to those labels than what meets the eye, here's important information for you. Before you go on, remember: Don't let this stuff drive you crazy. Take it for what it is, and take action when and where you can. Every purchase at the grocery store is a choice. Getting closely involved with understanding what we are really adding to our cart is one of the best steps you can take toward better health. Increasing awareness is key. And once you know, it's hard to ignore what you have learned.

What's on the Label?

When I was growing up, my folks would always flip the product over and read the label. Always. My parents were the only ones *reading* in the grocery aisle. It was embarrassing. They made me do it too. For all that it made me want to rebel against every move they made, I find myself grateful for guidance I received against my will, because now, I am also an avid label reader. Let folks think I'm counting calories or something equally pointless. I'm just being smart. I like to feel good. Bad food makes me feel just the opposite. If I don't know what an ingredient is, I tend not to buy the product. I also know that simple ingredients I understand aren't always of the best quality.

Even diligent shoppers can be fooled. Unless you are a very close label reader each time you shop, it is likely you may go home with food products other than what you expected they would be. To this day, I sometimes end up with things in my shopping cart that I regret buying. I just commit to doing even better next time. If you aren't already label-savvy, here's a crash course, or a little review for the veterans.

Let's start with the basics.

The ingredients list on a label is a hierarchy: the ingredient listed first is the number-one substance in the container by weight. Is the first ingredient water? Well that's mostly what you are paying for. (My mom used to put hand lotions back on the shelf when "water" was the first ingredient. She figured water dried out her hands enough as it was.) Cheerios lists "oats" first. Second is "modified corn starch," an indigestible filler, then "sugar." I prefer food rather than fillers, so I avoid such ingredients whenever possible.

There are certain first ingredients you should try to avoid. Sugar, for example, unless you happen to be buying a bag of it. If you are, look for "pure cane" and go organic. Consider selecting alternative organic sweeteners like honey, molasses, or coconut palm sugar. I like to do my own baking for the family. Occasional treats help encourage the good food to go down. For example, if there is a cookie waiting after my kids eat a big salad, the salad is eaten all the more enthusiastically. I know that the treats I make in my kitchen contain ingredients I choose, and I am much more comfortable giving them home-baked goodies than grocery-aisle prepackaged confections.

If you are going to give your kids candy, I mean cereal, for breakfast, you will need to be a close label reader. The first ingredient in Kellogg's Apple Jacks is sugar. It sure as heck isn't apples. Some Mom somewhere must have read that and wondered about this. However, I doubt the folks who buy this particular cereal are label readers anyway. (Just a hunch.) If they were, they would probably buy actual apples for breakfast.

However, if you have been fooled into thinking that somehow Apple Jacks is part of a balanced breakfast (maybe if you only have a tablespoon's worth tossed into a spinach, yogurt, blueberry, and flaxseed smoothie—not that I'm suggesting you do), I would recommend leaving that one on the shelf where it belongs, along with all the other "kid" cereals, and the adult varieties too. Practically every cereal box on the market is adorned with flashy, misleading labels. Lucky Charms says "MORE WHOLE GRAIN than any other ingredient!" Oh, and a boatload of sugar. Here's one: how about the box of Cocoa Krispies that claims to "support your child's IMMUNITY"![24]

Bull.

I'm sure you've already figured that out.

If you find yourself buying a box of sugary cereal your kids will devour without complaint because you *want* to believe the box but have an inkling that other foods would be so much better for your kids, follow your instinct and skip the cereal.

What about other products? Ice cream, for example. What used to be the "all natural" black label on some containers of Breyer's now is confusing the ice cream connoisseur. Some containers contain ice cream, others do not. Is that ice cream really ice *cream* or a "frozen dairy dessert"?[25] Look at the label carefully. Near the bottom. In small print.

It's not only what the label says, but what it doesn't say that can be disconcerting. No artificial flavors? What about colors? Preservatives? Genetically modified ingredients? Speaking of which, hats off to Vermont. Starting in 2016, it will be the first state that will require GMO labeling on products sold in their retail stores. For those who like to know what is in their food, this is a step in the right direction. Until your state does the same, you can do what we do. It's simple: if it contains often-used GMO ingredients like soy, wheat, sugar (unless labeled "pure cane" sugar, as sucrose is often from GMO sugar beets, and even "pure cane sugar" can be sprayed with glyphosate,[26] the active ingredient in Monsanto's Roundup, unless labeled "organic"), rice, corn, canola, and it isn't labeled GMO free, we assume it *isn't* GMO free, and we don't buy it.

The big GMO foods are soy, corn, canola, papaya, alfalfa, zucchini, summer squash, and sugar beets.[27] Ingredients like soy can be hidden. For example, GM soy is feed to animals that we in turn eat (if they are not organic). GMO soy can also be in oil or other additives.

Much can be changed through public action, and perhaps the best way to make an impact is with your wallet. We simply do not buy products that contain ingredients we don't want to eat or that are farmed in a way that we don't support. We make phone calls to companies and tell them we won't buy their product because of the ingredients they use, and we tell them which we do buy because they are actually pure or actually natural. We ask if their products contain GMOs. Each time Monsanto, the maker of GMO seeds and the herbicide Roundup, cuts their workforce by thousands because of a loss in sales,[28] it shows that our shopping choices make an impact. Every voice counts. Every dollar counts. You can vote with your dollar each time you shop.

Intelligent consumers not only read the label, they put on their critical thinking cap and exercise common sense. We can all do this.

"Natural"

The word "natural" used to mean something. Now, natural can mean "laden with junk you wouldn't want to eat if you knew better." So much can be hidden in food items labeled "natural." For example, genetically modified ingredients can still be in a product labeled all natural. In fact, unless otherwise labeled, it's probably the case, since over 80 percent of our foods in North America contain GMOs.[29] Natural food can still be grown with synthetic pesticides and fertilizers. Natural food can still be stuffed full of sugar and refined flour, but so can organic food. Organic cookies may be better than nonorganic cookies, but that doesn't make cookies suddenly good for you.

Pesticides

Just because food is GMO free doesn't mean it is pesticide free. For those wishing to avoid toxins such as glyphosate, the active ingredient in Roundup, we must know that "GMO free" does not mean "Roundup free."

Once I bought a bag of whole-wheat bread thinking, well, wheat is not GMO. This could be okay. Of course, I wasn't a close label reader that day. If I had been, I would have put the product back because of other ingredients, not just potentially Roundup-treated wheat. Crops like wheat and sugar cane may be treated with a desiccant (a drying agent) before harvest.

Coloring

They sure are pretty, but they sure are not good for you. Green #3? Blue #1 and 2? Yellow #5 and 6? Red #3 and 40? It is paint, folks. Gross. If you would not eat a spoonful of semi-gloss, then do not buy painted food. Artificial colors are by name synthetic and likely toxic too.

People like their food to be the color they think it should be. Oranges should be orange. Yellow banana peppers should be yellow. Strawberry yogurt should be pink. Kids can expertly judge candy flavor based on color. Purple? Must be grape. Red? Cherry. Would clear, color-free candies sell? Certainly not as well. Food companies know this, and use this information to make their products visually appealing to customers. It is a simple matter of economics. Food is colored because it helps sell product.

A middle school science-fair project taught me this when I was eleven. A fellow classmate of mine did one on food coloring and flavor perception. They took plain milk and artificially colored it blue, red, green, purple, and so on. Then they asked other kids to tell them what flavor the unknown beverage was before they were allowed to taste it. Every child they asked gave the answers you would expect to hear: red would taste like cherries; purple like grapes; green would be apple flavored. They were all quite surprised when the colored milk tasted nothing of the sort; but some imagined that it did indeed taste of the fruit that donned the same color. Manufacturers are fully aware of how the color of their food affects our perception of how it tastes.[30]

There are plenty of natural colors that work as well as the artificial ones, and are not nearly as nauseating. For example, beta carotene, beet juice, turmeric, and paprika. For my daughter's first birthday, her carrot cake cupcakes had a beautiful purple-pink cream cheese frosting colored with fresh, raw beet juice. They were lovely.

Buffalo, New York's favorite Weber's horseradish mustard used to contain red #40. I guess good ol' turmeric just wasn't doing the trick. Interestingly, now that red #40 is no longer on the ingredients list. Has the color of the product suffered too? Nope. Still looks a whole lot like mustard. Perhaps some folks called to complain about the coloring. I often do. When my favorite products stray from the "natural" path, I make a phone call and let them know I noticed. They may as well know why I'm not going to buy the product anymore.

And let's not discuss Heinz's green or purple ketchup. OK, let's. (Remember that stuff?) Ugh. The shock factor sold a few million bottles to curious consumers, but the puke factor kept it out of our cart.

Coloring is added to make food look a certain way, but that is all it does. It is superfluous. It does not enhance flavor (even thought we might think it does) or nutritional content. Moreover, synthetic colorants are unhealthy.

In a randomized, double-blinded, placebo-controlled trial, artificial colors were shown to increase hyperactivity, namely impulsivity, inattention, and over-activity, in children with attention-deficit hyperactivity disorder (ADHD) and those in the general population.[31] The same was found true for preservatives, namely sodium benzoate.

Harmful additives have no place on our dinner tables. And remember, just because a product says "no artificial colors," does not mean the product is free of other junk like artificial flavors or preservatives.

Preservatives

We don't want to eat rotten, moldy, or unsafe microbial-laden food. Preservatives would seem essential, no?

Not exactly. If you eat fresh, whole foods, you don't need preservatives.

Sodium benzoate? Sodium nitrate? BHT? TBHQ? BHA? Avoid them whenever possible.

While it is always best to eat foods in season, we need and have overwhelming access to fruits and vegetables all year long. We can eat whole foods throughout the year. I think we should, and there are many who would agree. We don't have to eat food with unhealthy preservatives. There are plenty of preservative-free options for sale.

Organic

I did not like spiders when I was a kid. I don't exactly like them now, either. (We get those aggressive wolf spiders around here. They have no qualms about *rearing* at you if you come close.) But growing up in our house meant learning about pest control in our enormous backyard organic garden. So while I was content to smash them into oblivion, my father didn't want us killing the spiders. He wanted to use them. He would capture and transport the spiders from our house to the garden like some sort of twisted witness-relocation program. These exceptionally lucky spiders would, in turn, eat the aphids on our broccoli plants, feasting and growing hearty, healthy, and large. I wasn't too pleased with this arrangement. I often tended the garden, and I was petrified of their innate ability to successfully exercise the element of surprise. Gardening was truly terrifying work. Still, my brother and I learned about how to control pests naturally, just one way organic farming keeps produce growing strong.

"Organic" is a handy label for many reasons. If a product is certified organic, it will be free of genetically modified ingredients, grown without synthetic pesticides or fertilizers, and raised without antibiotics or growth hormones. Organic food will not contain artificial colors, flavors, or preservatives. It will not contain flavor-enhancing chemicals like MSG—maybe. Organic foods cannot be irradiated.

Look for the USDA organic seal on your food. "Made with organic ingredients" does not mean "made with 100 percent organic ingredients"; rather, at least 70 percent is (excluding water or salt), and the rest is likely not.[32] Similarly, "organic," which is made with at least 95 percent organic ingredients, is not 100 percent organic. The other 5 percent of ingredients that are not available organically are approved by the National Organic Program in order to sport the "USDA Organic" label.

No USDA Organic label? Read the ingredients label closely, and don't buy the product unless each ingredient that you care about—or that is present in quantity based on its location on the ingredients list—is marked as "organic" clearly on the label. You can also call the manufacturer and ask. For example, ask, "Is this product made with organic soy?" I particularly like products that list the word *organic* in front of every ingredient on the label. They take the guesswork right out of it.

Organic doesn't mean "perfect." In my mind, it's just the current standard of "acceptable." As my father says, "The standard is not perfection. The standard is the alternative." Organic items can still contain ingredients you might not want to eat. Food additives with health consequences such as carrageenan (used for thickening) or yeast extract (which contains free glutamate, in other words, MSG) are still allowed in organic foods. Yes, really. So while MSG is not allowed in organic food, a "natural" additive that *contains* the main active ingredient of MSG is allowed. Can you avoid hidden sources of MSG? You bet. We just have to be comfortable with label reading, even when the word "organic" is advertised.

Monosodium Glutamate (MSG)

If you aim to avoid it, you have to become a careful label reader indeed. According to Truth In Labeling.org, "Everyone knows that some people react to the food ingredient monosodium glutamate. What many don't know, is that more than 40 different ingredients contain the chemical in monosodium glutamate (processed free glutamic acid) that causes these reactions".[33] They have a handy chart available online to show you just where hidden MSG lies.

Organic food does not necessarily mean "free of pesticides and fertilizers." It means free of *synthetic* pesticides and fertilizers. Labels may say instead that the product has been grown without the use of "persistent pesticides." Pesticides and fertilizers from natural sources are allowed in organic farming,[34] although applying a "material" to crops has been described as a "last resort." There are plenty of other steps that take place instead and first. Every once in a while, you may hear something that may upset you about this process. For example, spraying the flowers of apple or pear trees with antibiotics is allowed in organic farming.[35] This isn't exactly in keeping with what folks expect from an organic label, yet organic is still the best thing going. Again, "The standard is not perfection. The standard is the alternative." We can only do the best we can.

To control pests and prevent disease, organic farmers must keep their soil healthy, which in turn keeps their plants healthy. According to the Organic Farming Research Foundation (OFRF), organic farmers build soil by "nourishing the living component of the soil," the "microbial inhabitants" that release, transform, and transfer nutrients." They use cover crops, compost, crop rotation, mulch, mechanical tillage, and even weeding by hand to keep soil healthy, weeds under control, and to ensure the ability of the soil to hold onto water. Organic farmers use "a diverse population of soil organisms, beneficial insects, and birds to keep pests in check" and "a variety of strategies such as the use of insect predators, mating disruption, traps and barriers." These things must be done first, before organic farmers are allowed to apply a "material" to control pests, weeds, or disease. "As a last resort," says OFRF, "certain botanical or other non-synthetic pesticides may be applied."[36] That is about as good as it gets, at least for now.

Buy products from local farmers who reduce pesticide use and instead employ creative, healthier ways of combatting pests and plant diseases. The more you know about your food and the farmers who grow it, the better. This is a wonderful benefit of joining a CSA. You can *ask.* There is immense peace of mind when you can speak directly to a farmer about his or her crops. Perhaps their own kids are munching away on the produce they grow. Perfect.

An organic label is still the best thing we've got going. "Way less toxic than everything else" is better than "really toxic" or "known to be dangerous," but I still wash conventional store-bought organic produce with soap and water. It's a good idea regardless. And this is reason yet again to take your vitamins to help your body cope with inevitable exposure to toxins and to support the health of your gut bacteria by eating fermented foods and probiotics.

Remember, you can still eat a not-good-for-you organic diet. Chips, cookies, crackers, cereals, overly processed foods, and sweets may be organic, but that doesn't make them good for you.

OH, WHAT TO DRINK

What we drink is just as important as what we eat. That's why we drink boatloads of water. The kids like water, too. We don't have soda in the house. My husband and I have a soda about twice a year. Our kids have never had soda, but they are only three and five. We know we won't be able to protect them forever, but we are going to keep them from it as long as possible. Occasionally we'll have some fresh apple cider. We have juice, but it is reserved to get vitamin C powder down. We have coffee and tea, milk, and I just bought some eggnog for a treat. ('Tis the season.) I make my own hot cocoa at Christmastime, and that's about it for beverages.

Since the most important liquid we put in our bodies is water, we want to know it is clean. All water is not.

Reasons to Say "No" to Fluoride and "Yes" to Vitamins

Fluoride is always toxic if enough of it is ingested. "When most people hear the word 'fluoride,' they generally think of their teeth and their dentist. Fluoride, after all, is added to some public water systems and many dental products for the purpose of preventing cavities. Less well known is that fluoride is a highly toxic compound, a major industrial air pollutant, a key ingredient in some pesticides and fumigants, the cause of a tooth defect that currently impacts over 40 percent of American teenagers, and the cause of a devastating bone disease that impacts millions of people throughout the world," says the Fluoride Action Network.[37] And there's more. "Over 30 studies have associated elevated fluoride exposure with neurological impairment in children, which may, in part, result from fluoride's affect [sic] on the thyroid gland."[38]

Vitamin C can lesson or eliminate the toxicity of fluoride, and may in itself provide some protection from tooth decay.[39] A combination of vitamin C, vitamin D, and calcium has been shown to reverse the earliest-grade dental fluorosis in children and significantly improve more advanced stages.[40] "Especially noteworthy was that the vitamin C protocol 'markedly reduced' the fluoride levels in the blood, serum, and urine," says Thomas Levy, MD. "It appears that "vitamin C supplementation would have some protective effect against dental decay" and "would be an excellent alternative to the existing water fluoridation programs already in place in so many communities."[41]

What's in Your Water?

"The people in the United States do not have the happiness that comes from drinking good natural water; instead, they drink dilute sewage containing chlorine and organic and industrial contaminants."

—LINUS PAULING, ASSOCIATED PRESS, FEB 6, 1976

The thought of leftover pharmaceuticals in our water supply could make anyone a bit queasy. An increasing population places higher demand on fresh water supplies. The "answer for pollution is dilution" is challenged by the increasing load of drugs flushed through our bodies and down our toilets. As people continue to take more drugs, they're bound to collide with our drinking water.

Think water contamination is a concern? New York State does. Last time I was driving on the New York State Thruway, large signs in the rest areas asked folks to please not flush their medications. But the drugs that are excreted in urine can't really be avoided, unless we can help folks avoid them entirely.

According to Harvard Medical School, "Our bodies metabolize only a fraction of most drugs we swallow. Most of the remainder is excreted in urine or feces (some is sweated out) and therefore gets into wastewater." And that's not all. "An increasing number of medications are applied as creams or lotions, and the unabsorbed portions of those medications can contribute to the pollution problem when they get washed off. It's been calculated, for example, that one man's use of testosterone cream can wind up putting as much of the hormone into the water as the natural excretions from 300 men."[42] If you think this is all filtered out of our water at the treatment facility before we drink it, think again.

"We are inundated with drugs. It begins with the tons of antibiotics used in animal farming, which run off into the water table and surrounding bodies of water and are conferring antibiotic resistance to germs in sewage that are also found in our water supply. Following that abuse are the tons of drugs and drug metabolites that are flushed down our toilets, making their way around the world and ending up in our drinking water."

—CAROLYN DEAN, MD, *DEATH BY MODERN MEDICINE*

Sure, our drinking water is cleaned and many containments are removed, but not all. "Approximately 170,000 public water systems are monitored for nearly 80 harmful substances," says Harvard. "The prohibited nasties include bacteria, viruses, pesticides, petroleum products, strong acids, and some metals." But that list does not include pharmaceuticals. "Sewage treatment plants are not currently designed to remove pharmaceuticals from water. Nor are the facilities that treat water to make it drinkable."[43] Small amounts of drugs still make it into our glass. And our bath. And our baby formula.

Are these small amounts of drugs a problem? We would be unlikely to ingest a cup of water if we knew someone had put a drop of poison in it. Should we ignore water with drugs, and just hope it will be okay? "At this point, there's really no evidence of pharmaceutical and personal care products in the water harming people, but studies are showing adverse effects on aquatic life," says Harvard.[44] Seems like tricky territory to me.

It's no fun to hear about a problem and feel helpless. We can "stay on the safe side" and filter our own water. I imagine if any company comes up with a proven filtration system that takes the drugs out, they will market it tirelessly and I'm sure we will hear about it. You can avoid toxin exposure by avoiding the obvious: Don't take drugs. Eat organic foods. Don't use fluoride toothpaste, fluoridated nursery water, fluoride mouthwash, or fluoride based drugs. (Fluoride-based fertilizers are prohibited on organic foods, by the way.[45]) And most importantly, in addition to drinking the cleanest water you reasonably can, take vitamin C and lots of it. Vitamin C, in large doses, is an effective antitoxin. Read the chapter on vitamin C to find out more. See also "How Doctors Use Vitamin C Against Lead Poisoning."

We simply cannot escape all pollutants, poisons, toxins, drugs, and chemicals. We can live the best we can. We can eat the best we can. And we can add our "vitamin armor" to offer extra protection.

CHAPTER 2 REFERENCES

1. Goldman, L. "Eat to Cleanse Your Body." *Natural Health Magazine* (Mar/Apr 2014): 24–28.

2. American Heart Association. "Meat, Poultry, and Fish." http://www.heart.org/HEARTORG/HealthyLiving/HealthyEating/Meat-Poultry-and-Fish_UCM_306002_Article.jsp.

3. Food and Agriculture Organization of the United Nations. "The State of Food and Agriculture. Rome, 2009." Per Capita Consumption of Livestock Products, 1995–2005. Table A3. http://www.fao.org/docrep/012/i0680e/i0680e00.htm (accessed June 2016).

4. Daniel, C. R., A. J. Cross, C. Koebnick, et al. "Trends in Meat Consumption in the United States." *Public Health Nutr* 14(4) (April 2011): 575–583.

5. Ibid.

6. American Heart Association. "Meat, Poultry, and Fish." http://www.heart.org/HEARTORG/HealthyLiving/HealthyEating/Meat-Poultry-and-Fish_UCM_306002_Article.jsp.

7. Food and Agriculture Organization of the United Nations. "The State of Food and Agriculture. Rome, 2009." Per Capita Consumption of Livestock Products, 1995–2005. Table A3. http://www.fao.org/docrep/012/i0680e/i0680e00.htm (accessed June 2016).

8. United States Department of Agriculture. "World Agricultural Supply and Demand Estimates Report." (WASDE) (August 12, 2014): http://www.usda.gov/oce/commodity/wasde/ (accessed May 2016).

9. National Hot Dog and Sausage Council. "Hot Dog Fast Facts." http://www.hot-dog.org/culture/hot-dog-fast-facts (accessed May 2016).

10. Mercola, J. "Raw Milk Versus Pasteurized—Which Is Safer?" (July 22, 2014): http://articles.mercola.com/sites/articles/archive/2014/07/22/raw-vs-pasteurized-milk.aspx (accessed April 2016).

11. Moss, M. "While Warning about Fat, U.S. Pushes Cheese Sales." *The New York Times* (Nov 6, 2010): http://www.nytimes.com/2010/11/07/us/07fat.html?pagewanted=all&_r=0 (accessed May 2016).

12. Ibid.

13. Cass, H., and K. Barnes. *8 Weeks to Better Health.* New York, NY: McGraw, 2005.

14. Ibid.

15. Ibid.

16. Ibid.

17. Moss, M. "While Warning about Fat, U.S. Pushes Cheese Sales." *The New York Times* (Nov 6, 2010): http://www.nytimes.com/2010/11/07/us/07fat.html?pagewanted=all&_r=0 (accessed May 2016).

18. Ibid.

19. Cass, H., and K. Barnes. *8 Weeks to Better Health.* New York, NY: McGraw, 2005.

20. AD. Davis, A. *Let's Get Well.* New York, NY: Signet Classics, 1965.

21. Hoffman, J., and D. Chaykin. *The Weight of the Nation.* "Part 2: Choices. Are All Calories Created Equal?" New York: HBO Home Box Office, 2012. Available online at: http://theweightofthenation.hbo.com (accessed May 2016).

22. Hyman, M. "The Key to Automatic Weight Loss!" (Last updated Nov 12, 2015): http://drhyman.com/blog/2014/05/19/key-automatic-weight-loss/ (accessed May 2016).

23. Casagrande, S. S., Y. Wang, C. Anderson, et al. "Have Americans Increased Their Fruit and Vegetable Intake? The Trends Between 1988 and 2002." *Am J Prev Med* 32(4) (Apr 2007): 257–263. Available online: http://www.ajpmonline.org/article/S0749-3797%2806%2900551-4/abstract (accessed May 2016).

24. Cereal Facts: Food Advertising to Children and Teens Score. "Cereal Box Claims." http://www.cerealfacts.org/media/Parents/Cereal_Box_Claims.pdf (accessed May 2016).

25. "Breyer's Converts Ice Creams to 'Frozen Dairy Desserts.'" (Jan 21, 2013): http://www.mouseprint.org/2013/01/21/breyers-converts-ice-creams-to-frozen-dairy-desserts/ (accessed May 2016).

26. Mercola, J. "USDA Claims Pesticide Residues in Food Is Safe: Here's Why They're Wrong." January 7, 2015. Available online: http://articles.mercola.com/sites/articles/archive/2015/01/27/glyphosate-gmo-pesticide-residue.aspx (accessed June 2016).

27. Non-GMO Project. "What Is GMO?" http://www.nongmoproject.org/learn-more/what-is-gmo/ (accessed May 2016).

28. The Associated Press. "Monsanto to Lay off 1,000 Employees to Counter Sagging Earnings." http://www.nola.com/business/index.ssf/2016/01/monsanto_to_lay_off_1000_emplo.html (accessed May 2016).

29. Non-GMO Project. "GMOs and Your Family." http://www.nongmoproject.org/learn-more/gmos-and-your-family/ (accessed May 2016).

30. DuBose C. N., A. V. Cardello, O. Maller. "Effects of Colorants and Flavorants on Identification, Perceived Flavor Intensity, and Hedonic Quality of Fruit-Flavored Beverages and Cake." *Journal of Food Science* 45(5) (1980):1393–1399 & 1415. Oram, N., D. G. Laing, I. Hutchinson, et al. "The Influence of Flavor and Color on Drink Identification by Children and Adults." *Dev. Psychobiology* 28 (4) (May 1995): 239–46.

31. McCann, D., A. Barrett, A. Cooper, et al. "Food Additives and Hyperactive Behaviour in 3-Year-Old and 8/9-Year-Old Children in the Community: A Randomised, Double-Blinded, Placebo-Controlled Trial." *Lancet* 370 (9598) (Nov 3, 2007): 1560–1567.

32. United States Department of Agriculture. USDA National Organic Program. Agricultural Marketing Service. "Labeling Organic Products." (October 2012): https://www.ams.usda.gov/publications/content/labeling-organic-products (accessed May 2016).

33. "Names of Ingredients That Contain Processed Free Glutamic Acid (MSG)" (last updated March, 2014): http://www.truthinlabeling.org/hiddensources.html (accessed May 2016).

34. United States Department of Agriculture. USDA National Organic Program. Agricultural Marketing Service. "Organic Regulations." https://www.ams.usda.gov/rules-regulations/organic (accessed May 2016).

35. Godoy, M. "A Battle over Antibiotics in Organic Apple and Pear Farming." National Public Radio. (Apr 10, 2013): http://www.npr.org/blogs/thesalt/2013/04/08/176606069/surprise-organic-apples-and-pears-aren-t-free-of-antibiotics (accessed May 2016).

36. Organic Farming Research Foundation. "Organic FAQs." http://ofrf.org/organic-faqs (accessed May 2016).

37. Fluoride Action Network. "Infant Exposure." FluorideAlert.org. http://fluoridealert.org/issues/infant-exposure/ (accessed Nov 2014).

38. Ibid.

39. Levy, T.E. *Vitamin C, Infectious Diseases, and Toxins: Curing the Incurable.* Philadelphia, PA: Xlibris Corporation, 2002.

40. Gupta, S.K., R.C. Gupta, A.K. Seth, et al. "Reversal of Fluorosis in Children." *Acta Paediatr Jpn* 38(5) (Oct 1996): 513–9.

41. Levy, T.E. *Vitamin C, Infectious Diseases, and Toxins: Curing the Incurable.* Philadelphia, PA: Xlibris Corporation, 2002.

42. Harvard Health Publications. Harvard Medical School. "Drugs in the Water." http://www.health.harvard.edu/newsletter_article/drugs-in-the-water (accessed May 2016).

43. Ibid.

44. Ibid.

45. Fluoride Action Network. "FAN's Grocery Store Guide: 7 Ways to Avoid Fluoride in Beverages and Food." http://fluoridealert.org/content/grocery_guide/ (accessed May 2016).

CHAPTER 3

That Diet Word

"If man made it, don't eat it."

—JACK LALANNE, FITNESS AND NUTRITIONAL EXPERT

It would appear that many of us like the idea of a "diet." We get excited about new research that will tell us what we need to eat and why. Our diet will trend with the changing tides. We will shun some foods and embrace others. We look for a name, a trend, an infomercial, a doctor who can tell us this stuff works. We want it to be easy, comfortable, and reassuring. We want to know beyond a shadow of a doubt that we will lose weight and/or keep weight off.

Unfortunately, there is plenty of money to be made from well-meaning people who want to put their faith in an idea and lay down their money for products with weight-loss claims. The old advice to "eat lots of vegetables" and "exercise" has never really appealed to the dieting type. So companies scramble to market something else, anything else, that avoids the very things we need to do, but often don't want to, but still fills their pockets full of our cash. Eating right is still a spectacular idea (just *try* to get fat eating fresh veggies—you can't). It always has been, but it's, well, boring. People want a *new* idea. A new approach. Or they simply want a diet that includes what they already like to eat. Ever try to convince the bacon lover not to eat bacon? Good luck. Tell the bacon lover that bacon is part of a healthy diet, and you sell a million books.

I've seen diets that claim "you can still eat what you want" and then proceed to tell you what you can't. Other diets conveniently contain food folks eat anyway and love, but we know full well they aren't a good idea.

THE COOKIE, CANDY BAR, AND BACON DIET

Some may think, "This diet lets me drink beer? Perfect! This diet doesn't? Forget it." I'm sure that's why someone came up with the pizza diet. And the cookie diet. You can try the candy bar diet right now, if you want to. Make any trip to the grocery store and you'll find a wall of "bars" advertised as meal replacements. (Boy, chocolate coconut caramel sure sounds yummy.) We want to believe it is a good idea—to do what seems to be the right thing and eat something delectable at the same time. Except that one bar won't leave you satisfied and you won't feel full and you won't be particularly well nourished, but the bar manufacturer isn't too worried as long as you keep buying more. Candy bar diets, and the like, exist because we will buy them. If you aren't gullible enough to buy into it, someone else is. We fork over our hard-earned dollars for a dream. It may not work for everyone, but it might work for me, right? Are we learning not to be fooled? Empty wallets indicate otherwise. We have put so much faith in advertisement, and many of us are simply desperate.

It seems that many of us subscribe to the idea that if it's called a "diet" and someone with a degree says it works, we are willing, at least temporarily, to put all of our faith, and a good deal of cash, into an alleged dieting miracle.

Even changing to an "easy" diet takes effort and will power. A bar at breakfast, another at lunch, and then a healthy dinner. If we all had that kind of self-control, we wouldn't be this overweight in the first place. The bars have little to do with it. Effort and taking responsibility have far more.

Still, there are others who are truly attempting to find the diet that is the healthiest. We want to eat what promotes weight loss or weight maintenance, exceptional health, and mental well-being, and also what tastes good. There are many of us who will read labels, prepare our own meals, chart our results, and all the while adapt and change what we do accordingly. But with so many mixed messages, conflicting stories in the media, and less than stellar government recommendations, it is no wonder that folks end up confused.

Frustrated dieters throw their hands up and wait for the next thing to come along. In the meantime, the weight-loss industry cleans up.

Why do fad diets become so popular? What is so great about them? What isn't? What can we learn? It turns out, plenty. Let's start with one that has been popular lately.

PALEO: EATING LIKE A CAVEMAN . . . SORT OF

The fastest land mammal in the wild, the cheetah, can run up to 70 miles per hour. A cheetah misses its prey more than half of the time. The red tail hawk is a killing machine. Just look at one. Armed with a razor sharp beak and deadly talons, a large number will still die due to food shortages on insufficient territory and starvation even though they will, according to the Raptor Institute, "eat anything they can catch."[1]

Animals in nature are hungry and dirty and tired all of the time. This is the rule rather than the exception. Many people nowadays have the incredible good fortune of access to an abundance of food. Our burden is to choose and eat wisely. And eat less. Want to make an animal sick? Overfeed it. Fish, cats, dogs, livestock: they will eat and eat and eat until overweight and sick. Want to make yourself ill? Overeat. Then do it again the next day. And the next. You will get fat and sick. Especially on the typical American diet. It's just that easy.

It would be impossible for us to eat like an *actual* caveman unless we wandered off to live in the wilderness, risked death, killed and ate our own meat, and gathered our own (hopefully edible) berries. It must have been pretty awful to be a hunter-gatherer. Our ancestors were likely hungry. And flexible. They were glad (if not relieved) to find food—any food—and eat it. Not poisonous? Perfect. Down it went, I imagine. Hungry animals aren't picky. Neither are hungry humans.

Like every diet, the Paleolithic (Paleo) diet is a guideline. Folks will apply that guideline to the extent that it is convenient and comfortable. It is hard to imagine prehistoric folks planning their meals like we do. Did they prepare recipes like boar and rabbit stir fry with fresh herbs and roots? Or did they just eat what they could obtain depending on where they were at the time and what was available because they were incredibly hungry? Remember, although Paleo argues against the food that comes from agriculture, agriculture made sense to the prehistoric people. It kept them alive and kept kids eating. And just because the modern Paleo diet attempts to mirror how prehistoric people had to eat, that doesn't make it the healthiest way to eat, especially when we attempt to apply this to your ordinary grocery shopper.

"Meat" to us normally means attractive, tasty muscle meats. Cavemen were not selecting their Paleo steak for their Paleo barbecue and discarding the rest of the animal. They didn't walk away once the steak was done. Most of an animal is not muscle meat. Hunger assured the ingestion of the less glamorous selections.

Viscera, organs, and glands contain the nutrients from the herbivorous animals that the carnivorous animals were eating. Cavemen ate these too. As for us? Not so much. I imagine there are many folks who don't have the stomach to go truly "Paleo."

We can mimic or mirror our ancestors, and I suppose that's the Paleo point, but it really isn't the same. It will never be. When it comes to our food, we have fewer limitations. And we have nice kitchens. We can get just about any food and any ingredient at any time and recipes in a snap. Additionally, the kind of food we eat is different. Our meat is raised somewhere in conditions many of us would find deplorable, fed a diet of genetically modified grains and growth hormones, and pumped full of antibiotics often because the animal is unhealthy. It is then butchered, shipped, cut or ground, packaged, and getting old well before we get to it. "Sell by" and "use by" have nothing to do with when the meat was placed in the package in the first place.[2] Of course, there is better meat. You can raise your own. You can buy 100 percent grass-fed organic meat. Paleo folks would do well to encourage this. However, I find that many Paleo people don't; rather they eat large quantities of Delmonico steak, regardless of origin, and choice cuts of highly processed bacon. Probably not the caveman way. 'Round these parts (the United States that is), most of us avoid eating nutrient-packed brains, tongues, livers, or hearts. Why? Because other cuts of meat are tastier and more appealing to us, and, while not necessarily inexpensive, are readily available. Those with means and who have access to an abundance of food, to the point of becoming overweight, haven't needed to develop a taste for organs. Hunger has not defined the typical American Paleo dieter's palate. (Haggis, anyone?) Plus, we can obtain the same essential nutrients in other ways; we don't have to rely on eating an entire animal for nutrition. The question is, do we seek out these other choices?

Picking Apart Paleo

More than just a bunch of yuppies at a pig roast, the Paleo theory is this: to take weight off and keep it off, eat a high-protein, low-glycemic diet high in fruits and veggies and omega-3 fatty acids. You can eat meat (don't forget the organs), nuts (not peanuts), and seeds (in moderation), fish and seafood, healthy oils (olive, coconut), and fruit or veggies (especially in season), honey, grass-fed butter. "Organic" should precede most, if not all, of these. (Good idea.) I noticed that the list of "approved" meats far outnumbers the list of approved vegetables.

On the other hand, Paleo would have you avoid legumes such as beans, peas, or lentils, and grains such as wheat, corn, or oatmeal. While Paleo restricts carbohydrates, it would appear that cavemen didn't, and they (and their descendants) were all the smarter for it.[3] Paleo smartly says no to refined sugar, processed food, excess salt, candy, and junk food. Some folks will do better eliminating dairy on the Paleo diet, which includes cheeses (cream, cottage, or otherwise), yogurt, or milk. Paleo also says no to soda, fruit juice, soy, artificial sweeteners, corn syrup, refined vegetable oil, hot dogs, ketchup, squash, potatoes, alcohol, beer, sweets.[4] Food can still be prepared, cooked, and spiced.

The Plus Side of Paleo

Paleo has a rather impressive list of things you shouldn't eat. Eliminating beer, alcohol, soda, processed food, additives, preservatives, hot dogs, junk food, and artificial sweeteners, as per the Paleo diet, would be a wonderful dietary shift for absolutely everyone. Restricting these alone would mean America would slim down and feel good. Add in more vegetables, and we'd all be doing even better. If going Paleo is what it takes for people to remove this toxic "food" from their tables, have at it.

But there is also a way to live healthy and still include banned foods, such as beans, for example. If you detect a sensitivity to dairy, skip the milk. You may still be able to eat some cheese and cultured yogurt.

Yogurt Is Awesome

Even if you are sensitive to lactose, give yogurt a try. You may find it easier to digest. Yogurt is loaded with probiotics that are super healthy and helpful. It can be dressed up six ways from Sunday, so you don't even have to buy the artificially colored or flavored stuff. A container of plain and some imagination, and you are all set. There are plenty of salespeople who would be thrilled if you would buy into their probiotic tablets or designer products. If you can afford it, and you want to do it, go ahead. But for the rest of us on budgets, a few tablespoons of yogurt every day is a great way to keep the gut bacteria normal and help prevent (and treat) bacterial imbalances. You can even use it topically for thrush or intravaginally to treat yeast infections. If you ever take an antibiotic, eat yogurt too. Reintroducing beneficial bacteria is essential. Antibiotics are not selective. They kill good and bad bacteria alike. The very term "antibiotic" means "antilife." Don't let antibiotics cause other opportunistic infections. Sure, there are lots of fermented foods that are loaded with probiotics and are really good for you. But I've found that yogurt is one of the most cost-effective and tasty as well.

When I was younger my folks would pick up yogurt at the health food store. That's where they could get the good stuff. They would buy all-natural, whole-milk yogurt with the layer of cream on top. To save some dough, my folks "grew" their own in an incubator at home. It was pure and tasty. There is nothing quite like fresh, homemade yogurt. If you haven't tried it, do. But for those who like it made for them, there are some wonderful organic yogurts available now. Thirty years later, I finally started finding my favorite brand at our local grocery store. Every day our kids get the good stuff too. Probiotics are also really good for kids. See Appendix 2 for more about the benefits of probiotics.

I see it this way: if you are sensitive to wheat, don't eat it. If you eat wheat, eat organic. Eat more veggies than grains. Avoid genetically modified food. All vegetables are good for you. Period. This includes potatoes and squash. If your idea of potato comes fried and loaded with fat and salt, then you are missing the heart of the matter. As the Gerson Institute says, "even kale's reputation might suffer a little" under those circumstances.[5] "In addition to vitamin C, potatoes are a good source of vitamin B_6 and niacin (vitamin B_3 and nicotinic acid). Potatoes are also rich in minerals, including iron, copper, manganese and tryptophan. In fact, potatoes contain all 21 amino acids, which are the building blocks of protein, thus forming complete proteins upon digestion" and "are naturally high in potassium and sodium."[6] Even Marty, the fictional character stranded on Mars in the book *The Martian,* knew that good ol' potatoes were the key to keeping himself alive. The quality of the potato is determined by how and in which soil it is grown. For the best taters, buy organic, buy local, or grow your own. Potatoes can be an inexpensive and satisfying replacement for meat in soups and tacos, and can certainly be part of a healthy diet. Squash too. While a strict Paleo diet says otherwise, I wouldn't worry so much about potatoes, squash, and beans. Worry about refined sugar. Not sugar from potatoes. Worry about processed starches. Not starch in squash. I maintain the American obesity epidemic is not because of eating fresh whole squash, or potatoes, or beans.

Health folks tend to argue with each other. A lot. I suppose I am arguing too. In the end, the diet that keeps you free of disease, happy, vibrant, energetic, and feeling great is the right one. That diet is *your* diet and it may look very different from someone else's. Do what works for you. As long as it includes lots of veggies. You can't get out of that one.

THE ATKINS DIET

Ah, the low-carb diet. Got a lot of attention, didn't it? Sure, it is a great idea to eat plenty of whole, unprocessed foods and omit refined sugar, which is exactly what this diet encourages folks to do. However, for people getting started on the program, it limits *which* vegetables and fruits to eat for fear of too many carbohydrates. Sure, low-carb veggies like leafy greens are very good for you. But folks, *all* vegetables are good for you. Fruit too. Any diet that says they aren't is wrong.

Now, let's talk bacon. Many folks see the Atkins diet as an opportunity to make this their "bacon diet." For years the diet encouraged people to "satisfy their hunger with liberal amounts of steak, eggs and other saturated fats."[7] In other words, have as much as you want. "In their consumer publications," says the *New York Times,* "Atkins officials have never set limits on saturated fat, and Atkins is widely known as the diet that lets you eat all the meat you want."[8] It appears the Atkins officials did not really feel the need to correct this misconception. Even today, bacon is viewed as part of a "healthy" diet,[9] and Atkins.com does not actively prohibit this food. "[E]ach of the food groups should be enjoyed in moderation,"[10] says Atkins.com. "Some processed meat, bacon, and ham is cured with sugar which will add to the carb count. Avoid cold cuts and other meats with added nitrates."[11] I see. So as long as your *carb* count is okay, bacon is okay. Hopefully bacon-lovers made a point to stay away from bacon cured with nitrates like Atkins recommends. Hopefully Atkins dieters know that they really shouldn't eat all the meat they want. The promoters of the Atkins diet now say that "people on their plan should limit the amount of red meat and saturated fat they eat."[12] That goes for bacon, too.

THE FIT FOR LIFE DIET

"Do not overeat" is great advice. Eat "living" (raw) food is great advice too. However, according to a review of the *Fit for Life* program in *Elle* magazine, one of the "key rules" of this diet plan is "everything, even vegetables, can be eaten in excess, and excess leads to weight gain."[13] Uh-huh. Who is getting fat from eating too many vegetables? Who?! This diet also focuses on when to eat, and which foods you can and cannot eat together, presenting a hassle for most folks who just want to eat right without having to think too much about it. However, its focus on a predominantly vegetarian diet would do most folks a lot of good.

THE DASH DIET

Right from the start, it gets one thing right: it discourages refined and processed foods and limits sweets. The diet encourages eating lots of fruits and vegetables as well as some lean meats, nuts, seeds, legumes, and low-fat dairy. It also recommends including "at least 3 whole grain foods each day" but says to eat six to eight servings of grains in total.[14] This means refined grains could account for a considerable amount of one's daily DASH diet. Refined grains are milled to remove the bran and germ, removing nutrients and fiber too. They are not as good for you as whole grains, which remain intact. All that aside, when compared to the Standard American Diet (SAD), this one is arguably an improvement.

AN ARGUMENT AGAINST EATING ANIMALS

And argue they do. After I wrote the following article, I was roundly accused of being a vegetarian. I'm not, but I was raised that way. Now, I eat a predominantly plant-based diet. Along with all those fruits and veggies, I also eat meat, dairy, and seafood. I eat a little red meat about once a week. I have good reason for not eating more.

In *Another Reader's Digest Absurdity: Red Meat Is Bad—No, Wait—Good for You!* I wrote about the mixed messages we often get from the media. While we can argue that eating fresh, organic, grass-fed red meat is better than eating conventionally raised meat, the majority of us aren't eating that kind of meat. It would appear, then, that a diet heavy in the red-meat department is to be avoided. Perhaps *Reader's Digest* would have done well to say so.

Another *Reader's Digest* Absurdity: Red Meat Is Bad—No, Wait—Good for You!

by Helen Saul Case

From the *Orthomolecular Medicine News Service*, June 19, 2012.

Browsing through the latest issue of *Reader's Digest*, it's not those witty "Laughter Is the Best Medicine" sections that are making me chuckle. It's the ridiculous, contradictory health advice that the magazine gives to the reader.

Let's start with what makes sense. In the article "Is Meat Good or Bad for You?"[1] the author explains that red meat might be killing us. He references a Harvard study[2] that tracked over 121,000 adults for up to 28 years and shares with us that "people who ate three ounces of red meat every day were about 13 percent more likely to die—often from heart disease or cancer—before the study ended than people who didn't eat meat."[3] And, folks who eat processed meat fared worse. They increased their risk of early death by 20 percent. This sounds like pretty important information, not to be taken lightly. He writes, "It's no wonder that many experts recommend reducing or eliminating red meat from your diet." That's certainly true.

Alas, the author's common sense ends there. As my grandmother often said, "Common sense isn't common." Well, Grandma is right again.

The author mentions in his rebuttal that regular eaters of lean beef get more protein, zinc, potassium, and B vitamins. Ah yes, protein. Good thing we have red meat! I mean, you can't find adequate amounts of protein in *anything* else but red meat. Except for beans, of course. Oh, and cheese. And it's also in tofu, nuts, lentils, eggs, yogurt, milk, seafood, and more. Still, how do those vegetarians survive?! Apparently they do, if the Harvard study is to be believed, and in greater numbers than the meat-eaters.

Okay, vitamins and minerals sure are important. You can't get them anywhere but in a steak. Yeah, right.

With all that evidence the author just provided, we still want to know the final verdict: is red meat good or bad? Apparently, "You can still fit a daily serving of red meat into a healthy diet."[4]

Really? A "daily serving" is considered to be about three ounces. Awesome! I get to eat three ounces of red meat a day!

Wait, didn't the Harvard study *just say* that three ounces of red meat a day was killing people? Did the author read his own article? Qualifying the eating of red meat by using the phrase "as part of a healthy diet" makes about as much sense as the huge bowl of sugar-laden breakfast cereal pictured on the front of the cereal box that boasts being "part of a complete breakfast." But this is only when presented next to a pile of whole-wheat toast, fresh fruit, orange juice, and a pound of spinach. Okay, I made up the spinach part.

So, red meat is bad for us. But, according to the article that said so, we're supposed to go ahead and eat it anyway.

Isn't that what the reader of the *Digest* takes from the article? Must be. In the oxymoron box (or maybe just the "moron" box) entitled "How Healthy Carnivores Eat," it recommends that the "perfect" portion of meat is about the size of a deck of playing cards. Perfect for what? A coronary? Goodness knows, when many people eat red meat, the serving is larger than any "deck of cards" outside of a novelty shop. Nor will this advice likely prevent Americans from consuming their 100 pounds or more of red meat a year, an amount way out of proportion to our intake of fruits and vegetables.[5] Oh, but if red meat is a part of a *healthy* diet, we'll be A-Okay, says *Reader's Digest.*

Uh huh. Because *that's* your average American: fit and healthy. Eating lots of vegetables every day to deliberately offset that chunk of red flesh. Oh, *please*. Only about 30 percent of us get either two servings of fruit *or* three servings of vegetables,[6] and only 11 percent of Americans are meeting U.S. Department of Agriculture (USDA) guidelines for both.[7] Surveys have found that there are a whopping 20 percent of folks out there who eat absolutely no veggies *at all*.[8]

Is it really so daring to recommend that we skip red meat altogether? Would the *Digest* lose subscribers? Would the *Digest* lose advertisers? Well, they must be losing somebody, because the advice in the article encourages continuing to consume red meat and risk death and disease.

Folks, we don't need to chow down on cow to obtain our daily dose of zinc and B vitamins. Vegetables have plenty. And though the carnivore in us may be quick to disagree, plenty of widely available plant-based protein-packed foods can be placed in the shopping bag. Healthy sources of potassium are easy to find. Virtually all fruits and vegetables are excellent sources of potassium. A vegetarian diet, selected with care, provides generous amounts of protein and all the other nutrients necessary for excellent health.

So, let's see . . . eat red meat and risk death. Or, skip the meat, and actually try to eat the healthy diet we *should* be eating anyway, packed with vegetables. And, while we are at it, take vitamins and eat fresh fruit. I think that's doable.

Do yourself a favor and don't "digest" the *Reader's Digest* ridiculousness. Toss it in the trash bin, and you'll actually be a whole lot healthier for it.

REFERENCES FOR "ANOTHER *READER'S DIGEST* ABSURDITY"

1. Woolston, C. Is meat good or bad for you? *Reader's Digest* July/August, 2012: 36–38.

2. Pan A, Sun Q, Bernstein AM, et al. Red meat consumption and mortality: results from 2 prospective cohort studies. *Arch Intern Med* 2012;172(7):555–563. doi: 10.1001/archinternmed.2011.2287.

3. Woolston, C. Is meat good or bad for you? *Reader's Digest* July/August, 2012: 36–38.

4. Ibid.

5. Putnam J, Allshouse J, Kantor LS. U.S. per capita food supply trends: more calories, refined carbohydrates, and fats. *Food Review* 2002;25(3):2–15. Available at: http://ers.usda.gov/publications/FoodReview/DEC2002/frvol25i3a.pdf.

6. Centers for Disease Control and Prevention. CDC Online Newsroom. Majority of Americans not meeting recommendations for fruit and vegetable consumption. Press Release, September 29, 2009. Available at: http://www.cdc.gov/media/pressrel/2009/r090929.htm.

7. Casagrande SS, Wang Y, Anderson C, et al. Have Americans increased their fruit and vegetable intake? The trends between 1988 and 2002. *Am J Prev Med* 2007;32(4):257–263. Available at: http://www.ajpmonline.org/article/S0749–3797%2806%2900551–4/pdf.

8. Balch JF, Balch PA. *Prescriptions for Natural Healing*. New York, NY: Avery Publishing Group, 1990.

THE MEDITERRANEAN DIET

Here is a diet that has been appealing to healthy eaters for some time. This article written for the *Journal of Orthomolecular Medicine* by Christopher Lam, MD, shows just how beneficial the Mediterranean diet could be for those aiming to be as healthy as possible.

THE TRADITIONAL MEDITERRANEAN DIET: LESSONS LEARNED

by Christopher Lam, MD

From *J Orthomolecular Med* 2011; 26 (3): 109–116.

Introduction

Historically, the term "Mediterranean diet" (MeDiet) was loosely derived from the concept of a diet of the peoples living in the Mediterranean basin. By no means homogeneous, the diet varies from one country to another; the commonalities include a plant-based diet with substantial amounts of greens, pulses, fruits, nuts, seeds, whole grains, and olive oil. The benefits of the MeDiet were shown in the renowned Seven Countries Study: over 12,000 healthy middle-aged (40–59 years old) men—agricultural or railroad workers—from Finland, the United States, Netherlands, Yugoslavia, Italy, Japan, and Greece were studied in 1958–1964. The results were published in 1970 by the physiologist Dr. Ancel Keys (aka "Mr. Cholesterol" of the University of Minnesota). It showed the lowest mortality rates due to cardiovascular disease (CVD) in Crete (Greece was subdivided into two regions), at nine per 100,000 population over ten years; the highest rates were in the U.S. and Finland, 424 and 466, respectively.[1,2] In 1993 the Oldways organization, Harvard School of Public Health, and World Health Organization introduced the concept of the Mediterranean diet, "a delicious, pleasurable, and very healthful way to eat" (www.oldwayspt.org).

A large and growing body of evidence links the MeDiet with lower risks of CVD,[3–5] stroke,[6] certain cancers,[7,8] obesity and diabetes,[9–11] depression,[12] cognitive impairment,[13,14] and benefits to general health and longevity.[15–19]

In the European Prospective Investigation into Cancer and Nutrition cohort (EPIC), Trichopoulou and others (2005) showed that greater adherence to the MeDiet was associated with a significant reduction in the mortality of individuals with coronary heart disease (CHD). A higher adherence by two units (out of a ten-unit diet score) was associated with a 27 percent lower mortality.[20] In the Spanish EPIC cohort study of 41,000 participants from five centers, over a mean follow-up of ten years, Buckland and others used an 18-unit relative MeDiet score. The study showed that high adherence, versus low adherence, can reduce the risk of a first cardiac event by 40 percent;

even a one-unit increase in the diet score was associated with a 6 percent reduction in risk of CHD. The study supported the role of the MeDiet in primary prevention of CHD.[21] Another EPIC cohort study of 485,000 subjects aged 35–70 from ten European countries, over a mean follow-up of 8.9 years, showed a significant reduction in the risk of incident gastric adenocarcinoma with a higher adherence to the MeDiet. A one-unit (out of an 18) increase was associated with a reduction in the risk of gastric adenocarcinoma by 5 percent.[22]

Components of the Mediterranean Diet

The Mediterranean Diet Pyramid was developed in 1993 according to numerous scientific studies on nutrition and health. "This preliminary concept of a pyramid to represent a healthy, traditional Mediterranean Diet is based on the dietary traditions of Crete, much of the rest of Greece and southern Italy circa 1960, structured in light of current nutrition research."[25] Oldways has since updated the original version by placing all plant foods together as the staple of most meals; increasing the frequency of fish and seafood to at least twice weekly; and adding herbs and spices to reflect their role in not only enhancing the palatability of the foods, but also health promotion. The main constituents are listed in Table 1.

TABLE 1. COMPONENTS OF THE TRADITIONAL MEDITERRANEAN DIET

Vegetables including leafy greens, pulses (peas, beans, and lentils), roots, tubers, and so on form the staple of the MeDiet. Aside from cooked vegetables, raw salads are often added daily.

Fruits are frequently ingested—more than once daily. They are plentiful in the Mediterranean basin.

Grains include whole grains from barley, wheat, oats, corn, and rice, and are mostly unrefined.

Nuts and seeds provide, as with legumes, fiber and protein.

Yogurt and cheese, especially from goat and sheep, are eaten in small to moderate quantities.

Eggs and seafood are also consumed fairly regularly and provide high-quality protein.

Meats, including poultry, are eaten only in small portions in the MeDiet. On special festive occasions, there may be goat or lamb added to the meal.

Herbs are important as condiments or for medical purposes.

Desserts may be served during celebrations; otherwise they are not eaten on a regular basis. Honey is often used as a sweetener instead of refined sugar.

Wine is consumed in some, though not all, of the Mediterranean countries, and generally in small quantities (here, a little may be good but a lot is definitely not better).

Olive oil—"liquid gold," as Homer called it—is an essential component of the Mediterranean diet.

Olive oil is an integral constituent of the MeDiet with numerous health-promoting benefits. It is high in monounsaturated fats and rich in antioxidant phytochemicals and micronutrients, which can be destroyed by heat and chemical refining. Therefore extra virgin "cold-pressed" olive oil, with its greenish-gold tint, is the best kind. Its many benefits include improving lipid profiles and endothelial function, as well as protection against proinflammatory states and some cancers.[7,8,23,24] Although most of the research has been on extra-virgin olive oil, consumption of whole olives is also likely beneficial. The olive tree (*Olea europaea*) is indigenous to the Mediterranean basin, and the production of olive oil likely started in the early Minoan period (circa 4000 BC). Greece is now the largest producer of extra-virgin olive oil in the world (and third in total olive oil production).

The Traditional Diet of Crete

Because of Crete's superlative health parameters, including the lowest CHD rates and highest longevity, the traditional diet of Crete can be considered the prototypical MeDiet. The earliest archaeological evidence of the systematic cultivation and use of large quantities of olives for oil dates back to the Middle Minoan period (2160–2000 BC).[36] Crete was an important olive-producing area and traded with the Aegean islands and beyond. The main livestock were sheep and goats. Hare and ibex were some of the wild species that supplemented the diet of the early people of Crete. Protein residues in the skeletal material of human bones from the Neolithic, Minoan, and Mycenaean periods have been subjected to stable radioisotope analysis, showing a mixture of plants and meats, with variable amounts of seafood.[37] Available evidence suggests that, through some five thousand years until the past few decades, the people of Crete, especially in the rural areas, maintained basically a similar traditional diet.[38]

Crete has the highest consumption of olive oil of all the Mediterranean countries (about a third of the total caloric intake comes from olive oil and olives). Vegetables, pulses, fruits, and whole grains are consumed in large quantities, whereas meat is used mainly for celebrations, and eaten in modest amounts. Depending on the location, dairy and fish are also consumed in moderate to small amounts (lactose intolerance is quite common in the adult population of Crete and Greece).[26] Wine (one to two glasses) is often included with dinner as part of socializing.[27]

Herbs are an important and indispensable daily fare because of their savory as well as medicinal value.[28] Their purported uses and characteristics are based mainly on tradition and custom. However, there are known antioxidant properties in a number of herbs (such as thyme, Greek sage, wild sage, and spearmint).[29] Herbal teas of dittany, sage, thyme, marjoram, and chamomile are popular, as are mint with lemon balm or basil. A "mountain tea" popular in western Crete containing ironwort (*Sideritis syriaca*) is often mixed with other herbs.

Nuts and seeds are consumed regularly. Sabaté and others (2010) pooled 25 nut-consumption trials conducted in seven countries among 583 people[30] and showed improvement in blood lipid levels in a dose-related manner based on nut consumption, especially among subjects with higher low-density lipoprotein cholesterol (LDL-C) or with lower body mass index (BMI). Frequent intake of nuts, then, can be protective against CHD; consumption of different kinds of nuts lowers total and LDL-C. It also lowers the ratio of low-density lipoprotein to high-density lipoprotein in healthy subjects or those with moderate hypercholesterolemia.[31] Nuts have a high unsaturated to saturated fatty acid ratio, as well as beneficial macro- and micronutrients, including phytosterols, protein, folic acid, alpha-tocopherol, and so on. Further, nuts can blunt the postprandial glycemic response of a high-carbohydrate meal, and thus may have a role in the glycemic control of patients with diabetes or prediabetes.[32] The intake of tree nuts, peanuts, and seeds is higher in the south of Europe compared to the north. Jenab, Sabaté, and others[33] also found that the most popular tree nuts were walnuts, almonds, and hazelnuts, which, in general, were more widely eaten than peanuts or seeds. In the Mediterranean region the annual per capita nut consumption was highest in Lebanon (averaging 16.5kg), Greece (11.9kg), and Spain (7.3kg), followed by Israel and Italy (FAO, 2001).[34] A systematic review by López-Uriarte and others[35] of *in vitro* and *in vivo* studies in animals and humans, on the effect of nuts on oxidation, found that although nuts are high in total fat, no harmful effects on oxidation were reported; on the other hand, the presence of antioxidant activity appeared to be beneficial. Thus, frequent nut intake is associated with a lowered risk of CHD, type 2 diabetes, and death by all-cause mortality.

The MeDiet vs. "Western" Food Habits

Bringing all this forward, much has changed since the 1950s and 60s. Those countries that have increased the consumption of vegetables and cut down on animal fats have improved health parameters such as CVD rates. Conversely, those countries that have wandered away from the MeDiet showed worsening parameters. Twenty-five years after the Seven Countries Study, almost 6,000 of the 12,763 men had died. The CHD mortality in Greece was 5 percent; that of Finland, 30 percent.[38] Although traditional lifestyles were maintained in some segments of the Greek population, they have, in the urban areas, given way to a "Western"-type of diet with a decrease in consumption of fruits by 31 percent and bread by 70 percent, and an increase in consumption of meat by 160 percent and cheese by 366 percent. Concomitantly their lifestyle became more sedentary and smoking prevalence rose. The average BMI, blood pressure, cholesterol level, and rate of diabetes also rose. CHD mortality saw an increase, as did the rate of cancer (especially of the lung). In the same period of time the USA and Finland saw a decrease in their CHD mortality.[40] Alcohol consumption in Greece increased by 15 percent between 1970 and 1981; still, it was 59 percent that of Italy and 50 percent that of France. With the mechanization of agriculture, physical activity among rural people saw a drop. In Crete between 1960 and 1982 the frequency of very overweight people (BMI □ 30 kg/m^2) increased ten-fold.[40] Four decades after the Seven Countries Study, even among the farmers of Crete, the "gold standard of health," mean weight gain was 20 kg.[41]

Mediterranean Diet Slashes Risk of Cardiovascular Disease

"The Mediterranean diet has long been associated with a relatively low risk of cardiovascular disease," says nutrition expert Jack Challem. "A recent large-scale study in the *New England Journal of Medicine* shows that adopting the diet can lead to a significantly reduced risk of disease. Ramon Estruch, MD, of the University of Barcelona and his colleagues focused on 7,447 Spanish residents, ages 55 to 80 years, who did not have cardiovascular diseases but were at a high risk of developing them. They were overweight, had diabetes, smoked, or had other risk factors for heart disease. ...The study was halted after a little less than five years because the results were so dramatic. People on either of the Mediterranean diets had approximately a 30 percent lower risk of a cardiovascular event, such as a heart attack or stroke."

From *The Nutrition Reporter* 24(5), 2013.

Discussion

More data have emerged showing the benefits of such a plant-based MeDiet on acid-alkaline balance,[42,43] BMI,[44] blood pressure, metabolic syndrome,[45] diabetes,[46] mental health (depression), cognitive function, and Alzheimer's disease.[47–49] Such a diet provides plant (phyto-) sterols, which can lower serum cholesterol,[50–52] and even increases the success of couples undergoing fertility treatment (in vitro fertilization/intra cytoplasmic sperm injection) in achieving pregnancy (odds ratio 1.4).[53]

The MeDiet is associated with a lower risk of cancer at several sites,[54] including prostate cancer.[55,56] Although some components of such a diet—olive oil, fiber, folate, carotenoids, and flavonoids—–show an inverse relation with cancer risk, other important nutrients and components with such a favorable effect remain as yet undefined.[57,58] Various nutrients and antioxidants may work in synergy.[59] Furthermore, higher intake of fish and omega-3 fatty acids is associated with beneficial effects on a number of diseases,[60,61] including a lower risk of CVD,[62,63] certain mental disorders,[64–67] and depression.[68,69]

Although CHD mortality in Canada has decreased over several decades, it remains the major cause—one-third—of deaths. With the increasing prevalence of the metabolic syndrome, obesity, diabetes, and so on, the burden of CVD is expected to rise in the next decade.[70] First Nations people, because of their significantly increased risk for obesity, diabetes, and CHD, require special attention. By targeting what is known to be associated with a high risk of such diseases, preventive measures can have a profound impact.

Based on thousands of years of history, the MeDiet, exemplified by the traditional diet of Crete, has evolved to become one of the healthiest diets in the world. In order to advocate, protect, and preserve the traditional Mediterranean diet, the United Nations Educational, Scientific and Cultural Organization (UNESCO), in November 2010, added it to the "intangible" Cultural Heritage List.[71]

Conclusion

It is recognized that in observational studies, association may not be equal to causality. Results based on questionnaires and recall of dietary patterns by study subjects can contain inaccuracies; further, it is difficult to control for other important lifestyle factors. Nonetheless, numerous studies on men and women in various countries over the past several decades, especially since the inception of the Seven Countries Study, have shown convincingly strong links between a plant-based diet of whole foods, and good health and longevity—not just longer lives but also more disease-free years. The closer the adherence to the traditional Mediterranean diet, the better the health outcomes: the data are compelling. The key determinant of health remains the habitual diet of the populace.

REFERENCES FOR "THE TRADITIONAL MEDITERRANEAN DIET"

1. Keys AB, Menotti A, Karvonen MJ, et al. The diet and 15 year death rate in the Seven Countries Study. *Am J Epidemiol* 1986; 124: 903–915.

2. Keys AB. *Seven Countries: A Multivariate Analysis of Death and Coronary Heart Diseases.* Cambridge, MA: Harvard U Press, 1980.

3. Trichopoulou A. Mediterranean diet: the past and the present. *Nutr Metab Cardiovasc Dis* 2001; 11(4 suppl): 1–4.

4. Lairon D. Intervention studies on Mediterranean diet and cardiovascular risk. *Mol Nutr Food Res* 2007; 51: 1209–1214.

5. Estruch R, Martínez-González MA, Corella D, et al. Effects of a Mediterranean-style diet on cardiovascular risk factors: a randomized trial. *Ann Int Med* 2006; 145: 1–11.

6. Fung TT, Rexrode KM, Mantzoros CS, et al. Mediterranean diet and incidence of and mortality from coronary heart disease and stroke in women. *Circulation* 2009; 119: 1093–1100.

7. Owen RW, Haubner R, Würtele G, et al. Olives and olive oil in cancer prevention. *Eur J Cancer Prev* 2004; 13: 319–326.

8. Colomer R, Menendez JA. Mediterranean diet, olive oil and cancer. *Clin Transl Oncol* 2006; 8: 15–21.

9. Schröder H, Marrugat J, Vila J, et al. Adherence to the traditional Mediterranean diet is inversely associated with BMI and obesity in a Spanish population. *J Nutr* 2004; 134: 3355–3361.

10. Champagne CM. The usefulness of a Mediterranean-based diet in individuals with type 2 diabetes. *Curr Dia Rep,* 2009; 9: 389–395.

11. Schroder H. Protective mechanisms of the Mediterranean diet in obesity and type 2 diabetes. *J Nutr Biochem* 2007; 18: 149–160.

12. Sanchez-Villegas A, Delgado-Rodriguez M, Alonso A, et al. Association of the Mediterranean dietary pattern with the incidence of depression. *Arch Gen Psychiat* 2009; 66: 1090–1098.

13. Scarmeas N, Stern Y, Mayeux R, et al. Mediterranean diet and mild cognitive impairment. *Arch Neurol* 2009; 66: 216–225.

14. Scarmeas N, Stern Y, Mayeux R, et al. Mediterranean diet, Alzheimer disease and vascular mediation. *Arch Neurol* 2006; 63: 1709–1717.

15. Sofi F, Cesari F, Abbate R, et al. Adherence to Mediterranean diet and health status: meta-analysis. *BMJ* 2008; 337: a1344.

16. Trichopoulou A, Costacou T, Bamia C, et al. Adherence to a Mediterranean diet and survival in a Greek population. *NEJM* 2003; 348: 2599–2608.

17. Roman B, Carta L, Martínez-González MA, et al. Effectiveness of the Mediterranean diet in the elderly. *Clin Interv Aging* 2008; 3: 97–109.

18. Pérez-López FR, Chedraui P, Haya J, et al. Effects of the Mediterranean diet on longevity and age-related morbid conditions. *Maturitas* 2009; 64: 67–79.

19. Hu FB. The Mediterranean diet and mortality—olive oil and beyond. *NEJM* 2003; 348: 2595–2596.

20. Trichopoulou A, Bamia C, Trichopoulos D. Mediterranean diet and survival among patients with coronary heart disease in Greece. *Arch Intern Med* 2005; 165: 929–935.

21. Buckland G, Gonzáles CA, Agudo A, et al. Adherence to the Mediterranean diet and risk of coronary heart disease in the Spanish EPIC cohort study. *Am J Epidemiol* 2009; 170: 1518–1529.

22. Buckland G, Agudo A, Luján L, et al. Adherence to a Mediterranean diet and risk of gastric adenocarcinoma with the EPIC cohort study. *Am J Clin Nutr* 2010; 91; 381–390.

23. Perez-Jiménez F, Alvarez de Cienfuegos G, Badimon L, et al. International conference on the healthy effect of virgin olive oil. *Eur J Nutr Invest* 2005; 35: 421–424.

24. Perez-Jiménez F, Ruano J, Perez-Martinez P, et al. The influence of olive oil on human health: not a question of fat alone. *Mol Nutr Food Res* 2007; 51: 1199–1208.

25. International Conference on the Diets of the Mediterranean, Jan 1993. Retrieved from: www.oldwayspt.org.

26. Kanaghinis T, Hatzioannou J, Deliargyris N, et al. Primary lactase deficiency in Greek adults. *Am J Dig Dis* 1974; 19: 1021–1027.

27. Psilakis M, Psilakis N. *Cretan Cooking.* Karmanor, Crete, Greece, 2000.

28. Psilakis M, Psilakis N. *Herbs in Cooking.* Karmanor, Crete, Greece, 2003.

29. Lionis C, Faresjö A, Skoula M, et al. Antioxidant effects of herbs in Crete. *Lancet* 1998; 352: 1987–1988.

30. Sabaté J, Oda K, Ros E. Nut consumption and blood lipid levels: a pooled analysis of 25 intervention trials. *Arch Intern Med* 2010; 170: 821–827.

31. Sabaté J, Wien M. Nuts, blood lipids and cardiovascular disease. *Asia Pac J Clin Nutr* 2010: 19: 131–136.

32. Kendall CW, Esfahani A, Truan J, et al. Health benefits of nuts in prevention and management of diabetes. *Asia Pac J Clin Nutr* 2010; 19: 110–116.

33. Jenab M, Sabaté J, Slimani N, et al. Consumption and portion sizes of tree nuts, peanuts and seeds in the European Prospective Investigation into Cancer and Nutrition (EPIC) cohorts from 10 European countries. *Br J Nutr* 2006; 96 suppl2: S12–23.

34. Aranceta J, Pérez-Rodrigo C, Naska A, et al. Nut consumption in Spain and other countries. *Br J Nutr* 2006; 96 suppl2: S3–11.

35. López-Uriarte P, Bulló M, Casas-Agustench P, et al. Nuts and oxidation: a systematic review. *Nutr Rev* 2009; 67: 497–508.

36. *Minoans and Mycenaeans: Flavours of Their Time.* In. eds. Tzedakis Y, Martlew H. Athens, Greece. National Archaeological Museum, Greek Ministry of Culture. 1999; 36–41.

37. *Minoans and Mycenaeans: Flavours of Their Time.* In. eds. Tzedakis Y, Martlew H. Athens, Greece. National Archaeological Museum, Greek Ministry of Culture. 1999; 210–229.

38. Warren P. Cretan food through five millennia. *Cretan Studies* 2003; 9: 271–284.

39. Kromhout D, Bloemberg BPM. Dietary saturated fatty acids, serum cholesterol and coronary heart disease. In. eds. Toshima H, Koga Y, Blackburn, Keys A (Hon. Ed.). *Lessons for Science from the Seven Countries Study: A 35-year Collaborative Experience in Cardiovascular Disease Epidemiology.* Tokyo, Japan, Springer. 1994; 35–41.

40. Dontas AS. Recent trends in CVD and risk factors in the Seven Countries Study: Greece. In. eds. Toshima H, Koga Y, Blackburn, Keys A (Hon. Ed.). *Lessons for Science from the Seven Countries Study: A 35-year Collaborative Experience in Cardiovascular Disease Epidemiology.* Tokyo, Japan, Springer. 1994; 93–111.

41. Vardavas CI, Linardakis MK, Hatzis CM, et al. Prevalence of obesity and physical inactivity among farmers from Crete (Greece), four decades after the Seven Countries Study. *Nutr Metab Cardiovasc Dis* 2009; 19: 153–155.

42. Welch AA, Mulligan A, Bingham SA, et al. Urine pH as an indicator of the dietary acid-base load, fruit and vegetables and meat intakes: results from the European Prospective Investigation into Cancer and Nutrition (EPIC)-Norfolk population study. *Br J Nutr* 2008; 99: 1335–1343.

43. Dawson-Hughes B, Harris SS, Ceglia L. Alkaline diets favour lean tissue mass in older adults. *Am J Clin Nutr* 2008; 87: 662–665.

44. Tyrovolas S, Bountziouka V, Papairakleous N, et al. Adherence to the Mediterranean diet is associated with lower prevalence of obesity among elderly people living in Mediterranean islands: the MEDIS study. *Int J Food Sci Nutr* 2009; 11: 1–14.

45. Kastorini CM, Milionis HJ, Esposito K, et al. The effect of Mediterranean diet on metabolic syndrome and its components: a meta-analysis of 50 studies and 534,906 individuals. *J Am Coll Cardiol* 2011; 57: 1299–1313.

46. Champagne CM. The usefulness of a Mediterranean-based diet in individuals with type 2 diabetes. *Curr Diab Rep* 2009; 9: 389–395.

47. Gu Y, Nieves J, Stern Y, et al. Food combination and Alzheimer disease risk. *Arch Neurol* 2010; 67: 699–706.

48. Scarmeas N, Luchsinger JA, Schupf N, et al. Physical activity, diet and risk of Alzheimer disease. *JAMA* 2009; 302: 627–637.

49. Sofi F, Macchi C, Abbate R, et al. Effectiveness of the Mediterranean diet: can it help delay or prevent Alzheimer's disease? *J Alzheimers Dis* 2010; 20: 795–801.

50. Escurriol V, Cofán M, Serra M, et al. Serum sterol responses to increasing plant sterol intake from natural foods in the Mediterranean diet. *Eur J Nutr* 2009; 48: 373–382.

51. Demonty I, Ras RT, van der Knaap HC, et al. Continuous dose-response relationship of the LDL cholesterol-lowering effect of phytosterols intake. *J Nutr* 2009; 139: 271–284.

52. Malinowski JM, Gehret MM. Phytosterols for dyslipidemia. *Am J Health Syst Pharm* 2010; 67: 1165–1173.

53. Vujkovic M, de Vries JH, Lindemans J, Macklon NS, et al. The preconception Mediterranean dietary pattern in couples undergoing in vitro fertilization/intracytoplasmic sperm injection treatment increases the chance of pregnancy. *Fertil Steril* 2010; 94: 2096–2101.

54. La Vecchia C. Association between Mediterranean dietary patterns and cancer risk. *Nutr Rev* 2009; 67suppl1: S126–129.

55. Itsiopoulos C, Hodge A, Kaimakamis M. Can the Mediterranean diet prevent prostate cancer? *Mol Nutr Food Res* 2009; 53: 227–239.

56. Chan R, Lok K, Woo J. Prostate cancer and vegetable consumption. *Mol Nutr Food Res* 2009; 53: 201–216.

57. Pelucchi C, Bosetti C, Rossi M, et al. Selected aspects of Mediterranean diet and cancer risk. *Nutr Cancer* 2009; 61: 756–766.

58. Kafatos A, Moschandreas J, Apostolaki I, et al. Mediterranean diet of Crete: foods and nutrient content. *J Am Diet Assoc* 2000; 100: 1487–1493.

59. Beliveau R, Gingras D. Role of nutrition in preventing cancer. *Can Fam Physician* 2007; 53: 1905–1911.

60. Simopoulos AP. Essential fatty acids in health and chronic disease. *Am J Clin Nutr* 1999; 70(Suppl 3): 560S–569S.

61. Uauy R, Valenzuela A. Marine oils: the health benefits of omega-3 fatty acids. *Nutrition* 2000: 16: 680–684.

62. Dorian P, Ramadeen A. Omega-3 polyunsaturated fatty acids (fish oils) and heart disease—clinical benefit or just a fad? *Cardiol Rounds* 2008; 13: 1–6.

63. Hu FB, Bronner L, Willett W, et al. Fish and omega-3 fatty acid intake and risk of coronary heart disease in women. *JAMA* 2002; 287: 1815–1821.

64. Stoll AL, Locke CA, Marangell LB, et al. Omega-3 fatty acids and bipolar disorder: a review. *Prostaglandins Leukot Essent Fatty Acids* 1999; 60: 329–337.

65. Vancassel S, Durand G, Barthélémy C, et al. Plasma fatty acid levels in autistic children. *Prostaglandins Leukot Essent Fatty Acids* 2001; 65: 1–7.

66. Richardson AK, Puri BK. A randomized double-blind, placebo-controlled study of the effects of supple-

mentation with highly unsaturated fatty acids on ADHD-related symptoms in children with specific learning difficulties. *Prog Neuro-Psychopharm Biol Psychiatry* 2002; 26: 233–239.

67. Sinn N. Nutritional and dietary influences on ADHD. *Nutr Rev* 2008; 66: 558–568.

68. Samieri C, Féart C, Letenneur L, et al: Low plasma eicosapentaenoic acid and depressive symptomatology are independent predictors of dementia risk. *Am J Clin Nutr* 2008;88: 714–721.

69. Bountziouka V, Polychronopoulos E, Zeimbekis A, et al. Long-term fish intake is associated with less severe depressive symptoms among elderly men and women: the MEDIS (MEDiterranean ISlands elderly) epidemiological study. *J Aging Health* 2009; 21: 864–880.

70. Genest J, McPherson R, Frohlich J, et al. 2009 Canadian Cardiovascular Society/Canadian guidelines for the diagnosis and treatment of dyslipidemia and prevention of cardiovascular disease in the adult—2009 recommendations. *Can J Cardio* 2009; 25: 567–579.

71. The Mediterranean Diet. Available at: www. unesco.org/culture/ich/indexphp?lg=en&pg=00011&RL=00394.

Dozens and Dozens of Diets

"Whatever it is, I'm against it!"

—GROUCHO MARX

Search the internet and see: there are dozens of diets out there. Most are for sale. I've just highlighted a few for the sake of discussion. No matter what the diet, the result you seek can only be obtained by taking responsibility for your own health. There is no way out of this.

AN ORTHOMOLECULAR DIET

"There is no magic bullet . . . but there is a lifestyle change that prevents, arrests, and reverses serious chronic disease."

—ANDREW W. SAUL, *Food Matters* (2008)

Let's start with the basics:

- Fruits and vegetables are good for you. Any diet that says they aren't is wrong.
- Drink water. Drink plenty.
- Don't eat junk.
- And take your vitamins.

This isn't a diet per se, but you will probably want to call it one. Any eating suggestion that promotes really good-for-you food and also says don't eat junk means that somewhere, somehow, we are going to have to say good-bye to some things we really like to eat, and therefore, we are "dieting."

There is no "diet" but rather a lifestyle change that can improve health, prevent disease, shed pounds, and maintain a fit body. Want to feel better? Be better? Look better? You have to change your whole life. This is the truth, but most diet books would like to convince you otherwise. True health is an ever-evolving process, involving taking steps both big and small continually over time until you have overhauled what wasn't working and have embraced what does. The work never ends. Effort is always required. If we are going to work so hard on our diet, we may as well choose the right things to eat.

"Orthomolecular" means "the right molecule." An orthomolecular approach to diet means we focus on giving the body the right nutrients in order to keep it healthy and free of disease and also to heal from illness.

Eat right, exercise, and take your vitamins is the mantra. Most of us have a pretty good idea what exercise is. Eating right may need some clarification, but ultimately we already know what to do. We just might need a reminder or some encouragement. "Take your vitamins" is likely the area needing the most clarification. The majority of this book will share information about vitamins and why it is so important to take them, even in high doses.

If you happen to be well on your way to your fitness goals and are comfortable with healthy eating, you will still find value in the information that follows. Many diets stop short when it comes to proper or optimal supplementation of vitamins and minerals. But why stop now, when we are so close to getting it right?

Eat Right to Lose Weight

If you want to lose weight and get well, you first have to look at your diet. It is the answer, and it is the only answer, whether we like it or not. What we eat, and what we don't eat, has everything to do with what we gain.

"Eat fresh vegetables" won't be promoted in trendy packaging. If it is, read the label more closely. Anything that proudly proclaims "Now with a whole serving of vegetables!" is likely employing a marketing tactic to get you to buy a product that is otherwise unhealthy and loaded with fillers, fats, sugars, chemicals, and/or salt. Actual servings of vegetables aren't as spectacular. There is nothing particularly glamorous about a green bean or a carrot. There is no hook. There is no lure. You won't see plain old leafy greens advertised on television.

Produce is produce. It's not exactly exciting. Substantial profits aren't made from folks who eat whole vegetables. It's the packaged, processed, advertised food we eat that is profitable for industry—at great cost to us. The only way around this is to do the work yourself. Buy (or grow) the boring, whole, raw produce, and do something amazing with it. There are plenty of fantastic recipes out there to make vegetables appealing. It is time that we *make time* to make food from scratch.

As we used to say about our dog when she didn't soak the rug or chew up anything in the house while we were away, she *knows* she's been good. A clean house was a clear indication of good doggie behavior. You, too, *know* when you've been good. Your body knows even better.

She Would Do Just *Anything*

A beautiful, curvy college student in want of an "A" goes to her professor's office one day.

"Professor," she says while batting her eyes, "I would do just anything to get an A in your class. Just ***anything.****"*

Her professor, with glasses lowered, looks at her for a long moment, slowly leans toward her, and says, "Then study."

It would be nice if excellent health were effortless. For most of us it isn't. There is no easy "A" in *this* class. You simply have to do the work.

It breaks down to this: Eat a varied diet of fresh, whole, minimally processed food free of artificial additives. Avoid refined sugar. Choose complex carbohydrates over simple ones, eat fermented foods, and choose organic whenever possible.

Eat Right and Eating Doughnuts?

"Eating right" may be harder to define. For many people, "eating right" means not eating wrong, which so many of us do. First, we can try to add in good food, along with the other stuff we are eating. Over time, as you feel better and are healthier, it will be second nature to select the healthy option over the other, unhealthy choices. It works with kids. It can work with adults too. My toddlers eat salads. Yay! Before they were willing to do that (and even now that they are) they drank fresh raw vegetable juice loaded with carrots, spinach, apples, cabbage, cucumbers, and a splash of lemon.

Healthy eating is a not a permanent condition. It is just a default setting. When in doubt, eat right. Occasionally, you won't, and it becomes more okay. This is because the majority of the time you will be eating right. But we are still human.

Case in point: I had a doughnut yesterday. And not just any doughnut. This was one of those enormous, half-pounder peanut-covered grocery store doughnuts. I just couldn't help it. It was fantastic. I probably have about four doughnuts a year. Most of those I get at a local farm where they hand-make batches, cook them in front of you, roll them in their own cinnamon-sugar topping, and hand them to you while they are still warm, along with some hot apple cider.

Yes, please.

But most of the time, I avoid junk food. By avoiding it I find that over time, I don't really want it. Offer me a doughnut right now and I wouldn't eat it. The more I avoid sugar, the less I want it. Some folks will have to avoid treats entirely. I have found that I can have an occasional treat and still stick to a good diet.

Eating right is not just about salads, of course. But they are a big part. Most things in our fridge are perishable. But we get to them before they go, and they usually end up in a salad. If a girlfriend of mine drops by for lunch or dinner, most times she will be served a gigantic family-size bowl loaded with field greens, peppers, mushrooms, celery, sunflower seeds, tomatoes, onions, shredded cabbage, cucumbers, with some cheese, croutons, and oil and vinegar dressing to make things interesting. My husband and I eat these for dinner at least twice a week. We mix it up and include apples, strawberries, spinach, pecans, and different dressings.

Should you for any reason want to read more about how our family eats and what our grocery list looks like, you can check out the chapter "Oh, What to Eat?"

Start Small

Diets don't work because they tend to be temporary and contrast so very sharply with what most people regularly eat. Cold-turkey diets that have you tossing out the door every tender morsel you've ever loved are likely to have you cheating very soon with a sign of relief. The only way to truly integrate all the healthy things you should be eating and eliminate the unhealthy ones you shouldn't is to do it gradually. Very gradually. But make a point to adhere to every small change you make. Make it small, but make it doable.

For example, a friend of mine used to drink five or six diet sodas each day. As you probably already know, diet soda is terrible for you.[15] Still, old habits are hard to change. In search of better health, she started to cut down her intake. For one week, she would drink one soda less per day. The next week, two. Over time, she got it down to one a day. For those of you already weaned off of artificial sweeteners and nonnutritious beverages, this may sound shocking. "Don't drink *any,*" you may be thinking. "It's not good for you!" But in the same way you can't tell a depressed person to just be happy, you can't tell someone who is so accustomed to certain foods that they just can't have them anymore. There is always more to it. Comfort, taste, enjoyment, routine may all play a part. As depression is often linked to nutrient deficiencies, so too can be the craving for sugary-tasting foods or beverages. Reduce the junk, and then introduce the nutrients. Try it the other way if you like. *Add* good food: I will eat X number of vegetables every day. Then work on eliminating the junk. Either way, it is a process. For it to be successful, for many folks it must also be gradual.

This was a huge improvement for our soda-drinking friend. She also cleaned up her diet in other ways and lost a lot of weight. Is there work yet to be done? Sure, she would say. No matter what shape we are in, *we all have work to do.* Every day I work at my health. Those who do the same know exactly what this means. If health sounds like a lot of work, I would argue that illness is more work. Far too many folks spend way too much time "working" on their sickness: doctor visits, specialists, blood work, waiting rooms, dealing with insurance companies, managing prescriptions, suffering side effects, experiencing poor results, or dealing with improper diagnosis or with a worsening or newly developing illness. This list does not include all the money it costs, how physically and mentally bad you feel when you aren't well, and all the things you could be doing if you weren't in this position. There is a way out. The door to good health does not lead into a doctor's office or a hospital room. It leads exactly the opposite way. The best part about working on health is the payoff: feel good, look better, and spend less time and money on disease care. It is a job with the very best of benefits.

Cut down your diet soda. Cut down the amount of processed meat you consume. Increase the number of vegetables. Increase the number of fruits. It is simplistic, but it is a start. Change is hard, but change must occur if there is a health problem in need of remedy. Want to lose weight? You will have to change what you do. Want to feel better? You will have to change what you do.

Changing Your Diet Is Hard. Let's Make It a Tad Easier.

1. Start small. Set a goal and take baby steps to get there. Make little changes you can stick to. Add more later.
2. Stay positive. You can do this. You are completely in charge of you. Remind yourself why you are doing this and why you want it. You are allowed to be proud of yourself.
3. Get help from others. Get the whole family on board. Great health comes easier when you have an active support system.
4. Write it down. What did you eat? Make yourself accountable for what goes in your mouth. (You may be surprised what that is after you start jotting it down.)
5. Share your successes. Call a friend who will listen and be happy for you and how far you have come.
6. Visualize the end of the race. Runners do it. You can too. And for diet-changers, the "end of the race" is the healthy you who enjoys the new foods you are eating along with the benefits therein, such as better health and the satisfaction that you did it all yourself.

The "Rules" of Food Selection

If you are bored when you open your fridge, maybe you are doing something right. I'm sure a few folks are about to argue with me, but sometimes it's hard to get excited about massive quantities of unprepared vegetables and fruits staring back and you. Look at all the work it is going to take to make these interesting. Cooking takes time and effort. And if cooked from these ingredients, the meal will probably be really nutritious.

Well, that's no fun.

I'm far more likely to grab and eat last night's leftover pizza order than whip up something from scratch. The trick is, then, to keep the junk food out of the fridge.

It is no surprise why we like takeout. It is no wonder we eat prepared and packaged foods. They are prepared already. There's no work. They taste good, and the box says they are pretty good for us. (We are supposed to believe the label, right?) Of course, we know full well that processed food is not good for us, and fresh whole foods are.

I've heard folks say that if you can't pronounce an ingredient, don't eat it. "Carrot" and "apple" and "kale" are pretty self-explanatory.

They are also boring.

Eating right involves a measure of creativity. We eat salads all the time in our house. Huge ones. Several dinners a week. But if we didn't mix up the ingredients on top of the lettuce and mix up the rest of the meals (and get the occasional pizza), we'd lose our minds. This means you have to cook. You have to try things you may not have wanted to in the past. You work at it. Over time, you find things you like. A good friend of mine tried pomegranate seeds for the first time. She liked them (you may too). Be brave. Challenge yourself to put the time and effort in to try new fruits and veggies and to discover how to make them tasty to you. When it comes to making collard greens tasty, perhaps "fry in bacon" is the only answer, but try to do better.

Ever order the vegetarian dish at a restaurant? It *has* to be good. Look what it's up against. Be inspired by these menu items. My husband, by the way, now makes a mean eggplant breakfast inspired by a local restaurant we like to frequent. He fries chopped eggplant, fresh chopped garlic, and chopped onion in butter or coconut oil until soft. Then he adds eggs, some feta cheese, chopped Greek olives, and hot cherry bell peppers, and serves it all with feta on top. Yum.

I get pretty excited about some fresh whole foods: summer tomatoes, the first watermelon, and peach season. But like most normal human beings, sometimes it is hard to get continually excited about healthy eating. You have to doll it up occasionally. Cook in butter. Add a little salt. Throw some cheese on it. Use salad dressing. Dieticians everywhere are cringing, but I'll tell you one thing: if you don't make the good food tasty, nobody eats it. And eventually, we get bored with the same healthy foods all the time. No wonder it is hard for some folks to stick to good eating habits. There is so much other stuff to eat out there that is yummy and we know it and the commercials keep telling us so. The trick is to eat it once in a while—and I emphasize once in a while—and spend the rest of your meals eating that nutritious food you are so diligently learning how to make delish.

So if what you have in your grocery cart and fridge does not really turn you on, good job. You won't be one of the many Americans eating cold cuts or pepperoni out of the package or heating up a microwaveable dinner. You won't be the one breaking into that bag of chips as soon as you get home or mowing down a few rows of cookies. You won't be able to drink a can of soda or enjoy some candy or pour a nice big bowl of sugary cereal *because you don't have any.* It isn't in your cart. It isn't in your fridge. It is also conspicuously absent from your cabinets. You eat right at home because, frankly, your food selection gives you no other choice.

Overcome the boredom. This is a lifelong challenge to eat right now, so we can avoid sickness and chronic disease. Being healthy is so worth it. You don't have to be a saint. You just have to try really hard. You have to make time to make the meals. And then eat them anyway.

FOOD ALLERGIES

"Wait! I can't eat that."

Allergies to certain foods may prohibit certain foods for certain people. However, orthomolecular physicians would have you look at this a slightly different way: you need vitamin C. "Most allergies usually disappear while you wait if you use the safest, most powerful, cheapest, and most effective antihistamine-antitoxin in existence: vitamin C," says Andrew W. Saul, PhD.[16] It can be this simple. Sort of. You may have to take a lot. A whole lot.

A friend once showed up at our door and immediately experienced an allergic reaction to our cats. Her face swelled, her eyes watered, and she was instantly miserable. While her symptoms surfaced, we casually mixed up a heaping teaspoon of ascorbic acid into some juice and asked her to drink it. Half an hour later, no sniffles. No red face. She was able to be around the cats just fine. So, every time she came over, she asked for C. Could the same thinking apply to food sensitivities? Could nutrients prevent and halt allergic reactions? My dad, Dr. Saul, thinks so:

> First of all, what we now label "allergies" could just as easily be called "undernutrition" and I think should be. The majority of Americans are demonstrably scorbutic, or on the very verge of scurvy. Insufficient vitamin C results in exaggerated sensitivity to even average levels of irritants, toxins, chemicals, pollution, and microorganisms. Deficiencies of vitamins A, B-complex, and E frequently manifest as skin problems or hypersensitivity to foods, stress, germs, or shock. Millions of vitamin-deficient but overstuffed persons are literally waiting to be allergic to something. Food that fills and fattens but doesn't fortify the body is like trying to build a wall with bricks and no mortar: it will hold up only until you lean upon it.[17]

How much vitamin C will you need? It depends. Vitamin C is a fantastic antihistamine, but you have to take enough. "'Allergic' tells you nothing more than any other symptom," says Dr. Saul. "Symptoms tell us that our body is not quite right. Naturopaths tell us that if our body is not quite right, we should take a good look at the way we take care of it. Check your diet first, not for the presence of allergens but rather for an absence of nutrients. You can start with a saturation test with vitamin C: take enough C to be symptom free, whatever the amount might be . . . but stay a few thousand milligrams under the amount that would cause loose bowels."[18] For more about getting to saturation of vitamin C, please see the chapter on vitamin C.

The following article is written by board-certified pediatrician Ralph Campbell, MD. It is about food allergies and sensitivity to gluten, and how high dose vitamin C is an effective, drug-free alternative for the treatment of allergic reactions.

Food Allergy, Gluten Sensitivity, and Celiac Disease

by Ralph Campbell, MD

From the *Orthomolecular Medicine News Service,* January 21, 2014.

What may have been called "food intolerance" or "food sensitivity" in the past may now qualify as "food allergy." On the other hand, certain conditions which mimic allergy symptoms should not come under that umbrella. We need an understanding of food allergy before successful management can be accomplished. There are no quick-fix remedies.

We tend to categorize by symptomatology, which accounts for the overlap of intolerance, sensitivity, and true allergy: 1) nasal symptoms of stuffy nose and sneezing; 2) bowel symptoms of intestinal cramping or gas; 3) lung symptoms of wheezing; and 4) skin that itches or produces a rash.

What Is an Allergy, Really?

For decades, allergists have considered what we might call an allergic reaction to be a true allergy only if it is of the Th2 type (a type of immune cell) that produces measurable IgE antibodies. The other type, Th1, produces tissue antibodies that protect against infection. When a baby is born, it no longer has the protection of mother's antibodies, making it vulnerable to infectious diseases. The infant's immune system can take either route: the allergy pathway or the "fight infection" pathway. Residing in our cell membranes are hormone-like substances called prostaglandins. Treatment will be addressed later, but for now we need to understand a bit about "good" fatty acids vs. "bad" to see how the choice is made. Omega-6 fatty acids (as derived from grains), incorporated in a prostaglandin, lead to the allergy pathway, whereas the omega-3 fatty acids (plentiful in fish oils) in a prostaglandin influence the development of the Th1 antibodies.

Heredity seems to play a part in the predisposition to develop allergies as well as the mechanism I just described, which is more "nurture" than "nature." The predisposed cell, upon exposure to a food allergen (antigen), produces IgE antibodies which attach to mast cells. With further exposure, the food antigen (a protein in the food) reacts with the IgE type of antibody, causing mast cells to break down and release histamine. It is the histamine, for the most part, that produces allergy symptoms. The food protein that remains intact by somehow escaping denaturing from heat or digestive processes, can become an antigen by sneaking into the blood stream via the "leaky gut syndrome" (the descriptive term for a porous gut), enabling distribution to cells in the nose, lungs, or skin. For the gut, symptomatology may include colic-like cramping, mucus (even bloody mucus) in the stool, or irritable bowel syndrome that can produce either diarrhea or constipation. Nasal mucosal-lining sensitization produces a stuffy, itchy nose or sneezing, while skin sensitization is manifest as eczema or topical dermatitis (both produce itching). Food allergens play a prominent part in wheezing; but so can irritants in the air, infection, and even exercise. The preservative, sodium sulfite, although certainly not a food itself, commonly contributes to wheezing and nasal symptoms.

I put allergy reactions into two categories: "rip-snortin'," and those fitting Dr. William G. Crook's description of "hidden allergies." (Dr. Crook was a pediatric allergist and a pioneer in the science of food allergy.) Under the first category, I would include sneezing, wheezing, vomiting, intestinal cramping, hives, and life-threatening, angioneurotic edema. The hidden allergies are manifest by a plugged-up, itchy nose, runny nose with postnasal drip causing a rattly cough, or mild abdominal cramping with mucus in the stool. Exposure to more than one allergen at the same time may create symptoms where a single exposure will not—the important concept of "allergy load."

The severe reactions are clearly IgE-antibody related, for which there are reliable tests. Even though there is documentation of milder allergies being on a different immune basis, this is given little attention, especially in infants with cow's milk allergy and the fact that they are often outgrown without the benefit of treatment.

Detection and Treatment

In one very detailed study,[1] a few workable, simple concepts came through among a maze of immunology jargon that only a few can comprehend. Researchers contend that food allergy is increasing due to taking the Th2 pathway. A September 17, 2013, Reuter's Health article by Lorraine L. Janeczko reports the findings of Dr. Peter Gillet, a gastroenterologist at the Royal Hospital for Sick Children in Edinburgh. He feels there has been a 64 percent rise in food allergy over a twenty-year period, there. Also America and several other countries are also showing large rises. The rate of rise is much greater in a more recent five-year period. However, the increase is attributed to more awareness and more testing in which only IgE-mediated allergy is accepted. This leaves me to believe there are many more undetected cases "out there."

The immunology study describes different types of tests, including the old standard of the prick or scratch skin test in which an antigen is scratched into the skin and the formation of a hive-like wheal is proof of allergy. They are taking new looks at old tests and treatment that were rejected in the past: oral specific, the "regular and gradual administration of escalating doses," and sublingual, in which the antigen rapidly enters the bloodstream. In desensitizing a patient to a potent antigen, such as peanut, these methods are undertaken in the presence of a doctor who is prepared for the worst. Intricate immune pathways are presented in the article. The good news comes from the admission that they are "far from understanding the complex mechanisms leading to the successful results in allergen-specific immunology." We don't need to hold our breath while waiting for the full development of the new paradigm, but rather, utilize what we already know works. A further admission is that the gold standard for testing for food allergy still is the oral challenge. This is strengthened by observing the shortcomings of some of the tests in which the test occasionally may be negative, but the patient can still have a bad reaction with future contact. The flip side is that the test may be positive, but the patient has no clinical signs of allergy after exposure.

I know that for the pediatric population the elimination-and-challenge test is totally adequate and reliable for detecting food allergies and reactions to items like food colorings and other food additives. Remember that:

- Symptoms arise within two hours after ingestion for most allergy problems, and that burning and itching sensations in the mouth or palate come immediately.
- Make a list of everything ingested that brings on those symptoms. Find commonality from your lists that leads to "suspects."
- Withdraw the suspects from the diet and note whether the allergy symptoms disappear.
- If adding back the suspect, one at a time, causes a return of symptoms, you have nailed a suspect. After a time of freedom from a reaction, periodically present a small, isolated challenge to see if the problem is still there. If not, reintroduce the food by gradually increasing doses.

Real Help with Vitamin C

Histamine, released in an allergic reaction, is the main chemical responsible for symptoms. Antihistamines are commonly prescribed. As with most medicines, there are side effects, most commonly drowsiness. Newer antihistamines claim to have less of this effect and to diminish symptoms better, but my personal experience does not bear this out. Response to these drugs is on an individual basis and varies. Fortunately, there is a natural remedy, without side effects, that really works. That is vitamin C, due to vitamin C's ability to neutralize histamine. The minimal amount in a daily multivitamin or an orange won't do the trick, but for many adults 2,000 mg every two hours until symptoms subside, will. I have had this experience with my patients. According to weight, scale down the amount, but don't hesitate to give repeated doses if the initial dose doesn't finish the job.

Not Allergy, but Allergy Look-Alikes

Certain foods, such as red wines (with or without sulfites) and moldy cheeses create histamine release that is not on an allergy basis. Infection in the respiratory tree can create similar symptoms. No one is allergic to running, but in some, exercise triggers wheezing.

Lactose intolerance may cause intestinal distress of gas and mild cramping, similar to that derived from food sensitization, and act much like irritable bowel syndrome. Interestingly, there is a strong familial tendency for its development. Those of Asian descent are much more susceptible. Although straight cow's milk is poorly tolerated, the good news is that milk treated with lactose-digesting probiotics, such as *Lactobacillus acidophilus,* is well tolerated. After weaning, many Asian infants go on to some form of fermented milk.

Gluten Sensitivity and Celiac Disease

Dr. Tom O'Bryan's article, "The Conundrum of Gluten Sensitivity," published in the National Health Federation's publication, *Health Freedom News,* showed that he had done his homework concerning the newer diagnostic tests that are providing a new look at gluten sensitivity as well as out-and-out celiac disease. He also described signs and symptoms of celiac disease outside the intestinal tract, which broadens its scope. I wish to provide a different slant on the subject that is derived from a pediatric point of view that extends from old time through current technological advances.

In my pediatric practice, I saw and successfully managed many cases of wheat allergy. At the same time, I had only one patient with classic celiac disease: a scrawny infant with the pathetic, heart-rending look of starvation and a flat area where his buttocks should be, a picture right out of the textbook. The best and only diagnostic tool for food allergy at that time was the food challenge. In the previously mentioned article in *Immunotherapy* by Enrique Gomez et al, the oral challenge was said to be the *current* gold standard as well. When positive, the infant/toddler was kept off of wheat for a time and periodically challenged, since wheat allergy, and the even more common cow's milk allergy, were known to clear spontaneously after a period of abstinence. Besides intestinal allergy symptoms, an infant with wheat allergy often exhibits nasal allergy signs, which appear very shortly after ingestion of the allergen, making the relationship obvious.

I see a continuum of simple allergy to the autoimmune condition of celiac disease. I can't agree that it isn't celiac disease until the intestinal villi are *completely* destroyed. It is a process. True, once the immune system response is under way, the only way to stop it is to refrain from intake of any of the gluten-containing grains. Intestinal biopsy that searches for destroyed villi is the only reliable test. Discovering the multiple double-, triple- or polypeptides of gluten can lead to lots of tests. Since there are false negatives as well as false positives results to the tests, and all require bloodletting, even if I had had access to them, I would not have employed them.

Scientific curiosity drives us to look for the precise causes of disease. But if the motive for such specificity is to enable developing target patentable pharmaceuticals, it would be better not to look. Avoiding the antigen does the job well enough.

Diagnoses Increase

What I am seeing, especially in well-educated young people who have computer savvy, is self-diagnosis of gluten sensitivity derived from bombardment by the press, the Internet highway, and TV news. It seems to be the in vogue diagnosis to have. An industry (much like the cholesterol-avoidance industry) of gluten-free foods is springing up. It is difficult to motivate the "gluten-free" adherents to obtain differentiation between simple wheat allergy and celiac disease. What has happened?

Dr. O'Bryan's article and the Enrique Gomez article referred to above, agree that there has been a marked increase in incidence in the last few decades. A 2010 *Medscape* article referred to a Mayo study by Joseph Murray in which they analyzed stored blood samples of Air Force recruits in the 1950s for gluten antibodies. These antibodies were practically nonexistent in the 1950s samples, but the article mentioned a large increase in incidence in the last three decades. Autoimmune diseases, in general, are on the increase. I believe that at the heart of these problems is the way we abuse our immune systems by direct attacks and nutritional deficiencies. Both diets and exposure to environmental toxins have changed exponentially since the 1950s.

Most current diets are very deficient in the vitamins that are essential as cofactors of enzymes that keep our metabolic wheels turning. Recommended Daily Allowances (RDAs) are barely able to prevent classic deficiency diseases like rickets or beriberi. I could fill pages with citations about the effect of environmental toxins on the immune system. A recent boon for those who treat allergy problems has been the gain in knowledge of omega-3 fatty acids (FAs). Whether the young immune system takes the Th1 pathway or the Th2 pathway (which produces measurable IgE antibodies that mark "big time" allergies), is largely determined by the ratio of omega-6 FAs to omega-3 FAs. Rather than having closer to the ideal of 2:1, current diets create a ratio more like 20:1. The makeup of our prostaglandins (hormone-like substances in cell walls that areready to spring into action) is determined by the essential fatty acids in the mix: those provoking inflammation and clumping of platelets or those doing the opposite. The "leaky gut syndrome" concept is getting some new, deserved attention. Just what causes the gut permeability that can allow whole proteins to sneak from the gut into the bloodstream and promote the antibody formation of simple allergy or autoimmunity in which the antibodies mistake normal body cells as foreign invaders?

Conclusion

We might keep trying to satisfy our scientific curiosity by seeking to pinpoint the causes of food allergy and autoimmune diseases that can be documented by specific tests. But should we wait for, or expect to be able to rely 100 percent on, new tests while other, more straightforward, proven diagnostic tools are available? Let's not get bogged down with minutiae. Rather, let us attempt to get straight, understandable information to the public that possibly could get them on a helpful, less cumbersome and less expensive track. Immune systems aren't functioning like they used to. A tangible effect is noted with antibody levels in response to various vaccines that are producing antibody levels well below the expected. I feel that the rapid rise in autoimmune diseases is getting away from us. Too often, drugs are not meeting our expectations. Let us concentrate on ways to improve immune health while continuing to identify the agents that weaken our immune systems. Immune health cannot be isolated from general health. Since it is nearly impossible in our culture to achieve a completely healthy diet, the intake of optimal amounts of vitamin supplements is essential.

REFERENCE FOR "FOOD ALLERGY, GLUTEN SENSITIVITY, AND CELIAC DISEASE"

1. Gomez E, et al. Food allergy: management, diagnosis and treatment strategies. *Immunotherapy* 2013; 5(7): 755–768. doi: 10.2217/imt.13.63.

DODGING THE DIETS

Diet Diary: Day One

"I have removed all the bad food from the house. It was delicious."

—POPULAR INTERNET DIET QUOTE

All kidding aside, we are starting to figure it out: there is no "diet," in spite of the hopeful folks out there who would like to convince you and your wallet otherwise. There is no prescriptive food list that works for absolutely everyone. You must do what is right for you. But there are foods and beverages that are more nutritious than others.

The best thing about most diets is what they don't include. Eliminating disease-promoting foods and beverages would be a huge step for many people.

It turns out that there are all sorts of ways to do it right—and as many ways to do it wrong. You have to make the move to select the right foods, not matter what "diet" they are included in. Every time you eat, you can make a choice to select the best food possible. By following basic guidelines like "do not eat highly processed foods" and "limit refined sugar," you do yourself and your health a favor every time. There is no way around the good-food argument. But if you don't eat right, taking vitamins is still a huge positive step forward. Take it even further. Do both.

CHAPTER 3 REFERENCES

1. The Raptor Institute. "Red Tailed Hawk." http://raptorinstitute.org/our-birds/red-tailed-hawk/ (accessed May 2016).

2. Robinson, J. "What You Need to Know about the Beef Industry." *Mother Earth News* (Feb/Mar 2008): http://www.motherearthnews.com/homesteading-and-livestock/beef-industry-zmaz08fmzmcc.aspx?PageId=8#ArticleContent (accessed May 2016).

3. Hardy, K., J. Brand-Miller, K. D. Brown, et al. "The Importance of Dietary Carbohydrate in Human Evolution." *Q Rev Biol* 90(3) (Sept 2015): 251–268.

4. Ultimate Paleo Guide. "Paleo Diet Food List." (Sept 5, 2015): http://ultimatepaleoguide.com/paleo-diet-food-list/ (accessed May 2016).

5. The Gerson Institute. "A Nutritional History of the Potato (& Why It Doesn't Deserve Its Bad Reputation!)" (July 24, 2014): https://gerson.org/gerpress/a-nutritional-history-of-the-potato-why-it-doesnt-deserve-its-bad-reputation/ (accessed May 2016).

6. Ibid.

7. Burros, M. "Make That Steak a Bit Smaller, Atkins Advises Today's Dieters." Jan 18, 2004. http://www.nytimes.com/2004/01/18/nyregion/make-that-steak-a-bit-smaller-atkins-advises-today-s-dieters.html?_r=0 (accessed May 2016).

8. Ibid.

9. Gunnars, K. "The Atkins Diet: Everything You Need to Know (Literally)." Apr 2016. https://authoritynutrition.com/atkins-diet-101/ (accessed May 2016).

10. "Find Out the Facts." http://sa.atkins.com/new-atkins/the-science/truth-vs.-fiction/find-out-the-facts.html (accessed May 2016).

11. "How It Works: Phase One List of Acceptable Foods." https://www.atkins.com/how-it-works/atkins-20/phase-1/low-carb-foods (accessed May 2016).

12. Burros, M. "Make That Steak a Bit Smaller, Atkins Advises Today's Dieters." Jan 18, 2004. http://www.nytimes.com/2004/01/18/nyregion/make-that-steak-a-bit-smaller-atkins-advises-today-s-dieters.html?_r=0 (accessed May 2016).

13. FFL. Schott, J. "Don't Call it a Diet: 'Fit for Life' Changes Everything." Sept 10, 2015. http://www.elle.com/beauty/health-fitness/news/a30358/fit-for-life-diet/ (accessed May 2016).

14. U.S. Department of Health and Human Services. National Institutes of Health. National Heart, Lung and Blood Institute. "Description of the DASH Eating Plan." https://www.nhlbi.nih.gov/health/health-topics/topics/dash (accessed May 2016).

15. Nettleton, J.A., P.L. Lutsey, Y. Wang, et al. "Diet Soda Intake and Risk of Incident Metabolic Syndrome and Type 2 Diabetes in the Multi-Ethnic Study of Atherosclerosis (MESA)." *Diabetes Care* 32(4) (2009): 688–694. http://www.ncbi.nlm.nih.gov/pmc/articles/PMC2660468/ (accessed May 2016).

16. Saul, A.W. "Allergies." Available at: http://doctoryourself.com/allergies.html (accessed May 2016).

17. Ibid.

18. Ibid.

CHAPTER 4

Weight and Weight Loss

"And Leon's getting laaaarrrrger!"

—STEPHEN STUCKER AS "JOHNNY," *AIRPLANE* (1980)

Fat is on many of our minds these days, and it probably should be. The people of the United States are growing larger. So are our friends from abroad when they eat the way we do.

DO WE DESERVE AN "A" FOR EFFORT OR AN "F" FOR FAT?

More than two-thirds of American adults are overweight.[1] It's been this way for years. And things are getting worse.

According to the Gallup-Healthways Well-Being Index, in 2013 the obesity rate crept up to a new high of 27.1 percent, the highest rate measured since they began tracking weight in the United States back in 2008. The number of folks marked "morbidly obese" also reached a new high for Gallup: 3.8 percent. This didn't include folks they categorized as "overweight," another 35.7 percent of adults. This means, as of 2013, about 63 percent of adults in the United States have weight to lose. Only 35.2 percent of the population is considered to be at a "normal weight."[2] This is just what we'll admit to. Gallup relies on respondents' *self-reports* of their weight and height.

Our government says we are even fatter. Based on clinical measurements, the U.S. Department of Health and Human Services reports that 37.9 percent of adults are obese. Roughly another 33 percent are overweight. This means *over 70 percent* of Americans age 20 or older are fat.[3] We aren't setting the best example for our kids, and it shows. On average, 31.8 percent of our children ages two to19 are overweight or obese. Obesity alone accounts for nearly 17 percent.[4]

High BMI? Why?

Your body mass index (BMI) is a relatively good indicator of whether or not you are overweight. It is calculated using your height and weight to determine if you are underweight, normal weight, overweight, or obese. It doesn't work so well for very muscular athletes or folks who might be losing muscle (as may the elderly), but for most folks, their BMI can help them understand if they are of "normal" weight or not.

A BMI of 18.5–24.9 is considered normal. Less that 18.5 is "underweight." A BMI of 25–29.9 is considered overweight. Obesity is indicated as a BMI measurement over 30. "Morbidly obese" is defined as a BMI above 40 or anyone who is 100 pounds (or more) over their ideal weight.[5] A quick online search will put you in touch with a BMI calculator, if you are curious where you stand.

How does that compute into actual pounds? The calculation is the same for both men and women. According to the National Institutes of Health BMI chart, a person who is five feet six inches would want to weigh somewhere between 118 and 154 pounds. A person who is six feet would want to weigh somewhere between 140 and183 pounds.[6]

The range for "normal weight" is rather generous. The first individual has 36 pounds of wiggle room; the second has 43. Similar figures appear up and down the BMI chart; the taller you are the more generous they become. The range starts at 27 pounds if you are four feet ten inches, and expands to 48 pounds of wiggle room if you are six feet four inches.[7] It would seem that we should be able to manage our weight within such wide parameters. It's a large target. There is much room for movement: the objective is to aim and hit anything on the "normal weight" target board. We can gain some pounds; we can lose some pounds. We could fluctuate to the tune of *several dozen* pounds, and still be of "normal weight." Yet the facts say the majority of us are missing the target *completely:* 60 to 70 percent of our population does not fall within these wide ranges of "normal" weight.[8]

There is a great deal of leeway in the "overweight" category as well, before one would weigh enough to be classified as "obese." The same five-foot-six individual is considered overweight if she falls between 155 and 185 pounds. The six-foot person is overweight if he weighs 184 to 220 pounds.[9] These folks have another 30 to 36 pounds of wiggle room.

Let's say the five-foot-six-inch woman's ideal weight is somewhere around 136 pounds, keeping in mind the "normal" weight range for her height is 118 to154 pounds. If she actually weighs 185 pounds, she has nearly 50 pounds to lose, and still just falls within the "overweight" range.

This makes the weight numbers that classify people as "obese" even more shocking, especially considering that nearly 35 percent of our population is considered to be so.[10] If our five-foot-six-inch woman weighs 186 to 246 pounds, she is now considered "obese." The six-foot man would be obese if he weighed 221 to 293 pounds.[11] Tack on any more pounds, and now they would be considered morbidly obese.

We cannot blame a chart. It's actually rather reasonable. Some might argue it is too generous with its weight allowances in the "normal" category.

Reaching a "normal weight" in accordance with BMI is something we can all do. It is not a rigid rule. We need not obsess over ounces. If we do, we are missing the whole point. We should pay attention to pounds, especially when there are dozens of them that we should shedding.

Fat Is a Four-Letter Word

"[B]igger caskets sometimes won't fit in hearses, requiring families to rent flatbed trucks to transport their loved ones."

—CBS

Fat is a four-letter word, at least when it adorns your waistline. Many of us know full well the negative health effects of being overweight. Nearly one in five deaths in America is associated with obesity.[12] This doesn't make it any easier to change our habits. Weight is a sensitive topic. Many of us would rather avoid the conversation entirely.

In fairness, we do want to lose weight. At least we say we do. But are we doing it? While half of us acknowledge we want to shed pounds, only about a quarter of us say we are seriously doing anything about it.[13] It has been this way for decades.[14] By our own admission, we are eating worse[15] and exercising less.[16]

You don't really need stats to tell you things are amiss. Just look around you. You can see it. Many of us are overweight. Many of us are sick. Many of us are medicated. It affects us, it affects our friends, and it affects our children. Thin does not always mean healthy, but fat never does.

Overweight, Undernourished, and Underactive

"We can make a commitment to promote vegetables and fruits and whole grains on every part of every menu. And we can help create a culture—imagine this—where our kids ask for healthy options instead of resisting them."

—MICHELLE OBAMA

You might think that being rotund would be a sign of plenty: we have had enough to eat. Just look at all the nourishment we have enjoyed. Instead, we have bodies that are fat and literally starving for nutrients.

The proof is in the pudding or maybe in *all* that pudding. This sugary snack, amidst countless others, all too obviously remains on the average American dinner table. We really aren't doing enough to maintain good health.

"Enough" includes eating a healthy, plant-based diet, exercising, taking care of our emotional well-being, limiting sugar, red meat, refined carbohydrates, processed foods, alcohol, and caffeine, and, to the best of our ability, avoiding additives, genetically modified ingredients, and environmental pollutants. "Enough" means drinking fresh, raw vegetable juice, eating whole foods, drinking plenty of water, and detoxifying our bodies. "Enough" includes taking the vitamins we aren't and working to decrease or eliminate the pharmaceuticals we are. "Enough" means setting a healthier example for our children. The real answer to well-being and weight loss is not found in fad diets, drugs, surgery, or dust-gathering exercise equipment. This is the hard truth.

Is it all bad news? Well, it's hard to call it "good." For example, there are years when we make slight improvements in our exercise habits. But we just as easily drift backward. Short-lived trends of increased action do not deserve gold stars for effort. Overall, since 2008, roughly half of us report exercising at least 30 minutes three or more days per week.[17] (Many an Internet dating profile states the same. Surely, what we say we do doesn't necessarily translate into what we actually do.) But even if we take our own word for it, slight climbs in exercise rates are still not much cause for celebration. The current downtrend speaks volumes. The average over the years speaks even more. As obesity rates rise, you would think we should be doing more than ever to counter that trend. While diet is far more important when it comes to slimming your waistline, exercise is critical for keeping extra weight off.

Is There Room for Size Acceptance?

Shouldn't we love each other for who we are? We may want bigger seats, roomy clothing, and validation that "big is beautiful."

Perhaps we shouldn't look for approval for something that could very well kill us. Perhaps we shouldn't accept chronic overweight as the new norm. Perhaps we shouldn't expect others to adapt and change our world because of it. We are not stuck. We can do better. Weight is a modifiable life factor. This is no time to cater to our fatter nation. It is time for our fatter nation to take responsibility and take action. This may hurt our feelings, but being overweight hurts our health more.

We should seek the praise and support that comes with doing the right thing: eating well, exercising—and not making excuses. Weight loss is the beginning of a new life, new habits, and new experiences. There is a light at the end of the tunnel; there is light through the process. It doesn't have to be a miserable experience. As the pounds come down, you will eventually feel better. Health problems caused by obesity will fade: lessened, prevented, or alleviated. Being of a healthy weight reduces your risk for coronary heart disease, high blood pressure, cancer, stroke, type 2 diabetes, joint issues, reproductive problems, metabolic syndrome, gallstones, and sleep apnea—all problems that increase with an increased BMI.

Ladies, there is plenty of room to be curvy in the "normal weight" range on the BMI chart. Gentlemen, there is room for, as one of our friends would call it, "man size." We aren't looking to create a country full of stick people, contrary to some of the imagery in popular magazines. We are looking for people to be healthy and in shape. The goal is to be *fit.* Fit is synonymous with healthy, in shape, vigorous, well, and in top form.

For pretty much everybody, this will take some work.

YOU HAVE TO EAT RIGHT. EVENTUALLY.

Do it now, or do it later. That's your choice. You can take care of yourself now and stay well, or you can eat poorly, exercise none, ignore your weight gain, and doctor's orders and disease will compel you to address all of it later.

Diabetes

Fail to pay attention to your diet, and the results could kill you. Diabetes does that to nearly 70,000 people each year.[18] If you aren't dead, then you still have to live with the disease, and you still have to pay attention to your diet. I realize I am being quite harsh, but unfortunately this is the scary reality. Sometimes it takes a kick in the pants to get going, and this is no time to sit on our hands. We can choose to make a difference in our health right this very second.

People diagnosed with type 2 diabetes must eat healthy in order to keep their blood sugar in check. The U. S. National Library of Medicine defines a healthy diabetic diet as one that includes eating fruits and veggies every day, eating less salt, eating smaller portions, and limiting sugar and alcohol.[19] If you are going to have to do all of this anyway, why not do it now and prevent the disease in the first place? Why feel sick? Why *be* sick?

"The good news is," says the Harvard School of Public Heath, "that type 2 diabetes is largely preventable. About 9 cases in 10 could be avoided by taking several simple steps: keeping weight under control, exercising more, eating a healthy diet, and not smoking."[20] Healthy eating means avoiding processed carbohydrates in favor of whole-grain foods, avoiding sugary drinks, eating good fat, and avoiding bad fat. Additionally, limit red meat and avoid processed meat; switch instead to nuts, fish, poultry, or whole grains. "The evidence is growing stronger that eating red meat (beef, pork, lamb) and processed red meat (bacon, hot dogs, deli meats) increases the risk of diabetes, even among people who consume only small amounts."[21]

Think you can keep right on with bad habits and be spared? "If type 2 diabetes was an infectious disease, passed from one person to another, public health officials would say we're in the midst of an epidemic," says Harvard.[22] Nobody gets a "free eating" pass. Poor diet catches up with you eventually. If diabetes doesn't get you, heart disease, the leading cause of death in the United Sates, just might. You may want to read *The Vitamin Cure for Diabetes,* by Ian E. Brighthope, MD, and *The Vitamin Cure for Heart Disease,* by Hilary Roberts and Steve Hickey, PhD. These books fully explore both lifestyle changes and vitamin supplement use. Additional reading is suggested at the end of this book.

Heart Disease

Many of the risk factors for heart disease are modifiable: you have the power to change them. This is an important point: "Most people who develop heart disease—at least 8 in every 10—have one or more major risk factors that are within their power to change."[23]

How do you prevent heart disease? Health advice is pretty consistent: don't smoke, exercise, get to a healthy weight, and limit alcohol. A healthy, heart-disease prevention diet includes more fruits and vegetables, whole grains, unsaturated fat, and good protein from sources like beans, nuts, fish, and poultry, and some herbs and spices.[24] What you omit is as important as what you eat. Avoid processed foods, limit salt, avoid fast-digesting carbohydrates like those in white bread or white rice, avoid red meat, and stop drinking sugary beverages.[25]

We know what to do. We must make a point to do it. Every day, every meal.

> "Consider this provocative finding from the Nurses' Health Study.[26] Non-smoking women with a healthy weight who exercised regularly, consumed a healthy diet, and had an alcoholic drink every other day were 83% less likely to have had a heart attack or to have died of heart disease over a 14-year period, compared with all the other women in the study. The results were almost identical in a similar study in men.[27] In these two studies, more than two-thirds of all cardiovascular events could be chalked up to smoking, excess weight, poor diet, and drinking too much."[28]
>
> —Harvard School of Public Health

There's more. The root of heart disease is based in reversible vitamin deficiency. A book by Thomas Levy, MD, *Stop America's #1 Killer,* clearly shows that we all should be taking vitamin C, and plenty of it, not to mention eating right and taking many other helpful nutrients. However, large intakes of vitamin C specifically are key for prevention and treatment of heart disease.

Stomach Surgery

Folks who get bariatric surgery have to change their diet. They will need to avoid sugary foods and beverages. They must pay attention to portion size. They have to exercise. They will need to take vitamins for the rest of their lives. They must drink plenty of water.

After going through this dangerous surgery, a person still has to do all the things he or she needed to do anyway to lose the weight and maintain health. Yes, weight loss will happen quickly. This, I imagine, is surgery's grandest allure.

Could we cut out the middleman? (Bad pun, sorry.) What if folks about to go under the knife took steps to do now what they will have to do anyway after surgery? The same goes for diet pills. Have you ever noticed that many say they work best when combined with good diet and exercise?

Must we have this dramatic surgery to get ourselves to finally acknowledge that we need to eat right and exercise? If you are desperate enough for surgery, then be desperate enough to make active changes now. You will still have to make these changes after surgery.

Most of us have the ability to feed ourselves. We can control what goes in our mouths. We have to stop feeling sorry for ourselves and start taking action. Obesity is preventable and it is reversible. We can do it on our own. If that doesn't sound like any fun, find someone willing to do it with you. It is hard to stop those who unite toward a common healthy goal.

TOXINS IN FAT: LOSING WEIGHT AND GETTING SICK

You may notice that when you start losing weight you feel awful. Research suggests this may be due in part to the release of persistent organic pollutants (POPs) into the bloodstream that were once stored in fat cells.[29] Once you burn the fat, it is hypothesized that these toxins are released, making you feel rather lousy as well as contributing to numerous health problems. It sounds like a "damned if you do, damned if you don't" situation: excess weight contributes to numerous health problems, and so do pollutants in our bloodstream.

There is help. "Pesticides are diverse in chemical structure, but they are usually susceptible to neutralization by vitamin C," says Thomas Levy, MD. "Vitamin C also tends to readily repair the damage done by many pesticides."[30] Anyone on a weight-loss regimen should also be taking plenty of vitamin C. "[A]scorbic acid nutritional status markedly affects the toxicity and/or carcinogenicity of greater than 50 pollutants, many of which are ubiquitous in the air, water, and food environments," states a paper in the *Journal of Environmental Pathology, Toxicology, and Oncology*. This paper proposed that the recommend dietary allowance (RDA) should take into account our exposure to pollutants. However, it concluded, "[a]t the present time, the data do not warrant changing the ascorbic acid RDA in light of the knowledge of pollutant interactions."[31] I see.

In large enough doses, vitamin C is an effective antitoxin.[32] We simply cannot count on the modest RDA to be sufficient, especially when our need is greater. When you are losing weight, your need is greater.

Weight loss is a mental battle. We miss what we used to eat. We have to say no to food we have enjoyed, and we don't like doing it one bit. It may be helpful to know that vitamin C (3,000 mg per day) has been shown to improve mood.[33] It helps and certainly won't hurt.

EAT RIGHT TO STAY FIT

Our culture spends a lot of time talking about specific ingredients or nutrients that we should eat or avoid. The truth is all nutrients are important. A varied diet is important. Moderation is important with some foods. Others, like veggies, we can eat as much as we want.

My First Jelly Bean

I didn't have a jelly bean until I was in third grade. I remember it distinctly. I was at school at the time. It was purple. I knew I really wasn't supposed to eat colored candy, and that made the experience much more secretive and exciting. But instead of wanting to stuff my face with more, I found I didn't crave such fake flavors. Jelly beans just weren't as tasty as real food. Whenever I would eat one, I always hoped it would taste better than it actually did. I found that true of most candy the kids stuffed in their mouths on the bus rides to and from school.

The purple jelly bean wasn't my last. (I guess I always hoped the next one would taste better than the last.) Kids have plenty of access to junk food, even if their folks aren't buying it. My parents were whole-foods radicals. They weren't raised that way, but when newborn babes were placed into their arms, all of a sudden good health for the whole family was imperative. They made sure we ate good food. More noteworthy perhaps is what we *didn't* eat: soda, junk food, candy, processed foods, white bread, and deli meats were inconspicuously absent from our diet. By "inconspicuous" I mean we never noticed they were missing. By the time we were older and knew such foods existed, we still did not have access to them in our home. I clearly remember that first jelly bean, but I also remember picking my first apple off the tree and how wonderful it tasted. It was red. To this day, I prefer the flavor of real fruit over fake fruit flavor.

One of the best things you can do now for your children is to feed them an amazing diet, and eat one yourself. Albert Einstein said, "Example isn't another way to teach, it is the only way to teach." They will get used to good food. They will develop a taste for it. They will seek it out when they are older. Their health will be all the better for it.

The Right Fats Help You Stay Thin

"Let no one who has the slightest desire to live in peace and quietness be tempted, under any circumstances, to enter upon the chivalrous task of trying to correct a popular error."

—WILLIAM THOMS, DEPUTY LIBRARIAN FOR THE HOUSE OF LORDS, C. 1873

My folks never drank skim milk or blotted the oil off our cheese pizza. Despite the trend at the time while I was growing up, we ate fat. All my friends had to pour that bluish-white skim milk over their cereal. It looked awful. It tasted awful. I was happy to go home and drink the real stuff. We always had whole milk in the house, real butter, and full-fat cheese. We ate yogurt with the cream on top, actual "cream" cheese (not the low-fat cheese spreads), and for dessert, real ice cream. It was entirely convenient that Mom worked at a dairy factory.

My brother and I were raised lacto-ovo vegetarian until about the age of eight. Many of our fat calories came from dairy products, a relatively inexpensive source. We also ate nuts, seeds, and, when we could afford it, seafood. The ample amounts of vegetables in our plant-based diet tasted better with oils, butter, and cheese. While other people worried about how much dressing they misted onto their salad, we didn't worry about such details. We ate the dressing if it got the salad down. (Mom made some great homemade vinaigrettes.) Fat did not make us fat, contrary to some popular trends in food marketing still perpetuated even today.

My parents figured, and rightly so, that growing children need fat in their diet in order to grow and develop properly. This is still true. Interestingly, in 2009 a Swedish study found that kids who drank whole milk, as opposed to those who drank medium- or low-fat milk, had less weight gain. Specifically, they conclude, "Saturated fat and intake of full fat milk were inversely associated with BMI."[34] More fat in their diet meant slimmer kids.

How could this be? It would be convenient if fat made us fat, but it isn't so. Good fats from good whole foods actually help keep weight off. *Try* to eat a whole bowlful of nuts. Even if you manage to eat them all before feeling full, you won't have an appetite for much else. Food with good fat makes a meal more satiating, satisfying, and filling. Fats help you absorb nutrients in your food too.

Interestingly, when the fat content of foods went down, the numbers on

Americans' scales went up.[35] Why were we gaining weight? When people switched to low-fat options, many just replaced fat with sugar and refined carbohydrates. Any benefit we gained from reducing saturated fat in our diets went away when we chose to eat unhealthy substitutes instead. We may not have even noticed we were doing it. Blinded by proclamations of "NOW 1/3 LESS FAT!" on the label, foods that used to taste good because they contained fat now tasted good for some other reason. Those reasons included sugar, fillers, refined carbs, and chemicals. Yuck.

Eating some saturated fat is a normal, healthy thing to do. Eating the large amount of fat that some Americans do, especially from unhealthy animals and from junk food, is not. Don't have a stick of butter for a snack, but eat real butter instead of margarine. Steer clear of hydrogenated oils and trans fats. Cut back on your intake of fatty meats, especially red, especially nonorganic. Increase your intake of fats from vegetable sources, like avocados, and from olive oil, fish, and nuts.

Eating Carbohydrates

Avoidance of grains is the new trend. Maybe it is a good idea for some. Others may find that *whole* grains, properly prepared, fit nicely into a well-rounded healthy diet. (I'm one of those.) If you have celiac disease or gluten sensitivity, of course, you'll steer clear of certain foods. But don't make the mistake of lumping carbs into one group. Carbs (and calories) are not created equal. Never skip carbs when they are found in vegetables. Legumes are good for you. Nuts too. Good grains can be, too.

Carbohydrates also include sugars. Here, the delivery vehicle matters. For example, fruit naturally contains some sugar. (So do vegetables and dairy.) Fruit also contains fiber, water, and nutrients. This is not true of refined, nutrient devoid, sugar-dense sweet treats. "Plus," says Joy Dubost, RD, "whole fruit has a lot of fiber, which actually slows down your body's digestion of glucose, so you don't get the crazy insulin spike (and subsequent crash) that candy causes. That also means your body has more time to use up glucose as fuel before storing it—as fat."[36] Peach or cookie? Eat the peach. In season? Eat several. Eat one before you reach for dessert. Your sweet tooth will be satisfied, and your waistline will thank you for the substitution.

Don't lose sight of the goal if you start to head down the low-carb path. Avoiding carbohydrates like refined sugar is *always* smart. Obtaining carbohydrates from good whole food is smart, too.

MIRACLE SLIMMING SOLUTION! (PREPARE TO BE DISAPPOINTED)

"The FDA has approved a new device to treat obesity.
The amazing breakthrough is called a 'vegetable.'"
—CONAN O'BRIEN

Ah, the tummy tuck belt. Oh, and the cream. A self-proclaimed "miracle slimming system."[37] For just about 60 bucks, after shipping, you too can have your very own. And you still have to do all the work. Really.

The "keep your lifestyle" method claims "no added exercise" but includes smearing on cream every day, squeezing into the tummy belt and wearing it for ten minutes, doing "standing abdominal contractions" (kind of *sounds* like exercise), and then after a month you supposedly see some results. Oh, and *next* month you'll need more cream for another 25 bucks, plus shipping, which may be automatically placed on auto-ship to make it a pain to cancel just in case you wise up too soon.

Does anybody, besides me, find this laughable? And yet people are buying. The infomercials are still on TV. There are *hundreds* of bad reviews about the product on Amazon.com. The vast majority of ratings are a dismal one star. "Waste of money" and "scam" are commonplace phrases from customers who have tried it. And yet, according to its ranking in Amazon's health and personal-care items, people keep purchasing. And people will keep complaining. In the meantime, somebody is making a bunch of money. Kind of makes you wish you had thought of it first.

Of course, the tummy belt works a whole lot better if you stick to a diet and exercise program. They will tell you this. I will too. If you need a ribbon around your finger, or a belt around your waist, to help remind you of your health goals, so be it. But the ribbon around your finger will be a lot less expensive for sure, and probably just as effective.

If you are interested, as plenty of folks are, there are also numerous other "weight loss" creams on the market you can try. While you are at it, you could attempt to make your boobs bigger or penis larger too. A search on Amazon for "penis enhancement" or "breast enlargement" will bring you over 1,500 products—each—including soaps, creams, serums, and songs. Yes, there are hypnosis sessions and "subliminal" CDs to "program your subconscious mind to increase your breast size"[38] or "invigorate and promote growth of the penis."[39] Oddly, the only review there for the breast-enhancement hypnosis CD states that the CD would not play in the CD player. As for the customer seeking penis enlargement, his review was aptly titled "Short," and the verified consumer states the "penis enlargement mind journey" CD did not play for its entire recorded length.

I couldn't make this stuff up. Clearly, there are folks looking for products out there for any number of personal issues, and nearly as many folks willing to sell "solutions."

Speaking of which, an Amazon search for "weight loss" brings you over 168,000 products to buy. It is a growing business on both ends of the spectrum to be sure. Obesity rates have never been higher in the United States. The weight-loss industry is cleaning up. There are folks lining up to collect your hard-earned dollars just as fast as they can. I am reminded of Dr. Seuss's dear Sylvester McMonkey McBean who would like you and every other Sneetch to have a walk through his star-on (or star-off) machine.

Now why would I be here poking fun at weight-loss products? Losing excess weight is good, right? You bet. Except we all know that isn't the whole answer. Only diet and lifestyle changes have been the real answers to weight-loss problems. Do I really have to tell you that if something sounds too good to be true it probably is? We must always be smart consumers, and that means we should "follow the money." Who really stands to gain from our belief in weight-loss gimmicks? Weight-loss products are not required for weight loss, and some are just silly.

Making Sense, Not Money

"Good health makes a lot of sense,
but it doesn't make a lot of dollars."

—ANDREW W. SAUL, PHD, *FOOD MATTERS* (2008)

Health does not make money; sickness does. And more so, it is the sick who seek medical intervention and are willing to pay dearly for medical treatments either as willing participants, dutiful patients, passive recipients, or because they feel they simply have no other choice.

We *do* have a choice. We can know better. We can do better. And we must. We can rarely, if ever, rely on our doctors for nutritional counseling. We must look into vitamins and nutrition for ourselves.

Folks, there is no wealth to be made from good health. Not really. Hospitals are not funded because people are well. Surgeons are not employed because folks needn't be cut open. Doctors are not making money from the patients who don't go to see them. Health insurance companies do not pay you for wellness, although some are attempting to change that. Similarly, purveyors of whoop-de-do products selling wishful thinking are funded by hopeful consumers. Just because it is sold at a health food store doesn't mean it's good. We have to be careful, cautious, and informed consumers.

You will not see commercials plastered all over your television for spinach, broccoli, carrots, and cabbage. You will not be inundated with online advertisements and ads in popular magazines for sunshine, meditation, fresh air, or exercise without the equipment. Things we can do right now to feel better, to *be* better, cost very little, and yet we resist. It is time for a change.

Vitamins are no exception. The cost of vitamin supplementation to promote good health is vastly less than the cost of illness. This is not to say it is cheap, but it's *cheap-er.* Opponents will say that the dietary supplement industry (vitamins, herbs, and minerals included) is big business. Is the health supplement industry a large one? Well, at an estimated 30 billion in revenue a year in the United States,[40] and about 100 billion worldwide,[41] we might think so. If we do, then the pharmaceutical industry is positively gargantuan. Merck, just *one* drug company, makes nearly 40 billion a year in sales in the United States alone, which is 10 billion more than the entire US supplement industry. Globally, the pharmaceutical industry makes over *one trillion* dollars in sales.[42] That doesn't count the money spent on visits to the doctor or hospital, nor does it count repeat visits when drugs fail the consumer or there are side effects to contend with. Plus, you feel awful and you can't do the things you used to do. The cost of poor health goes well beyond a dollar value.

Good Nutrition Includes Vitamins

Vitamins are nutrients. They are *food.* It is darn near impossible to acquire even the tragically low doses of nutrients recommended by the RDA even in a carefully chosen, healthy diet. Vitamins are part of the solution to be healthy. The difference between vitamins and the fad health products du jour, is the decades of science-based research that has demonstrated time and time again the efficacy and safety of vitamins to prevent and treat illness.

Now perhaps I sound a bit like an advertisement for a tummy-tuck belt, except all I have for you here is information. There is nothing to buy, save a book. I don't have supplements to sell. I don't have brands to recommend. I do not endorse any health care products. Personally, I am skeptical of folks who talk up certain name-brand supplements and just so happen to sell them, as you may also be.

You can go for a walk down the street or at the beach; it doesn't much matter. What matters is that you are walking. Similarly, it doesn't matter so much what brand of vitamins you take, but that you take them. For more information about how to choose quality supplements, please read the chapter "Vitamin Questions and Answers."

I write about vitamins and good nutrition because I know they work. Numerous doctors and researches before me have proven the same, and yet you have likely not heard about them or their work. Information can take the desperation out of health care. You needn't make that knee-jerk purchase at two a.m. for the latest weight-loss gimmick. Pay attention to diet and get exercise, and the weight fades as a consequence. You can change your life with proper nutrition.

DEFINE "EXERCISE"

"The world cares very little about what a person knows; it is what the person is able to do that counts."

—BOOKER T. WASHINGTON

We don't have to be marathon runners and muscle-bound weight lifters. We already know this. We don't have to adhere to any rule or schedule. (Unless it helps, then do it.)

The best way to start exercising is to just start being more active:

- Take the shopping cart back to the store when you are done with it. It's a nice thing to do, too.
- Walk to your mailbox instead of driving the short distance there.
- Use a push lawn mower.
- Adopt a dog to play with and walk.
- My dad likes to suggest that your next vehicle purchase be a pickup truck. You will get all sorts of exercise when all your friends ask you to help them move.

In pain? Sore? Address it:

- Start by drinking fresh, raw, homemade vegetable juice every day.
- Take your vitamins.
- Drink plenty of water.
- Soak in a detoxing Epsom salt bath each week.
- Think about taking a few moments or fifteen to stretch or do some yoga. My body is rarely content to be idle, so I like to stretch while I'm just standing around. Flexing and releasing my muscles feels great. In airports, I'd much rather walk and stand than sit; goodness knows there's enough sitting on the plane.

Exercise is contagious. Once you start, you'll want to keep going. But this isn't always easy. Exercise is work. Many times, I have no interest whatsoever in going for a run or hauling around yard waste or climbing stairs. But I do it. After, I feel better. So I do it again. There is pride and satisfaction that comes when you use your body, challenge your muscles, make it move, make it work for you. You will feel all the better for it, and look better too.

There is an immense sense of accomplishment that comes with following through on a workout. The first step? Just put on your workout clothes, suitable for whatever activity you are about to embark on. Drink plenty of water. Stretch when necessary. Don't overdo it the first few days. There are ways to do it wrong, I suppose, but failure to do it at all would be the greatest mistake.

Here's the executive summary on exercise:

- If your goal is weight loss, it takes a long time to see results. There is no quick fix. Those who tell you there is probably have something to sell.
- The secret? Move. Anyhow, anyway. Just *move.* Do something you like to do. Gardening? Perfect. Walking? Take a friend and go. Carrying around your babies? Sounds fun for all involved.
- All the expensive equipment in the world does you no good unless you use it. Personally, I cannot tolerate being stuck inside on any machine. You'll find my activities are almost always outdoors.
- Exercise will give you more energy, not less. This is hard to believe, perhaps, but very true.

- The more you move, the better you will feel. Exercise does wonders for your state of mind, and your figure.
- You do have the time. Health should always be a priority. Skip the half hour of TV. Move instead.
- Define your "exercise." Do what you want to do.
- It is worth it. The short-term effects, the long-term health benefits—all are worth it.
- Have kids? Set an example. When they are young, they will imitate what you do. When they are older, they will have a life full of healthy habits to recall and turn to when they, too, see their benefits.
- Once again, just move.

Go ahead, do it! The next chapter can wait half an hour.

"Your choices are your own. You know your lifestyle, your body, and your level of determination better than anyone else."

—HYLA CASS, MD, *8 WEEKS TO VIBRANT HEALTH*

CHAPTER 4 REFERENCES

1. US Department of Health and Human Services. Centers for Disease Control and Prevention. National Center for Health Statistics. "Obesity and Overweight." Available at: http://www.cdc.gov/nchs/fastats/obesity-overweight.htm (accessed May 2016).

2. Riffkin, R. "U.S. Obesity Rate Ticks Up to 27.1% in 2013. Percentage "morbidly obese" rose slightly to a new high of 3.8%." Gallup Well-Being. (February 27, 2014): http://www.gallup.com/poll/167651/obesity-rate-ticks-2013.aspx (accessed May 2016).

3. US Department of Health and Human Services. Centers for Disease Control and Prevention. National Center for Health Statistics. "Obesity and Overweight." Available at: http://www.cdc.gov/nchs/fastats/obesity-overweight.htm (accessed May 2016).

4. Ogden, C. L., M. D. Carroll, B. K. Kit, et al. "Prevalence of Childhood and Adult Obesity in the United States, 2011–2012." *JAMA* 311(8) (Feb 2014): 806–14. doi: 10.1001/jama.2014.732.

5. University of Rochester. Highland Hospital Bariatric Surgery Center. "What Is Morbid Obesity?" http://www.urmc.rochester.edu/highland/departments-centers/bariatrics/right-for-you/morbid-obesity.aspx (accessed May 2016).

6. U.S. Department of Health and Human Services. National Institutes of Health. National Heart, Lung and Blood Institute. "Body Mass Index Table 1." http://www.nhlbi.nih.gov/guidelines/obesity/bmi_tbl.htm (accessed May 2016).

7. Ibid.

8. Ogden, C. L., M. D. Carroll, B. K. Kit, et al. "Prevalence of Childhood and Adult Obesity in the United States, 2011–2012." *JAMA* 311(8) (Feb 2014): 806–14. doi: 10.1001/jama.2014.732.

9. U.S. Department of Health and Human Services. National Institutes of Health. National Heart, Lung and Blood Institute. "Body Mass Index Table 1." http://www.nhlbi.nih.gov/guidelines/obesity/bmi_tbl.htm (accessed May 2016).

10. Ogden, C. L., M. D. Carroll, B. K. Kit, et al. "Prevalence of Childhood and Adult Obesity in the United States, 2011–2012." *JAMA* 311(8) (Feb 2014): 806–14. doi: 10.1001/jama.2014.732.

11. U.S. Department of Health and Human Services. National Institutes of Health. National Heart, Lung and Blood Institute. "Body Mass Index Table 1." http://www.nhlbi.nih.gov/guidelines/obesity/bmi_tbl.htm (accessed May 2016).

12. Mercola, J. "One in Five Americans Deaths Now Associated with Obesity." Mercola.com (Dec 21, 2013): http://articles.mercola.com/sites/articles/archive/2013/12/21/obesity-death-risk.aspx (accessed May 2016).

13. Brown, A. "Americans' Desire to Shed Pounds Outweighs Effort. Majority exceed ideal weight, 18% are at ideal weight." Gallup Well-Being. (November 29, 2013): http://www.gallup.com/poll/166082/americans-desire-shed-pounds-outweighs-effort.aspx (accessed May 2016).

14. "Personal Weight Situation." Gallup. http://www.gallup.com/poll/7264/Personal-Weight-Situation.aspx (accessed May 2016).

15. Sharpe, L. "Americans' Eating Habits Worsening in 2013. Produce consumption down in most months compared with 2012." Gallup Well-Being. (November 27, 2013): http://www.gallup.com/poll/166070/americans-eating-habits-worsening-2013.aspx (accessed May 2016).

16. Mendes, E. "Americans Exercising Less in 2013. Workout habits worsen this year after improving in 2012." Gallup Well-Being. (July 29, 2013): http://www.gallup.com/poll/163718/americans-exercising-less-2013.aspx (accessed May 2016).

17. Ibid.

18. Harvard School of Public Health. "Simple Steps to Preventing Diabetes." http://www.hsph.harvard.edu/nutritionsource/preventing-diabetes-full-story/ (accessed May 2016).

19. National Institutes of Health. MedlinePlus. U.S. National Library of Medicine. "Diabetic Diet." http://www.nlm.nih.gov/medlineplus/diabeticdiet.html (accessed May 2016).

20. Harvard School of Public Health. "Simple Steps to Preventing Diabetes." http://www.hsph.harvard.edu/nutritionsource/preventing-diabetes-full-story/ (accessed May 2016).

21. Ibid.

22. Ibid.

23. Harvard Medical School. Harvard Health Publications. "Diagnosis: Coronary Artery Disease." http://www.health.harvard.edu/special-health-reports/heart-disease-a-guide-to-preventing-and-treating-coronary-artery-disease? (accessed May 2016).

24. Harvard Health Publications. Harvard Medical School. "These Five Habits Can Save Your Heart — Here's How." (March 1, 2011): http://www.health.harvard.edu/healthbeat/these-five-habits-can-save-your-heart-heres-how (accessed May 2016).

25. Ibid.

26. Stampfer, M. J., F. B. Hu, J. E. Manson, et al. "Primary Prevention of Coronary Heart Disease in Women Through Diet and Lifestyle." *N Engl J Med* 343(1) (Jul 2000):16–22.

27. van Dam, R. M., E. B. Rimm, W. C. Willett, et al. "Dietary Patterns and Risk for Type 2 Diabetes Mellitus in U.S. Men." *Ann Intern Med.* 136(3) (Feb 2002):201–9.

28. Harvard Health Publications. Harvard Medical School. "These Five Habits Can Save Your Heart — Here's How." (March 1, 2011): http://www.health.harvard.edu/healthbeat/these-five-habits-can-save-your-heart-heres-how (accessed May 2016).

29. Lim, J. S., H. K Son, S. K. Park, et al. "Inverse Associations Between Long-Term Weight Change and Serum Concentrations of Persistent Organic Pollutants." *Int J Obes (Lond)* 35(5) (May 2011):744–7. doi: 10.1038/ijo.2010.188.

30. Levy, T. E. *Vitamin C, Infectious Diseases, and Toxins: Curing the Incurable.* Philadelphia, PA: Xlibris Corporation, 2002.

31. Calabrese, E. J. "Does Exposure to Environmental Pollutants Increase the Need for Vitamin C?" *J Environ Pathol Toxicol Oncol* 5(6) (Jul 1985):81–90.

32. "Antibiotics Put 142,000 into Emergency Rooms Each Year. U.S. Centers for Disease Control Waits 60 Years to Study the Problem." *Orthomolecular Med News Service* (October 13, 2008): http://www.orthomolecular.org/resources/omns/v04n14.shtml (accessed May 2016). Saul, A. W. "Notes On Orthomolecular (Megavitamin) Use of Vitamin C." http://www.doctoryourself.com/ortho_c.html (accessed May 2016).

33. Brody, S. "High-Dose Ascorbic Acid Increases Intercourse Frequency and Improves Mood: A Randomized Controlled Clinical Trial." *Biol Psychiatry* 52(4) (Aug 2002):371–4.

34. Eriksson, S. "Studies on Nutrition, Body Composition and Bone Mineralization in Healthy 8-yr-olds in an Urban Swedish Community." (Doctoral thesis, University of Gothenburg. Sahlgrenska Academy, 2009).

35. The Public Broadcasting Service. "Did the Low-Fat Era Make Us Fat?" http://www.pbs.org/wgbh/pages/frontline/shows/diet/themes/lowfat.html (accessed May 2016).

36. "Is Sugar from Fruit Better for You than White Sugar?" Youbeauty.com interview with Joy Dubost, R.D. (June 29, 2013): http://www.huffingtonpost.com/2013/06/29/fruit-sugar-versus-white-sugar_n_3497795.html (accessed May 2016).

37. http://www.tummytuckbelt.com/ (accessed May 2016).

38. Brainwave Mind Voyages. "BMV Quantum Subliminal CD Breast Enhancement: Enlargement Augmentation Aid (Ultrasonic Subliminal Series)" (CD)

39. Lordi, J. "Penis Enlargement" (CD Import) (Jan 9, 2009): http://www.amazon.com/Penis-Enlargement-John-Lordi/dp/B002N5KVPE/ref=sr_1_1?ie=UTF8&qid=-1462379286&sr=8-1&keywords=Penis+Enlargement+[Import]+John+Lordi+%28 (accessed May 2016).

40. Lariviere, D. "Nutritional Supplements Flexing Muscles as Growth Industry." *Forbes.* (April 18, 2013): http://www.forbes.com/sites/davidlariviere/2013/04/18/nutritional-supplements-flexing-their-muscles-as-growth-industry/#22ed58f64255 (accessed May 2016). "Retail Sales of Vitamins & Nutritional Supplements in the United States from 2000 to 2017 (in Billion U.S. Dollars)." http://www.statista.com/statistics/235801/retail-sales-of-vitamins-and-nutritional-supplements-in-the-us/ (accessed May 2016).

41. Thomas, A. "Global Nutrition and Supplements Market: History, Industry Growth, and Future Trends by PMR." *Globe Newswire.* (January 27, 2015): https://globenewswire.com/news-release/2015/01/27/700276/10117198/en/Global-Nutrition-and-Supplements-Market-History-Industry-Growth-and-Future-Trends-by-PMR.html (accessed May 2016).

42. "Statistics and Facts about the Pharmaceutical Industry Worldwide." http://www.statista.com/topics/1764/global-pharmaceutical-industry/ (accessed May 2016). "Statistics and facts about the Pharmaceutical Industry in the U.S." http://www.statista.com/topics/1719/pharmaceutical-industry/ (accessed May 2016).

CHAPTER 5

Vitamin Questions and Answers

"It is rare that anyone addresses the most important question: 'What works best?'"

—W. TODD PENBERTHY, PHD

When it comes to vitamins, folks tend to get hung up on the details. I understand. There is so much conflicting information out there about supplements. It is time to sort fact from fiction. Answered here are some of the most common questions I am asked about vitamins.

Which Brand of Vitamins Do You Buy?

I do not endorse or recommend any particular brand of supplements. I do not sell any nutritional supplements, nor am I paid by any health products or supplement company.

If I just happened to sell the very vitamins I recommend, I believe it would take away a great deal of credibility from my message. There are plenty of good vitamin sellers out there. Like you, I just sat down and did a lot of reading and made the best choice for my family based on some straightforward guidelines that I can share with you. Ultimately, you have to learn as much as you can and make your own best choice.

Here's what I look for when I buy supplements:

- They are free of artificial colors and flavors and fake sweeteners.
- They are high-potency, pure, fresh, natural, and inexpensive.
- The serving size is acceptable. Some vitamins will have you taking three tablets to get what is indicated on the label. This is not very cost effective.

I am a very close label reader when it comes to supplements, especially the ones I give my kids. I buy in bulk and I buy on sale, mostly online. I check expiration dates, and I store vitamins properly to help maintain freshness and potency. And most importantly, I make sure to actually take them.

There is a lot of infighting between brands claiming theirs is the best, and by comparison, others cannot possibly be as good. This is substantially untrue. I have found that those proclaiming to be the "best" often sport a hefty price tag. Go ahead and buy them if you can afford to do it. But careful label readers may find that low-cost vitamins can be just as good.

If I have questions about sourcing, purity, or any ingredients on the vitamin label, I call the company. If the product label says NSF International, US Pharmacopeia, or carries a Consumer Lab seal, it verifies that the supplement actually contains the ingredients that the label says it does. This can save some time.

However, *all* supplements are regulated. The US Food and Drug Administration (FDA) can, at any time, pull any supplement off the shelves for any reason. In addition, do not confuse FDA approval with FDA regulation. Just because a dietary supplement is not FDA approved does not make it "bad." Pharmaceutical drugs that are FDA approved are not automatically "good." Supplement companies are responsible for ensuring the safety of their products and for providing accurate labeling. If they don't, the FDA has always had the power to take dangerous or falsely labeled supplements off the market. Make no mistake, they use this power. Health and Human Services (HHS) Secretary Tommy G. Thompson stated, "[T]he FDA will not tolerate the marketing of dietary supplements that are more likely to harm health than help it."[1] This has always been the case.

Are Vitamins from Genetically Modified (GMO) Sources Okay?

You may be concerned about taking vitamins derived from GMO sources. Yes, I am against GMOs. We make a point to avoid them.

But when it comes to vitamins, I look at things like my father, orthomolecular educator Andrew W. Saul, PhD, does: "Vitamin C is ascorbic acid, $C_6H_8O_6$, and that's pretty much all there is to it," he says. "Even if this molecule comes from GMOs, which I disapprove of, it is still molecularly OK. You cannot genetically modify carbon, hydrogen, or oxygen atoms."[2]

When in doubt take C. If you can afford vitamins sourced from GMO-free ingredients, go for it. For the rest of us, it is far more important that we take the C in the first place. The same is true with other supplements.

Should I Take Natural or Synthetic Vitamins?

I have found that quite a few folks are against synthetic vitamins, but even high-potency whole-food vitamins contain synthetic ingredients or, as my dad would say, the tablet would have to be the size of a football to pack in all the nutrients. If you prefer whole-foods vitamins, take them. If you aim to take large, therapeutic doses of nutrients, whole-food vitamins are going to cost you a small fortune. To learn more, you'll want to look at the following article.

What's the Difference between Natural and Synthetic Vitamins?

by Andrew W. Saul, PhD

From http://www.doctoryourself.com/synthetic.html (accessed June 2016).

Nobody really likes what I have to say on this subject. And, to be fair, the answer is an inherently awkward one.

Most vitamin products, even those sold in health food stores or by distributors, contain synthetic vitamin powders. There are only a few manufacturers of vitamin powders, and they are almost always large pharmaceutical companies. Generally:

a. Laboratory-made vitamins are far cheaper than whole-food concentrates;

b. Synthetic vitamins *usually* work quite well;

c. High potency can be achieved with a nice, small tablet size.

One of the chief differences in "health food store" vs "drugstore" brands is what is *not* in the tablet. For example, the natural brands leave out artificial chemical colors, which is a good thing to do. Just about all brands contain tablet fillers and excipients (inert substances), needed to physically hold the pill together. Since these will vary, the only way to find out exactly who uses what is to write to the company and find out.

Some tableting ingredients are pretty standard, such as magnesium stearate or stearic acid, sodium citrate, dicalcium phosphate, cellulose, and silica. I consider these harmless fillers to be natural enough for me.

Vitamins can legally be called "natural" even if made in a laboratory. You would not think so, but it is true. Vitamin C, for example, is factory-made from starch. Starch is certainly natural, so the product can be termed "natural." Is this starch-based vitamin C identical to orange-juice vitamin C? Most biochemists say yes, because:

1. they appear to have identical molecular structure,
2. vitamin C in animal bodies is made from carbohydrates anyway, and
3. the product is clinically effective.

But the actual molecular construction process is *not* identical. Factories do not use L-gulonolactone oxidase from animal liver to make vitamin C. Nor do they copy the orange tree's plant metabolism. Can one get an identical product from a different process? Probably; there is more than one way to skin an enzyme. But the real test must be, does the vitamin in front of you prevent and cure disease?

Linus Pauling, Ewan Cameron, Robert Cathcart, and others have established that very high doses of factory-made ascorbic acid vitamin C work just fine against viral and bacterial illness. It is possible that food-concentrate vitamin C may be superior. Let's say it was twice as good. But to use 40,000 milligrams (mg) of orange juice C, instead of 80,000 mg of synthetic ascorbic acid, is impractical, bordering on the impossible. It would be too expensive, either to manufacture from oranges, or to eat from the oranges. It would take roughly 600 oranges to obtain 40,000 mg of vitamin C. Even if natural C were ten times as effective, which I sincerely doubt, it would still take well over 100 oranges a day to do the job.

My recommendation? When you are sick, eat as many oranges (and other vitamin C-rich fruits) as you can, *while you also take* tens of thousands of milligrams of cheap, supplemental ascorbic acid vitamin C.

In some cases, the natural form of a vitamin IS clearly superior to the synthetic form. The best example is vitamin E. The natural form of vitamin E is called "D-alpha tocopherol" and is made from vegetable oil. The synthetic form is DL-alpha tocopherol. Not a big difference in name, is it? There is considerable evidence that the natural "D" (dextro-, or right-handed) molecular form of vitamin E is far more useful to the body than is the synthetic. The natural form is also more expensive, but not much more. In choosing a vitamin E supplement, you should carefully read the label—the *entire* label. It is remarkable how many natural-looking brown bottles with natural-sounding brand names contain the synthetic form.

To learn more about natural versus synthetic vitamins, please see the article titled: "Supplements: The Real Story."

What Vitamins Do You Take?

For the most part, I, H. S. Case, take the following supplements every day:

A (preformed)	10,000 international units (IU)
A (beta-carotene)	25,000 IU
B_1, B_2, B_6	100–125 milligrams (mg)
B_3 inositol nicotinate (flush free)	1,000 mg
B_3 nicotinic acid	250–500 mg
B_{12} and pantothenic acid	50–100 micrograms (mcg)
Biotin	50–250 mcg
Vitamin C (ascorbic acid)	8,000–10,000 mg
Calcium (citrate)	100–200 mg
Chromium picolinate	400 mcg
D_3 (cholecalciferol)	5,000 IU
E (d-alpha with mixed tocopherols)	400 IU
Folic acid	800–1,200 mcg
Iron (ferrous fumarate)	18 mg
Magnesium (citrate)	450 mg
Omega-3	340 mg
Selenium	100–200 mcg
Zinc	15–30 mg
Manganese	4 mg
CoQ_{10}	100 mg

This list is not meant to be prescriptive. Just because this is what I take doesn't mean you should too. I'm not a doctor. Of course, you should always look into things for yourself. Be sure to talk to your doctor. (If he or she is an orthomolecular physician, all the better.)

My husband's list is different; so is the children's. The amount of each nutrient we take may change on a daily basis, seasonally, and when we get sick. I take much more vitamin D in the winter: 5,000–10,000 IU per day. In the summer I see to it that I get 15 to 20 minutes or so of midday sun exposure instead. I take far more vitamin C when I am sick (8,000 to 10,000 an hour) and more niacin (nicotinic acid) if I am under stress, feeling anxious, or trying to abort a migraine headache. I also take magnesium sulfate (Epsom salt) baths weekly for an additional dose of magnesium, delivered transdermally (through the skin). I apply a patch of iodine to my skin about once a month. Since I do not always eat a lot of animal products, I dissolve a sublingual 5,000 mcg B_{12} tablet under my tongue about once weekly. The same is true for biotin. I eat a couple of tablespoons (13 grams [g]) of lecithin granules a couple of days a week, or swallow three (1.2 g) capsules each day if I don't get to the granules. My list of vitamins was a little different when I was pregnant, and I have included it in my book *Vitamins & Pregnancy: The Real Story.*

Helpful Hints for Vitamin Takers

1. Take supplements with food, and divide the dose throughout the day.
2. Always read labels carefully. Take supplements free of artificial sweeteners, artificial colors, and artificial flavors.
3. Just because a supplement label says "whole foods" does not mean it is made from whole foods, but rather synthetic vitamins in a whole-food base.
4. Synthetic vitamins are more okay than you might think. Some vitamins, however, like vitamin E and vitamin A, should be taken in natural form.
5. Avoid taking zinc on an empty stomach. It may make you feel queasy.
6. If you have a hard time swallowing pills, perhaps try this: put the pill in the front of your mouth and tip your head forward. With your head in this position, take a drink, and swallow.
7. Take magnesium on an empty stomach: in the morning before any meals, in the afternoon, and before bed. You'll absorb more and reduce magnesium's laxative effect. Avoid magnesium oxide, which does not absorb well at all. Take, for example, magnesium citrate or glycinate instead.
8. Take iron separately from vitamin E. For example, take vitamin E in the morning and iron in the afternoon to enhance absorption. Also, take iron separately from calcium.

9. Take natural vitamin E: D-alpha tocopherol. Avoid synthetic E (DL-alpha tocopherol), indicated by that little "L" after the "D." Natural E is worth the extra money since your body can utilize natural E (not synthetic) best. For more about vitamin E, please see the chapter on vitamin E.

10. Take natural vitamin A from fish oil or from carrots (i.e., beta-carotene).

11. Avoid iron in the form of ferrous sulfate. It will probably make you puke. (I am always astonished to see this form of iron in prenatal vitamins or children's supplements.)

12. If you get adequate sunshine, you can skip your vitamin D supplement that day.

13. Avoid taking CoQ_{10} late in the day. It may cause insomnia. I like to take it first thing in the morning.

14. I avoid taking a B-complex vitamin late in the day, as it tends to energize me. However, niacin (B_3), taken alone, has a wonderful calming effect before bed.

15. Regular, immediate-release niacin will cause a flush, a reddening, and sometimes an itchy sensation that usually begins to be felt in the face. It won't hurt you, but it can be unnerving and/or uncomfortable. If you are new to niacin, start with a small dose (25–50 mg). As you become more at ease with its use, increase your dose depending on your therapeutic goals and what works best for you. The benefits I get from niacin outweigh the temporary flush.

16. If you suffer constipation with iron supplementation, take more vitamin C. Vitamin C helps you better absorb the iron you're taking (which may mean you won't have to take as much), and in large doses, vitamin C keeps the bowels moving along, as do eating plenty of veggies and drinking fresh, raw homemade veggie juice and lots of liquids in general.

17. Children's vitamins are convenient and formulated especially for growing kids, but sometimes adult vitamins can be modified for kid use. For example, you will not find "children's niacin." We take an adult tablet and shave off a tiny smidgen, perhaps 10 mg, crush it between two spoons, and give it to them with a little honey or ice cream. Why we give our kids niacin is discussed in the article "Tips from a Megavitamin Mom."

Can Supplements Help You Sleep?

Yes. Taking immediate-release niacin (B_3) before bed helps me relax and fall asleep, especially if I'm experiencing any anxiety about the day (or the next one). The warming feeling of a niacin flush is calming to me, but I usually feel relaxed and fall asleep in advance of a flush. I usually take 100–200 mg, but you may wish to start smaller. When you first start taking niacin, or if you take it after you haven't taken any in a while, you may experience a strong flush. Some folks find this very disconcerting. Before you say "no" to niacin, remember that a niacin flush is temporary. The flush won't hurt you, but some may find the redness and itchiness to be very uncomfortable, especially at first. If your flush feels too intense, you can always take less niacin. You may find that you "hold" more when you are under stress. Additional aspects of niacin therapy are thoroughly discussed in *Niacin: The Real Story*, by Abram Hoffer, MD, PhD, Andrew W. Saul, PhD, and Harold D. Foster, PhD.

Periodically, I also take 3 mg of melatonin an hour or so before bed.

L-tryptophan is an amino acid that converts into serotonin, a neurotransmitter that improves mood and can help you fall asleep and feel more rested in the morning. It is found in dairy, such as yogurt, milk, and cheese, and also in beans, cashews, chicken, and turkey.

Magnesium can combat irritability, nervousness, anxiety, adrenaline rushes, muscle spasms, and cramps. This is why I like to soak in Epsom salt (magnesium sulfate) baths. A warm bath is soothing even without the magnesium, and even better with it.

Choline, found in phosphatidyl choline (found in lecithin), can help you *stay* asleep. Choline is also found in wheat germ, eggs, soy, meat, milk, seafood, quinoa, broccoli, cauliflower, nuts, seeds, and lentils.

Turn off media, and read a book instead. Check your e-mail tomorrow.

Make sure your room is dark, or wear an eye mask, and keep noisy or active pets out.

When Do You Take Vitamins?

Our family takes vitamins at every meal and every snack. My husband and I fill up large pill cases with the larger morning and afternoon doses, and then just go straight to the bottles for any doses in between. Pill cases allow us to prepare everything assembly-line style so we don't spend each meal opening up a dozen different bottles. We have travel bottles too, for us and the kids, for when we are on the road or at a restaurant. If we are sick, we may take vitamin C every 15 minutes to every hour to get to bowel tolerance.

Keep in mind, there is no magic bullet nutrient. They are all important, and they need each other. Nutrients work well together. Therefore, take them together.

What Form of Vitamins Do You Take?

Most supplements my husband and I take are in pill form. A couple, including B_{12} and biotin, are in the form of sublingual tablets and simply dissolve under the tongue for better absorption. Magnesium we take orally, and transdermally in weekly Epsom salt baths. We take vitamin C in powder form when we wish to achieve especially high doses. We take lecithin in the form of granules and capsules.

My husband and I both have also received vitamin C intravenously (IVC). About a year after my second child was born, stress, sleepless nights, breastfeeding, and trying to balance my career as an author with my husband's intense business-travel schedule meant I was run down and a prime target for serious infection. And that is exactly what happened. If you have children, you know what a toll parenthood takes on your body. There is no good time to be sick when you have children. There is no replacement for sleep, which I simply needed to get more of, but I suspected that my oral nutrient intake could really use a boost to combat this infection. I turned to IVC to jump-start the healing process, which is exactly what it did.

Intravenous vitamin C is incredibly effective and safe. We are fortunate: we do not live far from an alternative health care office that regularly sees patients for treatments such as IVC. This is great news for folks who are really sick and would benefit from a safe, natural alternative or adjunct to drug therapy. Along with lifestyle changes, for about a year and a half after my first IVC treatment, I continued to receive periodic IVs as preventive treatment. Taking large, oral doses of vitamin C worked well. But IVC worked even better at keeping me well during this difficult time.

The downside is this: intravenous vitamin C is very expensive. As of 2016, the clinic we visit charges about $150.00 for a 30,000 mg dose. The IV takes over an hour to do, not to mention drive time to get there. There is also the cost of gas to and from the office. Oral C is vastly cheaper. A pound of vitamin C powder (45,000 mg of ascorbic acid) costs about ten dollars, delivered to my door. Last winter, I bought it on sale for just five dollars a pound. If IVC is cost prohibitive or unavailable in your area, you can simulate IVC therapy by taking frequent, smaller, oral doses of vitamin C. Take 500 to 1,000 mg of vitamin C every ten minutes or so. Once bowel tolerance is reached, take less C, less often.

You don't need as much C when you can bypass the digestive system and get it straight into the bloodstream. Still, the high-cost factor of IVC makes it difficult to recommend it for daily, or even semi-regular use, unless *you really need it.* Practically speaking, we can't have everyone walking around hooked up to IVs all day. However, for patients who have cancer or other chronic disease, or for those who are hooked up to IVs anyway, the proven benefit of IVC treatment is worth it, and the cost pales in comparison to the price of conventional drug treatments.

Bio-individuality is the rule rather than the exception. Your optimal vitamin dose depends on you and your needs.

CHILDREN AND VITAMINS

How do you get your kids to take vitamins? Which vitamins do they take? How often do they take them? What brands do you buy? How do you get them to take so much vitamin C? What if they don't want to take it? I get these questions often. In the following article, I answer them and more.

TIPS FROM A MEGAVITAMIN MOM: GETTING KIDS TO TAKE VITAMINS AND LOTS OF THEM

by Helen Saul Case

From the *Orthomolecular Medicine News Service,* April 9, 2016.]

Born and raised in a household where we used vitamins and nutrition instead of drugs, I am very familiar with utilizing high-dose nutrients to prevent and cure illness. I remember taking all those vitamins when I was a kid. And I still take them. I know how well they work. Now, I see how optimal doses of vitamins help keep my children, ages three and five, healthy and free of pharmaceuticals. You can do this for your family, too.

How Do You Get Your Kids to Take Vitamins?

The number one rule is: keep 'em tasty. For younger children, find a liquid C they like and will swallow. Start young to get them used to it. We started in the hospital within hours of birth. When they were infants, we gave them liquid vitamin C with a dropper. When they got older, we used a medicine spoon. For kids who chew, chewable tablets work well on a day-to-day, meal-to-meal basis.

Multivitamins also can be given in liquid form. We administered multivitamins this way until the children could eat chewables.

How Do You Get Kids to Saturation of Vitamin C?

It is winter: the kids have runny noses (at the very least). If they don't have a cough, some other kid does and it seems like there is a perpetual wave of illness afflicting your home. It is high time for high-dose vitamin C.

Bowel tolerance: an indicator of oral dose vitamin C saturation. Bowel tolerance is indicated by gas, a rumbling stomach, or slightly loose stool. If you take way too much C, very loose stool will result, but it goes away once doses are reduced. When bowel tolerance is reached, back off the extra C.

Cathcart RF. Vitamin C, titrating to bowel tolerance, anascorbemia, and acute induced scurvy. *Med Hypotheses.* 1981 Nov;7(11):1359–76. Free full text: http://www.doctoryourself.com/titration.html.

Large doses are needed in order to achieve therapeutic, saturation levels of vitamin C. We do this only when kids get sick, are about to get sick, or are receiving immunizations. We start with a larger "loading dose" in the morning, then continue to give C throughout the day. Once bowel tolerance is reached, we cut back how much C we give and how often we give it, but we continue to give C regularly. We do not allow children to get diarrhea. If symptoms of sickness persist, we do it again the next day, and the next. My brother and I were raised into adulthood without a single dose of any antibiotic. So far, my children have not needed to take an antibiotic, either. We use vitamin C instead.

When we get our kids to saturation, we make sure they stay hydrated with plenty of water. Since high-dose C can take their appetite away, we make sure that during this process, they eat good-for-them food that they enjoy. We also have them drink plenty of fresh, raw, homemade vegetable juice every day. This is exactly what my parents did with me when I was young.

Remember, if you have a really sick kid, you should go to the doctor. Diagnosis is a valuable tool. However, my husband and I know that if our children's pediatrician hands us a prescription for an antibiotic, antiviral, antihistamine, or antipyretic, high-dose vitamin C can be used in place of all of them.

> *"I was always known as a vitamin C nut, but I won many converts, especially during a virus infection. A segment of the population 'gets' nutrition issues but a larger segment doesn't understand."*
>
> —RALPH CAMPBELL, MD

What Forms of Vitamin C Do You Give Your Children?

Chewable tablets are not very practical for saturation dose C administration. Liquids come in handy here. We add extra vitamin C crystals to presweetened, store-bought liquid vitamin C to increase the potency in order to give high doses, and because C in liquid naturally loses potency as it sits.

Or, when it is time for a dose, we scoop vitamin C powder into their favorite juice and have them drink it down right away.

We add a combination of approximately 80 percent vitamin C as ascorbic acid crystals and 20 percent vitamin C calcium ascorbate as a buffer to the juice or liquid C. The more ascorbic acid in the liquid, the more bitter it becomes. Therefore, we follow each dose with a tasty "chaser." Now that they're a little older (over age one) we follow really potent (and therefore more bitter) doses of vitamin C with an unbelievably tasty chaser. They get a small bite of organic ice cream, a little honey, a raisin, more juice, even chocolate: anything to get the job done.

For toddlers and older kids, when they are not getting C in liquid, they can also be given chewable tablets to mix up the form of C to keep it interesting (and more likely to go down the hatch). We offer more than one flavor of chewable C tablets.

We also give liposomal vitamin C. Liposomal C is expensive, but so are doctor's visits. When we want to get lots of C into our kids, we give any form of C that they will take, and vary the form frequently. When my daughter came down with a swollen sore throat, she could swallow liposomal C when she would not, or could not, easily swallow other forms of C. After each dose, we would let her slurp a homemade frozen juice bar, which she looked forward to having.

What If Kids Don't Want to Take All That Vitamin C?

Sometimes our kids will take C like champions. No complaints. They even ask for it when they are not feeling well.

Other times, they fight it tooth and nail. This is when creativity and patience and bribery and love and persistence pay off.

When you are a new parent and are breastfeeding or giving a bottle, you don't just give up if your child does not eat and get the nutrition he or she needs. You do it *until*. This is how we feel about vitamin C. We insist they take the C. This is not negotiable. It is that important. But if, for example, they want to watch TV, we say, "Take C, and then you can." Anything they want to do can be used as a motivator. Sometimes kids don't want to do what is good for them, so we make it worth their while. I said to our daughter one day, "You have to take your vitamins if you want chocolate ice cream in the morning."

There's more. We cuddle them. We praise them. We agree with them that it is hard to take C all the time. And when all else fails, straight-up bribery works wonders. At vaccination time, our daughter takes saturation-level vitamin C to earn presents.

Giving them C when they wake up at night almost ensures protest, but nobody sleeps if a child coughs until morning. Our daughter will wake up very upset and nearly inconsolable. One night I simply said, "You can cough all night or you can take the C. Your choice." My daughter chose the C. Other nights, we have to choose for her. We wait it out. Her desire to go back to sleep is often enough reason to come around and take the C.

Toddlers are notoriously contrary. These are the tricks we have employed to get high-dose C into our kids. Infants are not as likely to tell you "no." Toddlers suffer no such inhibition. Making certain that vitamins are tasty (and seeing to it that you give small doses regularly, throughout the day, with meals) helps them take vitamins without much fuss. When my kids were breastfeeding, I would give them C before nursing and feed them immediately afterwards. If they needed more C, I would give them small doses more often. I would also get to bowel tolerance myself, which in turn, would provide vitamin C for them in my breast milk.

Older kids, who have done this for a while, may be more used to taking, and therefore more willing to take, high-dose vitamin C. When I was eight and older, I took the C because I knew it worked. I would do it on my own.

How Often Do Your Kids Take Vitamin C?

At every meal and every snack. We have travel bottles too, for when we are on the road or at a restaurant. If we are sick, we may take vitamin C every 15 minutes to every hour to get to bowel tolerance.

Days before, the day of, and for several days after immunizations, we give saturation-dose vitamin C to minimize the risk of side effects from the vaccination, and to help the shot work better. You may notice that your child's bowel tolerance will be much higher at this time. To learn more about vitamin C and vaccinations, please see the articles "Don't Vaccinate Without Vitamin C" and "Vaccinations, Vitamin C, and 'Choice.'"

How Much Vitamin C Do You Give to Your Children?

On a day-to-day basis, we follow board-certified chest physician Dr. Frederick R. Klenner's dosing protocol: they get 1,000 mg of vitamin C per year of age. We started the day they were born with 50 milligrams (mg) per day of vitamin C. As the months went by, we gradually increased the dose. By age one, they were getting 1,000 mg per day. Now our three-year-old gets 3,000 mg per day; our five-year-old gets 5,000 mg per day. We will continue to increase the dose until they are ten, for a routine dose of 10,000 mg per day. And this is when they are in ***good*** health.

They get *far more* when bowel tolerance doses are needed due to stress, sickness, or shots. For example, after her last immunization, our four-year-old daughter, who weighed about 33 pounds at the time, comfortably held 15,000 to 20,000 mg of vitamin C a day, and had no negative side effects from the shot.

> *"What a wonderful world it would be for children if there were more parents following this routine."*
>
> —KEN WALKER, MD

What about Getting Vitamins from Their Diet?

One of the best ways to get vitamins into kids is to juice and serve fresh, raw vegetables and fruit, preferably organic. Our kids love homemade vegetable juice. They chug it. I'm not kidding. We make sure they will by blending in sweeter fruits and veggies with the ones that are less so. For example, a family favorite starts with a carrot base, eight or so, an apple or two, a handful of cabbage, a few handfuls of spinach, and several stalks of celery and a beet, leaves included.

My kids are getting far more vegetables (and therefore nutrients) in their diet than most. Sure, we get them to eat vegetables and fruit, too. But we also juice three to five times every week to ensure the good food gets into their growing bodies. And we make a point to keep refined sugar out of their diet, which limits the sugar to primarily what comes naturally in their plant-based diet.

What Brand of Children's Vitamins Do You Buy?

That's one question I don't answer. I do not endorse any vitamin company. Nor will I. In my opinion, if I tell folks to take vitamins, and then I just happen to sell them the very ones they need, it may detract from my message. But I can help a little.

We take (and give to our kids) vitamins free of artificial colors and artificial sweeteners. Remember that a *little* sugar gets the vitamins down. The ends justify the means. Vitamins have to be tasty or kids just won't eat them. The goal is to get the nutrients in them; don't worry about the bit of extra sugar in vitamins or the chaser you give them after they take them. (Just keep it out of the rest of their diet.)

Vitamins need not cost a fortune. There are plenty of folks who will tell you otherwise, but we buy the cheapest vitamins we can that are free of junk and give us the results we seek. Read labels. Check potency. Sometimes it takes two or even three tablets to get the amount indicated on the label. This can be confusing, and pricey. If you have questions about purity or sourcing, call the company. I do.

What Vitamins Do You Give Your Children in Addition to Vitamin C?

We buy two different multivitamins for our kids. (One is actually for adults.) They each contain some vitamins and minerals the other does not, and in varying concentrations, so we mix it up every other day so they can get the benefits of both. Basically, we look for multivitamins that include, among other things, 5,000 IU (international units) of vitamin A, at least 30 IU of vitamin E, 500 to1,000 IU of vitamin D, all the B's, and a variety of minerals, including 5 mg of iron and 100 mcg (micrograms) of iodine. We don't worry about the amount of vitamin C in their multi because we supplement with far more than is present in any multivitamin on the market.

As for minerals, they take chewable calcium and magnesium tablets in addition to the minerals they get in their multivitamin. We also throw a handful or two of unscented Epsom salt in their bath water one to two times per week. Occasionally, they get trace mineral drops in their water. Our efforts are to ensure that they get, in particular, enough magnesium.

There are nutrients in their multivitamin that we give them more of as needed. We use our higher-potency adult vitamins and find a way to administer them in a child-friendly manner. Here are some examples:

It may be no surprise that when the kids aren't getting some sun, they are getting a cold. In the winter, we give the kids additional doses of vitamin D to the tune of about 5,000 IU weekly, and if they get sick. I open the capsule and drip it onto something they like. Ice cream works well. Really well.

We do the same with vitamin A. When they are sick, I give them a dose of 10,000 IU of vitamin A on ice cream as soon as they show symptoms. I do this only for a day or two. They continue to get their regular dose of A in their multivitamin.

If they are about to have a tantrum-inducing dose of sugar, like ice cream in the summer or a piece of birthday cake, I crush up a tablet of about 10 to 20 mg of flush-inducing, immediate-release niacin, put the dust on a spoon with some raw honey, or right in the ice cream or bite of cake. It works remarkably well. It has also come in handy when the kids get a case of, what my father-in-law calls, "the can't help its" due to exhaustion, overstimulation, or some other factor. When kindness, reasoning, hugs, understanding, distractions, time-outs, rest, and patience do not bring a toddler down from the brink of an irrational breakdown, we have found that a little flush niacin does. The results can be incredible to behold, and it is safe.

Remember, niacin may cause a flush. Your child may feel warm, look a little red, and feel itchy. This is saturation of niacin. It means they have had enough niacin, for now. We give the *minimal* amount of niacin that helps them be calm, and not so much that they experience a strong, uncomfortable flush. Work out the right dose for your child in cooperation with your physician.

Doesn't Taking Vitamins Just Make Expensive Urine?

Kids are expensive. Some people may think that giving kids vitamins just makes for more expensive kids. That is certainly one way to look at it. Here is another: Nutrients in urine may indicate that our children are well-nourished and have some to spare. It also means nutrients have been through the kidneys. What has been in the kidneys has been in their blood. What has been in their blood their bodies have absorbed. What has been absorbed is available for their bodies to use. Vitamin deficiency is the problem. Abundance, however, is not.

It is a good idea to see that children eat right and take vitamins. Give their bodies the *opportunity* to absorb essential nutrients. The body cannot absorb what simply is not there.

Like a good meal, vitamin sufficiency does not last forever. Their bodies will be "hungry" for these nutrients again. In the same way a baby needs nourishment many times each and every day, kids (and adults) should be taking vitamins in several intervals throughout each day.

Vitamins are very safe and, when compared to drugs, vitamins are not only vastly safer but remarkably inexpensive. Pharmaceuticals make for far more expensive urine.

Are Vitamins Safe?

Yes. Far safer than any drug on the market, prescription or over-the-counter.

Doing It Yourself

Bear in mind, I am not a physician. You should always look into vitamins and nutrition for yourself, and do what is best for you and your family. Talk it over with your doctor. However, I do not believe you have to be a doctor in order to take control of your own health or your children's health. Doing it yourself does not mean it will be easy. It is an incredible amount of work to keep kids healthy. But it is worth it. Sure, take your kids to their pediatrician. But wouldn't it be nice not to *need* to go?

CHAPTER 5 REFERENCES

1. HHS. U.S. Food and Drug Administration. U.S. Department of Health and Human Services. "FDA Acts to Remove Ephedra-Containing Dietary Supplements From Market" (November 23, 2004): http://www.fda.gov/NewsEvents/Newsroom/PressAnnouncements/2004/ucm108379.htm (accessed May 2016).

2. Saul, A.W. "Ascorbic Acid Vitamin C: What's the Real Story?" (Dec 6, 2013): *Orthomolecular Medicine News Service.* http://orthomolecular.org/resources/omns/v09n27.shtml (accessed May 2016).

PART TWO

Vitamins: The Real Story

"No one dies from vitamins."

—ABRAM HOFFER , MD

What is the real story when it comes to supplements? Yes, vitamins are effective. Yes, vitamins are safe. And we've known it for a long time.

DOCTORS SAY VITAMINS ARE SAFE AND EFFECTIVE

From the *Orthomolecular Medicine News Service,* March 13, 2012.

The news media proclaim that taking vitamin supplements is of no value and, somehow, actually dangerous. You have heard an earful from reporters. Now let's hear from doctors.

Michael Janson, MD:

The standard American diet does not provide even the Recommended Dietary Allowance (RDA). Two-thirds of all meals are eaten outside the home, and nearly half of them are in fast-food joints. You can't expect this sort of diet to provide all the necessary nutrients, and many studies show that it does not. A large number of people admitted to hospitals are found to have deficiencies, and the problems worsen in the hospital. Those given supplements have a lower rate of complications, faster discharge from the hospital, and fewer deaths. Vitamin companies do not send doctors on expense-paid vacations or "seminars," as do the drug companies for prescribing their drugs, and vitamins are safe and cheap. But surely this does not influence pharmaceutical-advertising-paid-for media!

Vitamin E in high doses (800 international units [IU]) enhances immunity in healthy elderly subjects. Vitamin C in doses (2,000 milligrams [mg]) far above the RDA (90 mg) significantly reduces allergic rhinitis and asthma and speeds the recovery from airway constriction induced by histamine. Vitamin B_1 (thiamine) was used successfully to treat trigeminal neuralgia, as described in an article published in the *Journal of the American Medical Association* way back in 1940.

Many people are losing their faith in the medical profession because many doctors are unwilling to accept what is becoming common knowledge: nutrition and nutrient therapies are safer, cheaper, and more effective than most other medical treatment. It is clear that most media reporters do not know the current nutrition literature, they do not know the old literature, and they do not know the middle-aged literature. If they do not know the literature, they should not be writing articles.

Martin Gallagher, MD, DC:

I have been a practicing physician for 37 years. During that time, I have directly treated and supervised over 12,000 patient encounters per year. With each patient, I have prescribed a variety of vitamins, minerals, homeopathic medicines, and herbs. I have to date not encountered a single complication, anaphylactic reaction, or death. The doses have been well above the RDA's for vitamins and minerals. In fact, the IV treatments include doses of ascorbate (vitamin C) that vary from 10,000 to over 100,000 mg per treatment session.

At a time when the leading cause of death in the U.S. is correctly prescribed medication, we need to embrace, not chastise, nutritional supplements.

Robert G. Smith, PhD:

Most people in modern societies have vitamin and mineral deficiencies because these nutrients are removed by industrial food processing. Vitamin and mineral supplements are effective in preventing deficiencies that cause major illness, such as heart disease, cancer, diabetes, arthritis, osteoporosis, dementia, and many others. Supplements of vitamins and minerals, when taken in proper doses large enough to work (for example: vitamin C for an adult at 3,000 to 6,000 mg per day, and much more when stressed or sick), are safe and effective—and far less expensive than taking prescribed drugs overblown by the medical profession and media.

Michael J. Gonzalez, PhD:

Research in Europe has shown that long-term users of antioxidant vitamin supplements have a 48 percent reduced risk of cancer mortality and 42 percent lower all-cause mortality.[1] The media did not bother to mention it. There is in fact overwhelming clinical evidence to justify the use of nutritional supplements for the prevention of disease and the support of optimal health. The Lewin Group estimated a $24 billion savings over five years if a few basic nutritional supplements were used in the elderly.[2] On the other hand, prescription medication kills over 100,000 people a year.[3]

Thomas E. Levy, MD:

There are more politics in modern medicine than in modern politics itself. Today's average physician deserves even less trust than today's average politician, as doctors continue their refusal to allow the scientific data on the profound benefits of vitamins and other antioxidant supplements to reach their eyes and brains. And the staunch support of a press, which collectively no longer has a shred of journalistic or scientific integrity, completes the framing of today's colossal medical fraud. Money always rules the day: properly dosed vitamins would eliminate far too much of the profit of prescription-based medicine.

William B. Grant, PhD:

Modern lifestyles, including wearing clothes and sunscreen and working and living largely indoors, have led to widespread vitamin D deficiencies. Numerous ecological and observational studies have found correlations between higher solar UVB doses and vitamin D concentrations and reduced risk of many types of cancer, cardiovascular disease, diabetes mellitus, bacterial and viral infectious diseases, autoimmune diseases, falls and fractures, cognitive impairment, and many more types of disease. To compensate for lack of sun exposure, 1,000 to 5,000 IU per day of vitamin D_3 should be taken to raise serum 25-hydroxyvitamin D concentrations to at least 30 to 40 ng/ml (nanograms per milliliter) or 75–100 nmol/L (nanomoles per liter). These amounts are safe for all but those with granulomatous diseases, who can develop hypercalcemia. Vitamin D in doses of 1,000 to 5,000 IU per day is effective in reducing risk of many types of diseases, as shown in a number of randomized controlled trials, such as cancer, falls and fractures, type A influenza, and pneumonia.

W. Todd Penberthy, PhD:

Niacin in particular has been shown to provide exceptional benefit in treating cardiovascular disease in clinical trial after clinical trial.[4] By comparison, the popular diabetes drug Avandia was found to cause a 43 percent increase in heart attacks in diabetics.[5] This came out only *after* Avandia had already become the most popular diabetes drug in the world. Never underestimate the power of market-driven forces to sell drugs, and books, such as *The End of Illness* by Dr. Agus, instead of proper information regarding what actually works best.

People are amazed by how quickly simply taking supplemental niacin corrects high cholesterol, high triglycerides, low high-density lipoprotein (HDL, the "good" cholesterol), and very low-density lipoprotein (VLDL). All of these parameters are pushed in the healthier direction because niacin ultimately functions inside the body in over 450 reactions. There is a reason niacin continues as a preferred therapy for doctors in the know, who have been using niacin therapy for over 50 years now. Niacin works better than any drug to correct dyslipidemia.

One thing to always remember is this. You can "prove" that any drug or vitamin does not work if you are not using high enough doses to achieve the correct concentration of the molecule. Furthermore, all biochemical pathways rely on more than one molecule to function properly, so generally one drug or vitamin is not enough for optimal health. Our bodies rely on vitamins, not drugs, to routinely stave off illness by means we often take for granted. Sometimes we need much more of these essential molecules. This is common sense, and it is known as orthomolecular medicine.

James A. Jackson, PhD:

For over twenty years, I was the laboratory director of a federally approved clinical reference laboratory. We accepted samples from all the United States and foreign countries. We measured all the fat-soluble and water-soluble vitamins in blood and urine. It was common to find vitamin deficiencies in both males and females, whether children or adults. The most common vitamin deficiencies were of vitamin C and vitamin D_3. The clinic's physicians treated the patients with the appropriate vitamins the patients and were monitored by our laboratory. Many were helped by the vitamin replacement treatment, including those with complaints such as headache, joint and muscle pain, chronic fatigue syndrome, and attention-deficit hyperactivity disorder (ADHD). We published many of these cases in the *Journal of Orthomolecular Medicine*. (See: http://orthomolecular.org/library/jom/index.shtml.)

Ian Brighthope, MD:

Over 70 percent of Australians consume vitamins on a regular basis. A search of the department of health's database reveals that no serious adverse reactions or deaths have occurred in the Australian population over the past ten years from the use of complementary medicines. There is an extreme bias against very low- to extremely low-risk products by government regulators and health professionals working within and outside the establishment institutions.

Robert Jenkins, DC, MS:

I have been in practice for 52 years and have treated thousands of patients with diet and nutritional supplements for numerous health conditions ranging from hypertension to diabetes, hypercholesterolemia, metabolic syndrome, irritable bowel syndrome, and many others. I have yet to experience adverse patient reactions from taking nutritional supplements. I have lectured second-year medical students at two medical schools in the Philadelphia, PA area. When I asked those students how much nutritional training they had received, they all held up their hands with the sign of zero. The pharmaceutical industry makes sure medical students are trained in how to prescribe their drugs, while no positive mention is made of nutritional supplements. Why would anyone think that our modern medical doctors are to be considered authorities on nutritional supplementation for health conditions when they are not trained to be? When this lack of nutritional education is combined with the news media's ignorance of supplements and their benefits, we have "the blind leading the blind."

Gert Schuitemaker, PhD:

In the Netherlands, a report of the Dutch Health Council states that less than 2 percent of the population is eating according to official dietary guidelines.[6] Moreover, the authorities state that, even if a person is eating according to the dietary guidelines, he is not getting enough vitamin A, D, folic acid, iron, selenium, and zinc.[7] Research in a Dutch hospital showed that 40 percent of patients at the time of admission were malnourished.[8] So, dietary supplements are necessary. Usually, chronic diseases, which develop with increasing age, are treated with medicines, inevitably accompanied by the risk of severe side effects and unnecessary deaths. Because the basis of many chronic diseases is a metabolic disturbance and nutritional deficiencies, the best treatment approach is good nutrition, including the use of dietary supplements. The "danger" of vitamins and minerals lies in chronic deficiencies, not in alleged toxic effects. Following the scientific literature on a daily basis, in 30 years, I have not seen any harmful effect from supplements.

Damien Downing, MD:

The more toxins you are exposed to, the more nutrients you will use up in dealing with them. Every year, we are exposed to more and more toxins, and our DNA has had no time to adapt. These include heavy metals such as lead, mercury, fluorine; pesticides, including the newer ones like glyphosate (found in Roundup); flame retardants that are even contaminating the Arctic; and hundreds of thousands of other new-to-nature molecules that every human has to deal with. And like it or not, pharmaceutical medications are mostly toxins too.

At the same time, intensive farming, soil depletion, and poor diets (often foisted on us for spurious reasons such as fear of cholesterol) mean that it's normal to be deficient now. We are deficient in vitamins, minerals, and other nutrients as well.

What chance does a human have? A much better one if she doesn't buy the hype from big companies, the dogma from pharma-paid scientists, and the bullying from governments. Take your vitamins.

Steve Hickey, PhD:

Over the past three centuries, the frequency of deficiency and infectious diseases has been reduced, through improved nutrition and better hygiene. Throughout this time, however, the role of nutrition has been belittled by the authorities. These same authorities now reject the idea that nutritional supplements can prevent our current chronic diseases. Thus, as a result of such authoritarian medicine, we may have replaced the horrors of pellagra, scurvy, and rickets with those of dementia, heart disease, and cancer. If so, it is likely that people in the future will look back with similar dismay on the current and needless destruction of health. How will we answer them, when they ask how we could have allowed this to happen?

Dean Elledge, DDS, MS:

The high-carbohydrate, nutrient-poor diet is a primary contributing factor in dental diseases.[9] Vitamin D and vitamin C are safe to use in dentistry to help the patient recover from dental diseases. Vitamins in general help reduce inflammation, and antioxidant vitamins reduce the inflammation in periodontal disease. Vitamin supplements improve antioxidant reserves.

Michael Ellis, MD:

I see so many patients in conventional general practice who are deficient in vitamins. I had one patient who had ended up in a hospital neurosurgical unit only to be found to have severe B_{12} deficiency. The foods that most people eat are high in sugar, processed, and denatured of essential nutrients. All patients need, at the very least, daily multivitamins.

Ralph Campbell, MD:

We have had lots of talk of the alleged "toxicity" of vitamins over the decades I have been in pediatric practice. I remain leery of the validity of such accusations. Most are just uninformed regurgitation of poorly designed studies. If alert, a clinician can easily detect vitamin deficiencies, and with experience, quickly spot suboptimal vitamin levels. The medical establishment seems to be increasingly aware of vitamin D, B_{12}, and folic acid deficiency. What is taking the media so long?

Karin Munsterhjelm-Ahumada, MD:

I have been a physician for 35 years. For the last 20 years, I have combined general medicine with nutritional (orthomolecular) medicine, the practice of preventing and treating disease by providing the body with optimal amounts of substances which are natural to the body, principally vitamins and minerals. I have had good opportunity to *compare* the results of my work as a GP from the time *before* I got knowledge of vitamins and minerals as therapeutic substances with the time *after* I had learned to integrate them in my work with patients. I can today certify that I have seen a great number of very positive results after beginning to integrate vitamins in my clinical work. The results have been particularly fine in neurologic and psychiatric conditions, including schizophrenia, and in hormonal and infectious diseases. During these last 20 years I have not seen severe side effects from orthomolecular substances. On the contrary, I have often been able to decrease the dosage of strong pharmaceutical drugs that carry severe side effects. This has led to a completely new and better quality of life for my patients, and for myself as a doctor.

Conclusion

The old saying remains true: the person who says it can't be done should not interrupt the person successfully doing it. Progressive doctors prescribe vitamins because they work. If your doctor doesn't "believe" in vitamins, maybe it is time for him or her to change such an antiquated belief system in favor of the true clinical evidence.

REFERENCES FOR "DOCTORS SAY VITAMINS ARE SAFE AND EFFECTIVE"

1. Li K, Kaaks R, Linseisen J, et al. Vitamin/mineral supplementation and cancer, cardiovascular, and all-cause mortality in a German prospective cohort (EPIC-Heidelberg). *Eur J Nutr* 2011; 51(4):407–413.

2. Suh DC, Woodall BS, Shin SK, et al. Clinical and economic impact of adverse drug reactions in hospitalized patients. *Ann Pharmacother* 2000;34(12):1373–1379.

3. Lazarou J, Pomeranz BH, Corey PN. Incidence of adverse drug reactions in hospitalized patients: a meta-analysis of prospective studies. *JAMA* 1998 15;279(15):1200–1205.

4. Carlson LA. Nicotinic acid: the broad-spectrum lipid drug. A 50th anniversary review. *J Intern Med* 2005; 258: 94–114.

5. Nissen SE, and Wolski K. Effect of rosiglitazone on the risk of myocardial infarction and death from cardiovascular causes. *N Engl J Med* 2007; 356: 2457–2471.

6. Significant trends in food consumption in the Netherlands. The Hague: Health Council of the Netherlands, 2002; publication no. 2002/12.

7. Voedingscentrum. Richtlijnen goede voedselkeuze. [The Netherlands Nutrition Centre. Guidelines Good Nutritional Choice] 2011.

8. Naber TH, Schermer T, de Bree A, et al. Prevalence of malnutrition in nonsurgical hospitalized patients and its association with disease complications. *Am J Clin Nutr* 1997; 66(5):1232–1239.

9. Elledge DA. Effective hemostasis and tissue management. *Dentistry Today,* Oct 2010, p. 150.

SUPPLEMENTS: THE REAL STORY

From the *Orthomolecular Medicine News Service,* January 17, 2012.

It's a nutritional "Catch 22": The public is told, confusingly, *"Vitamins are good, but vitamin supplements are not. Only vitamins from food will help you. So just eat a good diet. Do not take supplements! But by the way, there is no difference between natural and synthetic vitamins."*

Wait a minute. What's the real story here?

One study reported that the risk of heart failure decreased with increasing blood levels of vitamin C.[1] The benefit of vitamin C (ascorbate) was highly significant. Persons with the lowest plasma levels of ascorbate had the highest risk of heart failure, and persons with the highest levels of vitamin C had the *lowest* risk of heart failure. This finding confirms the knowledge derived over the last 50 years that vitamin C is a major essential factor in cardiovascular health.[2,3] The study raises several important questions about diet and vitamin supplements.

Was It Food or Supplements?

The report discussed vitamin C as if it were simply an indicator of how many fruits and vegetables were consumed by the participants. Yet, ironically, the study's results show little improvement in the risk for heart failure from consuming fruits and vegetables. This implies that the real factor in reducing the risk was indeed the amount of vitamin C consumed. Moreover, the study appears to utterly ignore the widespread use of vitamin C supplements to improve cardiovascular health. In fact, out of four quartile groups, the quartile *with the highest plasma vitamin C had six to ten times the rate of vitamin C supplementation* of the lowest quartile, but this fact was not emphasized. This type of selective attention to food sources of vitamin C, while dismissing supplements as an important source, appears to be an attempt to marginalize the importance of vitamin supplements.

Many medical and nutritional reports have maintained that there is little difference between natural and synthetic vitamins. This is known to be true for some essential nutrients. The ascorbate found in widely available vitamin C tablets is identical to the ascorbate found in fruits and vegetables.[3] Linus Pauling emphasized this fact, and explained how ordinary vitamin C, inexpensively manufactured from glucose, could improve health in many important ways.[4] Indeed, the above-mentioned study specifically measured the plasma level of ascorbate, which was shown to be an important factor associated with lower risk of heart failure.[1,2] The study did not measure blood plasma levels of the components of fruits and vegetables. It measured vitamin C.

A known rationale for this dramatic finding is that vitamin C helps to prevent inflammation in the arteries by several mechanisms. It is a necessary co-factor for the synthesis of collagen, which is a major component of arteries. Vitamin C is also an important antioxidant throughout the body that can help to recycle other antioxidants like vitamin E and glutathione in the artery walls.[2,3] This was underscored by a report that *high plasma levels of vitamin C are associated with a 50 percent reduction in risk for stroke.*[5]

Yes, Synthetic Vitamin C Is Clinically Effective

Synthetic vitamin C works, in real people with real illnesses. Ascorbate's efficacy has little direct relation to food intake. A dramatic case of this was that of a dairy farmer in New Zealand who was on life support with lung whiteout, kidney failure, leukemia, and swine flu.[6] He was given 100,000 milligrams (mg) of vitamin C daily, and his life was saved. We have nothing against oranges or other vitamin C-containing foods. Fruits and vegetables are good for you for many, many reasons. However, you'll need to get out your calculator to help you figure out how many oranges it would take to get that much vitamin C, and then also figure how to get a sick person to eat them all.

It is established that liver function improves with vitamin C supplementation, and it is equally well known that adequate levels of vitamin C are essential for the proper functioning of the immune system. Vitamin C improves the ability of the white blood cells to fight bacteria and viruses.

Deficiency of vitamin C is very common. According to US Department of Agriculture (USDA) data,[7] nearly half of Americans do not get even the US Recommended Dietary Allowance (RDA) of vitamin C, which is a mere 90 mg.

Synthetic Vitamin E Is Less Effective

For some other nutrients, there is a significant difference in efficacy between synthetic and natural forms. Vitamin E is a crucial antioxidant, but it also has other functions in the body, not all well understood. It comprises eight different biochemical forms: alpha-, beta-, delta-, and gamma-tocopherols, and alpha-, beta-, delta-, and gamma-tocotrienols. All of these forms of vitamin E are important for the body. Current knowledge about the function of vitamin E is rapidly expanding, and each of the eight forms of natural vitamin E is thought to have a slightly different function in the body. For example, gamma-tocotrienol actually kills prostate cancer stem cells better than chemotherapy does.

Synthetic vitamin E is widely available and inexpensive. It is DL-alpha-tocopherol. Yes, it has the same antioxidant properties in test tube experiments as does the natural D-alpha-tocopherol form. However, the DL- form has only 50 percent of the biological efficacy, because the body utilizes only the natural D isomer, which comprises half of the synthetic mix.[8] Therefore, studies utilizing DL-alpha-tocopherol that do not take this fact into account are starting with an already-halved dose that will naturally lead to a reduction in the observed efficacy.

Then there are the esterified forms of vitamin E such as acetate or succinate. These esterified forms, either natural or synthetic, have a greater shelf life because the ester protects the vitamin E from being oxidized and neutralized. When acid in the stomach cleaves the acetate or succinate component from the original natural vitamin E molecule, the gut can then absorb a good fraction and the body receives its antioxidant benefit. But when esterified vitamin E acetate is applied to the skin to prevent inflammation, it is ineffective because there is no acid present to remove the acetate ester.

Based on USDA data[9] an astonishing *90 percent of Americans do not get the RDA of vitamin E,* which is, believe it or not, under 23 IU (15 mg) per day.

Magnesium Deficiency Is Widespread

Magnesium is another example. *Over two-thirds of the population do not get the RDA of magnesium.*[10] Deficiency can cause a wide variety of symptoms, including osteoporosis, high blood pressure, heart disease, asthma, depression, and diabetes. Magnesium can be purchased in many forms. The most widely available form is magnesium oxide, which is not very effective because it is only about 5 percent absorbed.[11] Magnesium oxide supplements are popular because the pills are smaller—they contain more magnesium, but they won't help most people. Better forms of magnesium are magnesium citrate, magnesium gluconate, magnesium malate, and magnesium chloride.

It's always good to consult your doctor to determine your ideal intake. Testing may reveal unexpected deficiency.[12]

Well, Which? Natural or Synthetic?

While the natural form of vitamin E (mixed natural tocopherols and tocotrienols) is at least twice as effective as the synthetic form, this is not true of vitamin C. The ascorbate that the body gets from fruits and vegetables is the same as the ascorbate in vitamin C tablets. On first thought, this may sound confusing, because there are many so-called "natural" forms of vitamin C widely available. But *virtually every study that demonstrated that supplemental vitamin C fights illness used plain, cheap, synthetic ascorbic acid.* Other forms of ascorbate, for instance, the sodium or magnesium salt of ascorbic acid, are digested slightly differently by the gut, but once the ascorbate molecule is absorbed from these forms, it has identical efficacy. The advantage of these ascorbate salts is that they are nonacidic and can be ingested or topically applied to any part of the body without concern about irritation from acidity.

Further, it is known that essential nutrients are symbiotic; that is, they are more effective when taken as a group in proper doses. For example, vitamin E is more effective when taken along with vitamin C and selenium, because each of these essential nutrients can improve the efficacy of the others. Similarly, the B vitamins are more effective when taken together.

Food Factors

Natural food factors are also important. Bioflavonoids and other vitamin C-friendly components in fresh fruits and vegetables (sometimes called "vitamin C complex") do indeed have health benefits. These natural components are easily obtained from a healthy, unprocessed, whole-foods diet. However, eating even a very good diet does not supply nearly enough vitamin C to be effective against illness. A really good diet might provide several hundred milligrams of vitamin C daily. An extreme raw food diet might provide 2,000 or 3,000 milligrams of vitamin C, but this is not practical for most people. Supplementation, with a good diet, is.

The principle that "natural" vitamins are better than synthetic vitamins is a widely quoted justification for actually avoiding vitamin supplements. The argument goes: because vitamins and minerals are available from food in their natural form, somehow one might suppose that we are best off by ignoring supplements. Apparently this is what the authors of the above-mentioned study had in mind, because the report hardly mentions vitamin supplements.

Conclusion

In the real world of today's processed food, most of us don't get all the nutrients we need in adequate doses. Most people are deficient in *several* of the essential nutrients.

These deficiencies are responsible for much suffering, including heart disease, cancer, premature aging, dementia, diabetes, and other diseases such as eye disease, multiple sclerosis, and asthma. The above-mentioned study showing the efficacy of vitamin C in reducing heart failure is but one of the many studies showing the value of vitamins.

For vitamin E, the natural form, taken in adequate doses along with a nutritious diet, is the best medicine. However, for most vitamins, including vitamin C, the manufactured form is identical to the natural one. Both are biologically active and both work clinically. It all comes down to dose. Supplements enable optimum intake; foods alone do not.

Don't be fooled: nutrient deficiency is the rule, not the exception. That's why we need supplements. When ill, we need them even more.

REFERENCES FOR "SUPPLEMENTS: THE REAL STORY"

1. Pfister R, Sharp SJ, Luben R, et al. Plasma vitamin C predicts incident heart failure in men and women in European prospective investigation into cancer and nutrition: Norfolk prospective study. *Am Heart J* 2011;162(2):246–253. doi: 10.1016/j.ahj.2011.05.007. See also: http://orthomolecular.org/resources/omns/v07n14.shtml.

2. Levy TE. *Stop America's #1 Killer: Reversible Vitamin Deficiency Found to Be Origin of All Coronary Heart Disease.* West Greenwich, RI: Livon Books, 2006.

3. Hickey S, Saul AW. *Vitamin C: The Real Story.* Laguna Beach, CA: Basic Health Publications, 2008.

4. Pauling L. *How to Live Longer and Feel Better.* Corvallis, OR: Oregon State University Press, 2006.

5. Kurl S, Tuomainen TP, Laukkanen JA, et al. Plasma vitamin C modifies the association between hypertension and risk of stroke. *Stroke* 2002; 33:1568–1573.

6. http://www.dailymotion.com/video/xh70sx_60-minutes-scoop-on-new-zealand-farmer-vit-c-miracle_tech.

7. Patterson BH, Block G, Rosenberger WF, et al. Fruits and vegetables in the American diet: Data from the NHANES II survey. *Am J Public Health* 1990; 80(12): 1443–1449. Available at: http://www.ncbi.nlm.nih.gov/pmc/articles/PMC1405127/pdf/amjph00225–0021.pdf.

8. Papas A. *The Vitamin E Factor: The Miraculous Antioxidant for the Prevention and Treatment of Heart Disease, Cancer, and Aging.* New York: HarperCollins, 1999.

9. Linus Pauling Institute. Micronutrient Information Center. Oregon State University. Vitamin E. Available at: http://lpi.oregonstate.edu/infocenter/vitamins/vitaminE/.

10. http://www.jacn.org/content/24/3/166.full.pdf+html (no longer available). See instead: Mercola, J. Magnesium: An invisible deficiency that could be harming your health. Jan 19, 2015. Available at: http://articles.mercola.com/sites/articles/archive/2015/01/19/magnesium-deficiency.aspx.

11. Dean, C. *The Magnesium Miracle.* Updated Edition. New York: Ballantine Books, 2007.

12. Saul, AW. Epilepsy. Available at: http://www.doctoryourself.com/epilepsy.html.

A TIMELINE OF VITAMIN MEDICINE

by Andrew W. Saul, PhD

From the *Orthomolecular Medicine News Service,* February 15, 2014.

Don't get bogged down by silly claims that multiple vitamins kill, or that antioxidants are bad for you. It is high time to take a look at the record and review what published medical research actually has been saying for eight decades.

Year Research

1935 Claus Washington Jungeblut, MD, professor of bacteriology at Columbia University, first publishes on vitamin C as prevention and treatment for polio; in the same year, Jungeblut also shows that vitamin C inactivates diphtheria toxin.

1936 Evan Shute, MD, and Wilfrid Shute, MD, demonstrate that vitamin E-rich wheat germ oil cures angina.

1937 Dr. Jungeblut demonstrates that ascorbate (vitamin C) inactivated tetanus toxin.

1939 William Kaufman, MD, PhD, successfully treats arthritis with niacinamide (vitamin B_3).

1940 The Shute brothers publish that vitamin E prevents fibroids and endometriosis, and is curative for atherosclerosis.

1942 Ruth Flinn Harrell, PhD, at Columbia University, measures the positive effect of added thiamine (B_1) on learning.

1945 Vitamin E is shown to cure hemorrhages in the skin and mucous membranes, and to decrease the diabetic's need for insulin.

1946 Vitamin E is shown to greatly improve wound healing, including skin ulcers. It is also demonstrated that vitamin E strengthens and regulates heartbeat, and is effective in cases of claudication, acute nephritis, thrombosis, cirrhosis, and phlebitis; also, William J. McCormick, MD, shows how vitamin C prevents and also cures kidney stones.

1947 Vitamin E is successfully used as therapy for gangrene, inflammation of blood vessels (Buerger's disease), retinitis, and choroiditis; Roger J. Williams, PhD, publishes on how vitamins can be used to treat alcoholism.

1948 Frederick R. Klenner, MD, a board-certified specialist in diseases of the chest, publishes cures of 41 cases of viral pneumonia using very high doses of vitamin C.

1949 Dr. Kaufman publishes *The Common Form of Joint Dysfunction.*

1950 Vitamin E is shown to be an effective treatment for lupus erythematosus, varicose veins, and severe body burns.

1951 Vitamin D treatment is found to be effective against Hodgkin's disease (a cancer of the lymphatic system) and epithelioma.

1954 Abram Hoffer, MD, PhD, and colleagues demonstrate that niacin (vitamin B_3) can cure schizophrenia; the Shutes' medical textbook *Alpha Tocopherol in Cardiovascular Disease* is published; and Dr. McCormick reports that cancer patients tested for vitamin C were seriously deficient, often by as much as 4,500 milligrams.

1955 Niacin is first shown to lower serum cholesterol.

1956 Mayo Clinic researcher William Parsons, MD, and colleagues confirm Dr. Hoffer's use of niacin to lower cholesterol and prevent cardiovascular disease; Dr. Harrell demonstrates that supplementation of the pregnant and lactating mothers' diet with vitamins increases the intelligence quotients of their offspring at three and four years of age.

1957 Dr. McCormick publishes on how vitamin C fights cardiovascular disease.

1960 Dr. Hoffer meets Bill W., cofounder of Alcoholics Anonymous, and uses niacin to eliminate Bill's long-standing severe depression.

1963 Vitamin D is shown to prevent breast cancer.

1964 Vitamin D is found to be effective against lymph-nodal reticulosarcoma (a non-Hodgkin's lymphatic cancer).

1968 Linus Pauling, PhD, publishes the theoretical basis of high-dose nutrient therapy (orthomolecular medicine) in psychiatry in *Science,* and soon after defines orthomolecular medicine as "the treatment of disease by the provision of the optimum molecular environment, especially the optimum concentrations of substances normally present in the human body."

1969 Robert F. Cathcart, MD, uses large doses of vitamin C to treat pneumonia, hepatitis, and, years later, acquired immune deficiency syndrome (AIDS).

1970 Dr. Pauling publishes *Vitamin C and the Common Cold,* and Dr. Williams publishes *Nutrition Against Disease.*

1972 Publication of *The Healing Factor: "Vitamin C" Against Disease* by Irwin Stone, PhD.

1973 Dr. Klenner publishes his vitamin supplement protocol to arrest and reverse multiple sclerosis; so does H. T. Mount, MD, reporting on 27 years of success using thiamine. Also, Ewan Cameron, MD, and Dr. Pauling publish their first joint paper on the control of cancer with vitamin C, two years after Cameron began using high-dose intravenous vitamin C.

1975 Hugh D. Riordan, MD, and colleagues successfully use large doses of intravenous vitamin C against cancer.

1976 Ewan Cameron, MD, and other physicians in Scotland show that intravenous vitamin C improves quality and length of life in terminal cancer patients.

1977 Alfred Libby, MD, and Dr. Stone present findings that the use of high doses of vitamins hastens and eases withdrawal from highly addictive drugs.

1981 Dr. Harrell and colleagues demonstrate that very high doses of nutritional supplements help overcome learning disabilities in children, and bring about highly significant improvement in those with Down syndrome.

1982 In Japan, Murata, Morishige, and Yamaguchi show that vitamin C greatly prolongs the lives of terminal cancer patients.

1984 Robert F. Cathcart, MD, publishes on the vitamin C treatment of AIDS.

1986 Publication of *How to Live Longer and Feel Better*, by Linus Pauling.

1988 Dr. Lendon H. Smith publishes *Vitamin C as a Fundamental Medicine: Abstracts of Dr. Frederick R. Klenner, M.D.'s Published and Unpublished Work*, now known as *Clinical Guide to the Use of Vitamin C*.

1990 American doctors successfully use vitamin C to treat kidney cancer, and in 1995 and 1996, other cancers.

1993 Large-scale studies show that vitamin E supplementation reduces the risk of coronary heart disease in men and women.

1995 Dr. Riordan and colleagues publish their protocol for intravenous vitamin C treatment of cancer.

2002 Vitamin E shown to improve immune functions in patients with advanced colorectal cancer, by immediately increasing T-helper-1 cytokine production.

2004 Doctors in America and Puerto Rico publish more clinical cases of vitamin C successes against cancer.

2005 Research sponsored by the National Institutes of Health shows that high levels of vitamin C kill cancer cells without harming normal cells.

2006 Canadian doctors report intravenous vitamin C is successful in treating cancer.

2007 Harold D. Foster, PhD, and colleagues publish a double-blind, randomized clinical trial showing that HIV-positive patients given supplemental nutrients can delay or stop their decline into AIDS.

2008 Korean doctors report that intravenous vitamin C "plays a crucial role in the suppression of proliferation of several types of cancer," notably melanoma. And, natural vitamin E is demonstrated to reduce risk of lung cancer by 61 percent.

2009, 2010, 2012 Intravenous Vitamin C and Cancer Symposiums are filmed and made available for free access online at: http://www.riordanclinic.org/education/symposium/s2009 (twelve lectures), http://www.riordanclinic.org/education/symposium/s2010 (nine lectures), and http://www.riordanclinic.org/education/symposium/s2012 (eleven lectures).

2011 Each 20 micromole per liter (µmol/L) increase in plasma vitamin C is associated with a 9 percent reduction in death from heart failure. Also, B-complex vitamins are associated with a 7 percent decrease in mortality, and vitamin D with an 8 percent decrease in mortality.

2012 Vitamin C shown to prevent and treat radiation-damaged DNA.

2013 B-vitamin supplementation seen to slow the atrophy of specific brain regions that are a key component of the Alzheimer's disease process and are associated with cognitive decline.

2014 In patients with mild to moderate Alzheimer's disease, 2,000 international units (IU) of vitamin E slows the decline compared to placebo. Data from 561 patients showed that those taking vitamin E function significantly better in daily life, and required the least care; vitamin C greatly reduces chemotherapy side effects and improves cancer-patient survival.

2015 Vitamin C decreases complications, intubation time, and length of hospital stays in intensive care unit patients. And another large-scale study found a 26–55 percent risk reduction for pancreatic cancer in persons who consume more vitamin C.

2016 Supplementation with vitamin C improves insulin-mediated glucose disposal in people with type 2 diabetes. Other research shows that antioxidants reduce aggressive prostate cancer risk by 64 to 72 percent. And incredibly, the dose to do so was equivalent to a daily dose of only 1,500 mg of vitamin C.

For specific references on these subjects, just copy and paste or type any of the brief descriptions above into a search engine and press "enter." Doctors and reporters who say they "have not seen any good evidence that vitamins cure disease" are telling you the truth: yes, they have never seen it. That's not because it isn't available; it's because they have never done even this simple step.

Copy, paste, or type, and search. There is a whole body of knowledge out there. Take a look and decide for yourself.

"No amount of evidence will persuade someone who is not listening."

—ABRAM HOFFER, MD, PHD

NO DEATHS FROM VITAMINS, SUPPLEMENTS, MINERALS, AMINO ACIDS, OR HERBS. ABSOLUTELY NONE.

by Andrew W. Saul, PhD

From the *Orthomolecular Medicine News Service,* January 3, 2016.

There were *no deaths whatsoever from vitamins* in the year 2014. The 32nd annual report from the American Association of Poison Control Centers shows zero deaths from multiple vitamins. And, there were no deaths whatsoever from vitamin A, niacin, vitamin B_6, any other B vitamin. There were no deaths from vitamin C, vitamin D, vitamin E, or from any vitamin at all.[1]

Zero deaths from vitamins. Want to bet this will never be on the evening news? Well, have you seen it there? And why not?

After all, over half of the US population takes daily nutritional supplements. If each of those people took only one single tablet daily, that makes about 170,000,000 individual doses per day, for a total of well over 60 billion doses annually. Since many persons take far more than just one single vitamin tablet, actual consumption is considerably higher, and the safety of vitamin supplements is all the more remarkable.

Abram Hoffer, MD, PhD, always said, "No one dies from vitamins." He was right when he said it, and he is still right today.

No Deaths from Any Supplement

Not only are there no deaths from vitamins; there are also zero deaths from *any* supplement. The most recent (2014) information collected by the US National Poison Data System, and published in the journal *Clinical Toxicology,* shows *no deaths whatsoever* from dietary supplements across the board.

No Deaths from Minerals

There were zero deaths from any dietary mineral supplement. This means there were no fatalities from calcium, magnesium, chromium, zinc, colloidal silver, selenium, iron, or multimineral supplements. Reported in the "Electrolyte and Mineral" category was a fatality from the medical use of "sodium and sodium salts" and another fatality from nonsupplemental iron, which was clearly and specifically excluded from the supplement category.

No Deaths from Any Other Nutritional Supplement

Additionally, there were zero deaths from any amino acid or single-ingredient herbal product. This means no deaths at all from blue cohosh, echinacea, ginkgo biloba, ginseng, kava kava, St. John's wort, valerian, yohimbe, Asian medicines, ayurvedic medicines, or any other botanical. There were zero deaths from creatine, blue-green algae, glucosamine, chondroitin, or melatonin. There were zero deaths from any homeopathic remedy.

But When in Doubt, Blame a Supplement. Any Supplement.

There was one death attributed to a "Multi-Botanical without Ma Huang or Citrus Aurantium." It is interesting that they knew what was not in it but did not know what *was* in it. This is hearsay at best, and scaremongering at worst. There was one death alleged from some "Unknown Dietary Supplement or Homeopathic Agent." This, too, indicates complete lack of certainly as to what may or may not have been involved. One fatality was attributed to "Energy Products: Unknown." First of all, energy drinks or "products" are not nutritional supplements. But more importantly, how can an accusation be based on the unknown? Equally unscientific are the two deaths attributed to "Energy Products: Other." Well, what products were they? These are no more than vague, unsubstantiated allegations. Claiming causation without even knowing what substance or ingredient to accuse is baseless.

The Truth: No Man, Woman, or Child Died from Any Nutritional Supplement. Period.

If nutritional supplements are allegedly so "dangerous," as the FDA, the news media, and even some physicians still claim, then *where are the bodies*?

REFERENCE FOR "NO DEATHS FROM VITAMINS"

1. Mowry JB, Spyker DA, Brooks DE, et al. 2014 Annual Report of the American Association of Poison Control Centers' National Poison Data System (NPDS): 32nd Annual Report. *Clinical Toxicology* 2015; (53)10: 962–1147. Available at: http://dx.doi.org/10.3109/15563650.2015.1102927.

"Safe Upper Levels" for Nutritional Supplements: One Giant Step Backward

by Alan R. Gaby, MD

From *J Orthomolecular Med* 2003;18(3–4):127–130.

In May 2003, the Expert Group on Vitamins and Minerals (EVM), an advisory group originally commissioned in 1988 by the then Ministry of Agriculture Fisheries and Food, and subsequently reporting to the Food Standards Agency in England, published a report that set Safe Upper Levels (SULs) for the doses of most vitamin and mineral supplements. The establishment of SULs was based on a review of clinical and epidemiological evidence, as well as animal research and in vitro studies. For those nutrients for which the available evidence was judged insufficient to set an SUL, the EVM instead established Guidance Levels, which were to be considered less reliable than SULs.

This writer's analysis of the EVM report reveals that the dose limits were set inappropriately low for many vitamins and minerals, well below doses which have been used by the public for decades with apparent safety. While the release of this 360-page document would be of little import were it to be used solely as a manifesto for the pathologically risk-averse, preliminary indications are that it could be used very actively to support the arguments of those who are seeking to ban the over-the-counter sale of many currently available nutritional supplements. If the report is used that way, then the public health could be jeopardized.

On May 30, 2002, the European Union adopted Directive 2002/46/EC, which established a framework for setting maximum limits for vitamins and minerals in food supplements. The EVM report is seen by the UK government as the basis for its negotiating position in the process of setting these pan-European limits.

The apparent anti-nutritional-supplement, anti-self-care bias that permeated the process of setting safety levels is evident both in the way in which the SUL was defined and in the fact that the benefits of nutritional supplements were purposely ignored. The SUL was defined as the maximum dose of a particular nutrient "that potentially susceptible individuals could take daily on a life-long basis, without medical supervision in reasonable safety." In other words, it is the highest dose that is unlikely to cause anyone any harm, ever, under any circumstance. Furthermore, the EVM was specifically instructed not to consider the benefits of any of the nutrients, and not to engage in risk/benefit analysis.[1]

There is little or no precedent in free societies for restricting access to products or activities to levels that are completely risk free. Aspirin causes intestinal bleeding, water makes people drown, driving a car causes accidents, and free speech may offend the exquisitely offendable. Politicians and bureaucrats do not seek to ban aspirin or water or driving or free speech, because their benefits outweigh their risks. For vitamins and minerals, however, some authorities seem to believe that unique safety criteria are needed.

Moreover, the government's instructions to disregard the many documented benefits of nutritional supplements introduced a serious bias into the evaluation process. As the EVM acknowledged, determining safety limits involves an enormous degree of uncertainty and a fairly wide range of possible outcomes. The committee might have established higher safety limits than it did, had it been told to weigh benefits against risks. The government's instructions appeared to be an implicit directive to err on the side of excluding doses that are being used to prevent or treat disease. And that is what the EVM did, often by making questionable interpretations of the data, and doing so in what appears to have been an arbitrary and inconsistent manner.

Riboflavin Guidance Level

A typical example of the EVM's dubious approach to establishing safety limits is its evaluation of riboflavin (vitamin B_2). The committee acknowledged that no toxic effects have been reported in animals given an acute oral dose of 10,000 milligrams per kilogram (mg/kg) of body weight, or after long-term ingestion of 25 mg/kg/day (equivalent to 1,750 mg/day for a 70-kg [154-lb] human). Moreover, in a study of 28 patients taking riboflavin for migraine prophylaxis, a dose of 400 mg/day for three months did not cause any adverse effects. Despite a complete absence of side effects at any dose in either humans or animals, the EVM set the Guidance Level for riboflavin at 40 mg/day. That level was established by dividing the 400 mg/day used in the migraine study by an "uncertainty factor" of ten, to allow for variability in the susceptibility of human beings to adverse effects.

A more appropriate conclusion regarding riboflavin would have been that no adverse effects have been observed at any dose, and that there is no basis at this time for establishing an upper limit. If the EVM's recommendation is used to limit the potency of riboflavin tablets to 40 mg, then migraine sufferers will have to take 10 pills per day, in order to prevent migraine recurrences.[2]

Vitamin B_6 Safe Upper Level

Similar reasoning led to an SUL of 10 mg/day for pyridoxine (vitamin B_6), even though this vitamin has been used with apparent safety, usually in doses of 50 to 200 mg/day, to treat carpal tunnel syndrome, premenstrual syndrome, asthma, and other common problems. The SUL for vitamin B_6 was derived from an animal study, in which a dose of 50 mg/kg of body weight/day (equivalent to 3,000 mg/day for a 60-kg [132-lb] person) resulted in neurotoxicity. The EVM reduced that dose progressively by invoking three separate "uncertainty factors": 1) by a factor of three, to extrapolate from the lowest observed-adverse-effect level (LOAEL) to a no observed-adverse-effect level (NOAEL); 2) by an additional factor of ten, to account for presumed interspecies differences; and 3) by a further factor of ten to account for interindividual variation in humans. Thus, the neurotoxic dose in animals was reduced by a factor of 300, to a level that excludes the widely used 50- and 100-mg tablets.

The decision to base the SUL for vitamin B_6 on animal data (modified by a massive "uncertainty factor") was arbitrary, considering that toxicology data are available for humans.[3] Sensory neuropathy has been reported in some individuals taking large doses of vitamin B_6.[4,5] Most people who suffered this adverse effect were taking 2,000 mg/day or more of pyridoxine, although some were taking only 500 mg/day. There is a single case report of a neuropathy occurring in a person taking 200 mg/day of pyridoxine, but the reliability of that case report is unclear. The individual in question was never examined, but was merely interviewed by telephone after responding to a local television report that publicized pyridoxine-induced neuropathy.[6]

Because pyridoxine neurotoxicity has been known to the medical profession for 20 years, and because vitamin B_6 is being taken by millions of people, it is reasonable to assume that neurotoxicity at doses below 200 mg/day would have been reported by now, if it does occur at those doses. The fact that no such reports have appeared strongly suggests that vitamin B_6 does not damage the nervous system when taken at doses below 200 mg/day. As the EVM did with other nutrients for which a LOAEL is known for humans, it could have divided the vitamin B_6 LOAEL (200 mg/day) by three to obtain an SUL of 66.7 mg/day. Had the committee been allowed to evaluate both the benefits and risks of vitamin B_6, it probably would have established the SUL at that level, rather than the 10 mg/day it arrived at through serial decimation of the animal data.

Manganese Guidance Level

Chronic inhalation of high concentrations of airborne manganese, as might be encountered in mines or steel mills, has been reported to cause a neuropsychiatric syndrome that resembles Parkinson's disease. In contrast, manganese is considered one of the least toxic trace minerals when ingested orally, and reports of human toxicity from oral ingestion are "essentially nonexistent."[7] The neurotoxicity that occurs in miners and industrial workers may result from a combination of high concentrations of manganese in the air and, possibly, direct entry of nasally inhaled manganese into the brain (bypassing the blood-brain barrier).

In establishing a Guidance Level for manganese, the EVM cited a study by Kondakis et al. in which people exposed to high concentrations of manganese in their drinking water (1.8–2.3 mg/liter [L]) had more signs and symptoms of subtle neurological dysfunction than did a control group whose drinking water contained less manganese.[8] The committee acknowledged that another epidemiological study by Vieregge et al. showed no adverse effects among individuals whose drinking water contained up to 2.1 mg/L of manganese.[9] The EVM hypothesized that these studies may not really be contradictory, since the subjects in the Kondakis study were, on average, ten years older than were those in the Vieregge study, and increasing age might theoretically render people more susceptible to manganese toxicity. Based on the results of these two studies, the EVM established a Guidance Level for supplemental manganese of 4 mg/day for the general population and 0.5 mg/day for elderly individuals.

There are serious problems with the EVM's analysis of the manganese research. First, the committee overlooked that fact that in the Kondakis study the people in the high-manganese group were older than were those in the control group (mean age, 67.6 vs. 65.6 years). Many of the neurological symptoms that were investigated in this study are nonspecific and presumably age related, including fatigue, muscle pain, irritability, insomnia, sleepiness, decreased libido, depression, slowness in rising from a chair, and memory disturbances. The fact that the older people had more symptoms than did the younger people is not surprising, and may have been totally unrelated to the manganese content of their drinking water.

Second, the EVM broke its own rules regarding the use of uncertainty factors, presumably to avoid being faced with an embarrassingly low Guidance Level for the general population. In setting the level at 4 mg/day, the committee stated, "No uncertainty factor is required as the NOAEL [obtained from the Vieregge study] is based on a large epidemiological study." As a point of information, the Nurses' Health Study was a large epidemiological study, enrolling more than 85,000 participants. The Beaver Dam Eye Study was a medium-sized epidemiological study, enrolling more than 3,000 participants. In contrast, in the Vieregge study, there were only 41 subjects in the high-manganese group, making it a very small epidemiological study. In its evaluation of the biotin, riboflavin, and pantothenic acid research, the EVM reduced the NOAEL by an uncertainty factor of ten, in part because only small numbers of subjects had been studied. Considering that more subjects were evaluated in the pantothenic acid research[10] (n=94) than in the Vieregge study (n=41), it would seem appropriate also to use an uncertainty factor for the manganese data. Applying an uncertainty factor of ten to the Vieregge study would have produced an absurdly low Guidance Level of 0.4 mg/day for supplemental manganese, which is well below the amount present in a typical diet (approximately 4 mg/day) and which can be obtained by drinking several sips of tea. Parenthetically, in a study of 47,351 male health professionals, drinking large amounts of tea (a major dietary source of manganese) was associated with a reduced risk of Parkinson's disease, not an increased risk.[11] In changing its methodology to avoid reaching an indefensible conclusion, the EVM revealed the arbitrary and inconsistent nature of its evaluation process.

Niacin (Vitamin B_3) Guidance Level

Large doses of niacin can cause elevated liver function tests and, rarely, other significant side effects. The EVM focused its evaluation, however, on the niacin-induced skin flush, which occurs at much lower doses. The niacin flush is a sensation of warmth on the skin—often associated with itching, burning, or irritation—that occurs after the ingestion of niacin and disappears relatively quickly. It appears to be mediated in part by the release of prostaglandins. The niacin flush is not considered a toxic effect per se, and there is no evidence that it causes any harm. People who do not like the flush are free not to take niacin supplements or products that contain niacin. For those who are unaware that niacin causes a flush, an appropriate warning label on the bottle would provide adequate protection.

Granting, for the sake of argument, that the niacin flush is an adverse effect from which the public should be protected, the EVM's Guidance Level still is illogical. The committee noted that flushing is consistently observed at a dose of 50 mg/day, which it established as the LOAEL. That dose was reduced by an uncertainty factor of three, in order to extrapolate the LOAEL to a NOAEL. Thus, the Guidance Level was set at 17 mg/day, which approximates the RDA for the vitamin. The EVM also noted, however, that flushing has been reported at doses as low as 10 mg, so the true LOAEL is 10 mg/day. Applying the same uncertainty factor of three to the true LOAEL would have yielded a Guidance Level of a paltry 3.3 mg/day, which probably is not enough to prevent an anorexic person from developing pellagra. As with manganese, the EVM applied its methodology in an arbitrary and inconsistent manner, so as to avoid being faced with an embarrassing result.

Vitamin C Guidance Level

The EVM concluded that vitamin C does not cause significant adverse effects, although gastrointestinal (GI) side effects may occur with high doses. The committee therefore set a Guidance Level based on a NOAEL for GI side effects. It is true that taking too much vitamin C, just like eating too many apples, may cause abdominal pain or diarrhea. The dose at which vitamin C causes GI side effects varies widely from person to person, but can easily be determined by each individual. Moreover, these side effects can be eliminated by reducing the dose. Most people who take vitamin C supplements know how much they can tolerate; for those who do not, a simple warning on bottles of vitamin C would appear to provide the public all the protection it needs. Considering the many health benefits of vitamin C, attempting to dumb down the dose to a level that will prevent the last stomachache in Europe is not a worthwhile goal. However, as mentioned previously, the EVM was instructed to ignore the benefits of vitamin C.

Granting, for the sake of argument, that there is value in setting a Guidance Level for GI side effects, the EVM did a rather poor job of setting that level. The committee established the LOAEL at 3,000 mg/day, based on a study of a small number of normal volunteers.[12] An uncertainty factor of three was used to extrapolate from the LOAEL to a NOAEL, resulting in a Guidance Level of 1,000 mg/day. However, anyone practicing nutritional medicine knows that some patients experience abdominal pain or diarrhea at vitamin C doses of 1,000 mg/day or less, and the EVM did acknowledge that GI side effects have been reported at doses of 1,000 mg. It is disingenuous to set a NOAEL and then to concede that effects do occur at the no-effect level. To be consistent with the methodology it used for other nutrients, the committee should have set the LOAEL at 1,000 mg/day, and reduced it by a factor of three to arrive at a NOAEL of 333 mg/day. The EVM was no doubt aware of the credibility problems it would have faced had it suggested that half the world is currently overdosing on vitamin C. To resolve its dilemma, the committee used a scientifically unjustifiable route to arrive at a seemingly politically expedient outcome.

Conclusion

These and other examples from the report demonstrate that the EVM applied its methodology in an arbitrary and inconsistent manner, thereby arriving at "safety" recommendations that are excessively and inappropriately restrictive. While the directive to evaluate only the risks, and to ignore the benefits, of nutritional supplements created a rigged game, the members of the EVM appeared to be willing participants in that game.

If the EVM report is used to relegate currently available nutritional supplements to prescription-only status, then millions of people would be harmed, and very few would benefit. It would be of little consolation that the higher doses of vitamins and minerals could still be obtained with a doctor's prescription, because most doctors know less about nutrition than do many of their patients. Moreover, the overburdened health care system is in no position to take on the job of gatekeeper of the vitamin cabinet; nor is there any need for it to do so.

Ironically, as flawed as the EVM report is, its recommendations may ultimately prove to be "as good as it gets" in Europe. Other European countries are recommending that maximum permitted levels be directly linked to multiples of the RDA, which could result in limits for some nutrients being set substantially lower than those suggested in the EVM report. While some nutritional supplements can cause adverse effects in certain clinical situations or at certain doses, appropriate warning labels on vitamin and mineral products would provide ample protection against most of those risks.

REFERENCES FOR "'SAFE UPPER LEVELS'"

1. Expert Group on Vitamins and Minerals. Safe Upper Levels for vitamins and minerals, 2003, p. 28. Available at: http://www.food.gov.uk/multimedia/pdfs/vitmin2003.pdf.

2. Schoenen J, Jacquy J, Lenaerts M. Effectiveness of high-dose riboflavin in migraine prophylaxis. A randomized controlled trial. *Neurology* 1998;50:466–470.

3. Gaby AR. The safe use of vitamin B_6. *J Nutr Med* 1990; 1: 153–157.

4. Schaumburg H, Kaplan J, Windebank A, et al. Sensory neuropathy from pyridoxine abuse: A new megavitamin syndrome. *N Engl J Med* 1983; 309: 445–448.

5. Parry GJ. Sensory neuropathy with low-dose pyridoxine. *Neurology* 1985; 35: 1466–1468.

6. Parry GJ. Personal communication, July 14, 1986.

7. Nielsen FH. Ultratrace minerals. In: Shils ME, Olson JA, Shike M (eds.), *Modern Nutrition in Health and Disease,* 8th Edition, Philadelphia: Lea & Febiger, 1994, 276.

8. Kondakis XG, Makris N, Leotsinidis M, et al. Possible health effects of high manganese concentration in drinking water. *Arch Environ Health* 1989; 44: 175–178.

9. Vieregge P, Heinzow B, Korf G, et al. Long term exposure to manganese in rural well water has no neurological effects. *Can J Neurol Sci* 1995; 22: 286–289.

10. Calcium pantothenate in arthritic conditions: A report from the General Practitioner Research Group. *Practitioner* 1980; 224: 208–211.

11. Ascherio A, Zhang SM, Hernan MA, et al. Prospective study of caffeine consumption and risk of Parkinson's disease in men and women. *Ann Neurol* 2001; 50: 56–63.

12. Cameron E, Campbell A. The orthomolecular treatment of cancer. II. Clinical trial of high dose ascorbic acid supplements in advanced human cancer. *Chem Biol Interact* 1974; 9: 285–315.

CHAPTER 6

Vitamin C

"Vitamin C has already been researched more than any other supplement or pharmaceutical drug in the history of the planet. Don't allow another 70 years of research to transpire before its proper use begins."

—THOMAS LEVY, MD

Introduction to Vitamin C

When I was a kid, the first lesson I learned about good health was to look both ways before crossing the street. The second was to take vitamin C and lots of it. We took it all the time: at breakfast, at lunch in school, when we got home, and at dinner. We took it when we were well, and when we were sick we took more. If someone so much as sneezed in our house, my father's voice could be heard reverberating through the walls: "Take C!" And we would. We learned, at a very young age, when we *needed* extra C, and when we didn't. Most memorably, we learned that high-dose vitamin C made us feel better.

My parents weren't just making this stuff up. We were doing in practice what medical doctors like Robert F. Cathcart and Frederick R. Klenner, and Linus Pauling, PhD, knew to be true from clinical experience, and more recently, what doctors like Thomas Levy, MD, Suzanne Humphries, MD, and Steve Hickey, PhD, have confirmed.

Vitamin C Works

"Orthomolecular practitioners know that with therapeutic nutrition, you don't take the amount that you believe ought to work; rather, you take the amount that gets results. The first rule of building a brick wall is that you must have enough bricks."

—ANDREW W. SAUL, PHD

When you have kids, everything is an experiment the first time around. And while my dad knew about bowel tolerance of vitamin C, he had yet to give us such large doses. I was the honorary guinea pig.

It all started when I was four. Take one desperate dad (mine) and add one child coughing ceaselessly for hours into the night and ta da! "Bowel tolerance" of vitamin C became a part of our lives thenceforth.

I distinctly remember being awoken at night and walked to the kitchen to take C. Dad poured a heaping teaspoon of ascorbic acid crystals into orange juice, swirled it around a bit, handed it to me, and simply said, "Scarf it."

Down it went. We had always taken C, but not this much. It tasted kind of bitter, like lemonade, and soothed my sore throat. Shortly thereafter, my coughing stopped. And my fitful night's rest became deep sleep, and my father enjoyed the same.

Several hours later when coughing began again, down the hatch went more vitamin C. Then I slept until morning.

We were sick only occasionally (far less often than our friends), and when we took vitamin C to bowel tolerance, we got better more quickly. We were also more comfortable. Children can be downright miserable when they are sick. Adults too. Taking high doses of vitamin C made us feel better while we got better. As soon as we reached bowel tolerance, coughing would wane, body aches would be relieved, sneezing would stop, fevers would go down, and our moods would elevate. We kept our intake of vitamin C high, and for days if needed, and then without drugs and without antibiotics, we got better. In fact, we never needed any prescriptions or over-the-counter medicines. I never needed acetaminophen until I had my wisdom teeth out. I did not take a single dose of any antibiotic until I was a college student.

My family still takes high-dose vitamin C. My children know they will get it every day, several times a day, and when they're sick, they get it as often as every hour. The sensation of malaise (the feeling of something "coming on") is enough in our house to warrant increased doses of vitamin C.

Take C at the FIRST Sign of Sickness

"Few diseases become a problem when the nutrition is improved the minute the first symptom is noticed."

—ADELLE DAVIS, *LET'S GET WELL*

In our house, illness rarely ends up in a statement like "I have the flu." We like to target sickness before it is a problem. We take high-dose vitamin C at the first sign of sickness: a cough or sneeze, runny nose, sore throat, or feeling of malaise.

An important key to tackling illness is to get to it early. All nutrients are important when addressing illness, but especially vitamin C. Take C *before* there is a big problem. Don't wait to get to the point where you feel so awful you must finally resolve to go to the doctor and get a prescription. Ideally, we get on top of symptoms so fast with high-dose C, sickness doesn't stand a chance.

Taking vitamin C at the first sign of sickness has also taught us how to monitor and adjust to our own body's need for vitamin C based on how we feel. My husband takes more when he travels and is feeling stress. I take more if I feel overly lethargic or "off." Even my young children have a sense for when they need more C.

We take larger preventive doses of vitamin C, too. If we know we are going to be around someone else who is sick, we load up. We take C all the time. When in doubt, we take more. My kids have yet to need an antibiotic. We know that in large doses not only does high-dose C work like an antibiotic, but also as an antiviral, antihistamine, antitoxin, and antipyretic. Pretty much any illness you can readily think of improves with high-dose vitamin C. We have certainly found this to be true in our family.

Antibiotic-Resistant Pathogens? Take C!

"Massive doses of ascorbate assist the immune system to kill bacteria within the body but also have the ability to kill bacteria by some mechanism that does not seem to involve the immune system. These bacteria and L-forms of bacteria hide out in cells, especially when antibiotics are used, and explain some of the resis-

tance acquired by bacteria against antibiotics. I have yet to see bacteria that can become resistant to massive doses of ascorbate in combination with first- and second-generation antibiotics. Admittedly in a private practice, I do not see the most resistant bacteria, but this combination has been impressive and deserves to be tried against the most resistant bacteria. It may solve the impending problem of increasingly resistant bacteria."

—ROBERT F. CATHCART, MD

Getting to Saturation of C

"The most important factor in the treatment of any virus with vitamin C is to give enough, for a long enough period of time."

—THOMAS LEVY, MD

Normally, I take 8,000 to 10,000 milligrams (mg) of vitamin C every day. When I am sick I can take 8,000 to 10,000 mg an hour before I reach saturation or bowel tolerance, which means exactly what you think it means. Robert F. Cathcart, MD, explains: "Bowel tolerance doses are the amounts of ascorbic acid tolerated orally that almost, but not quite, cause diarrhea." When I'm not feeling well, first I start off with a loading dose of 8,000 to10,000 mg of vitamin C all at once. Then, I wait about an hour. If I still feel awful, and I haven't reached saturation, I take another 8,000 mg or so. Better yet, I take a smaller amount of vitamin C every fifteen minutes (2,000 mg or so) until I feel my stomach rumble, a sign that I'm getting close to saturation. Sometimes it takes several hours, or all day, before I start to get a rumbling tummy. I know that the longer it takes to get to saturation with high-dose C, the sicker I am, and the more I can hold. I don't quit after a couple of doses. I stay with it until I am completely better. This may take an afternoon, it may take days. But you continue to take enough C to get the job done.

If I were feeling fine, huge doses of C like that would have me on the toilet in no time. Sick bodies can hold an extraordinary amount of vitamin C. If you have been told differently, you have been told wrong. Once I do manage to get to saturation or loose stool, I throttle back the dose. I continue to take C, but I take less. At saturation, I generally feel better as some symptoms wane. But if they start to come back, I take more C. Once I get to saturation again, I take less. The symptoms of sickness are inversely related to how much C I am taking. The goal is to take as much C as possible without experiencing loose stool. If you do, it's not a problem. Take less C and make sure you drink plenty of water. This is the way I have been getting better from being sick for my entire life. It allows me to avoid taking antibiotics, antivirals, and antihistamines. I still go to the doctor. I just don't take the medication they prescribe. I use vitamin C instead.

How Much Vitamin C Should I Take?

How much vitamin C you should take depends on one thing: you. There is strong consensus among orthomolecular physicians that healthy individuals should take at least 1,000 to 2,000 mg of supplemental vitamin C each day. Frederick R. Klenner, MD, recommended that children get 1,000 mg of vitamin C per year of age up to a routine total dose of 10,000 mg per day. Double Nobel laureate Dr. Linus Pauling himself, author of *How to Live Longer and Feel Better,* took 6,000 to 18,000 mg of vitamin C per day. Far more is required when the body is sick or stressed. Robert F. Cathcart, MD, gave therapeutic doses of vitamin C up to 200,000 mg per day. Dr. Klenner gave up to an astounding 300,000 mg per day.

Oxidative Stress and Vitamin C

"In order to cure infections, an agent is needed to neutralize ongoing oxidative stress, repair oxidized molecules, and kill the pathogens, or at least render them more susceptible to eradication by a healthy immune system. Vitamin C does all of these things."

—THOMAS LEVY, MD

Among vitamin C's many benefits for maintaining a strong and healthy immune system, understanding oxidative stress may help us understand why vitamin C works so well to resolve illness. "At the cellular level, all chronic diseases are characterized by increased oxidative stress," says Dr. Thomas E. Levy. "No exceptions. And whenever there is increased oxidative stress, or oxidation, there is decreased antioxidant capacity." This is where nutrients come in, particularly vitamin C.

"At the molecular level, all quality nutrients share one common trait: they ultimately are antioxidant in nature, donating electrons or causing electrons to be donated to oxidized molecules," says Dr. Levy. "When increased oxidative stress is quenched in this manner, disease resolves. Vitamin C just ends up being especially important because its small size and biochemical nature allows it to reach so many cells by itself, along with its unique ability to regenerate (reduce) so many other important antioxidants after they have donated their electrons and become oxidized."

"However," says Dr. Levy, "even though increased oxidative stress is always the final common denominator in all chronic diseases, finding the ways to prevent and relieve this increased oxidative stress is not as simple. The reasons that the increased oxidative stress is present must be eliminated or severely curtailed, while balancing hormones and ingesting a wide range of antioxidant nutrients with enough biochemical variation that all tissues and cell types are affected."

When in Doubt, Take C

"Ascorbic acid is the safest and most valuable substance available to the physician."

—FREDERICK R. KLENNER, MD

I believe the most important thing you can know about orthomolecular medicine is how to use very high doses of vitamin C to cure illness. We all know about eating right, but precious few know about bowel tolerance of vitamin C. The word is getting out. There is a way to get better without drugs, and a safer way. There is a way to stay better without drugs. There is a way to not get sick in the first place.

You don't have to take my word for it. Robert F. Cathcart, III, MD, discovered how bowel tolerance works. Simply put, the sicker you are, the more vitamin C you can hold. Back in the 1940s, Frederick Robert Klenner, MD, was using massive doses of vitamin C to cure disease. It is time that everyone get to read about these physicians' important contributions to nutritional therapeutics.

If you haven't yet read the work of orthomolecular pioneers Dr. Klenner and Dr. Cathcart, here's your chance. Included in this chapter are what I and many people believe to be some of the most important papers ever written about high-dose vitamin C. Too few people have had access to them. It's time for a change.

THE THIRD FACE OF VITAMIN C

by Robert F. Cathcart, MD

From *J Orthomolecular Med* 1992; 7(4): 197–200.

Introduction

Clinical experience prescribing doses of ascorbic acid up to 200,000 or more milligrams (mg) per 24 hours to over 20,000 patients during the past 23-year period has revealed its clinical usefulness in all diseases involving oxidation damage from free radicals. The controversy continues over the value of vitamin C mainly because inadequate doses are used for most free-radical-scavenging purposes. Paradoxically, the non-controversial use of minute doses of vitamin C in the prevention and treatment of scurvy has set the minds of many against more creative uses.

Vitamin C has differing benefits in increasing dose ranges. Its usefulness is in three such distinct realms that I will describe them as the three faces of vitamin C.

Face 1. vitamin C to prevent scurvy (up to 65 mg per day)

Face 2. vitamin C to prevent acute induced scurvy[1,2] and to augment vitamin C functions (1,000 to 20,000 mg per day)

Face 3. vitamin C to provide reducing equivalents (30,000 to 200,000 or more mg per day)[3]

One might criticize the wisdom of my use of these massive doses but Frederick Klenner, MD, had previously used large doses intravenously.[4–7] The works of Irwin Stone, PhD, [8–10] Linus Pauling, PhD,[11–13] and Archie Kalokerinos, MD,[14] have supported many of my observations. In all published studies yielding negative or equivocal results, inadequate doses were used. In some studies, doses barely bordering on adequate tease the investigator with statistically significant but not very impressive beneficial results.

My early discovery was that the *bowel tolerance* to ascorbic acid of a person with a healthy GI tract was somewhat proportional to the toxicity of their disease.[15] Bowel tolerance doses are the amounts of ascorbic acid tolerated orally that almost, but not quite, cause a marked loosening of stools. A patient who could tolerate orally 10,000 to 15,000 mg of ascorbic acid per 24 hours when well, might be able to tolerate 30,000 to 60,000 mg per 24 hours if he had a mild cold, 100,000 mg with a severe cold, 150,000 mg with influenza, and 200,000 mg or more per 24 hours with mononucleosis or viral pneumonia.[1,2] Marked clinical benefits in these conditions occur only at the bowel tolerance or higher levels. I named the process whereby the patient determined the proper dose as "titrating to bowel tolerance." These increases in bowel tolerance in the vast majority of patients normally tolerant to ascorbic acid (perhaps 80 percent of patients) are invariable. The marked clinical benefits are noted only when a threshold dose, usually close to the bowel tolerance dose, is consumed. I call this benefit the "ascorbate effect."

Most patients are started at first with hourly doses of ascorbic acid powder dissolved in small amounts of water. Later, after the patient has learned to accurately estimate the dose necessary to achieve the ascorbate effect, comparable doses of ascorbic acid tablets or capsules are also used. Where patients are intolerant to adequate amounts of ascorbic acid orally and the severity of the disease warrants it, intravenous sodium ascorbate is used.

Failures are related to individual difficulties in taking the proper adequate doses. In patients who tolerate adequate doses, the results are almost invariably as described. I now have had 23 years to gather clinical experience and to reflect on this phenomenon.[16–19]

I want to emphasize the importance of increasing bowel tolerance with increasing toxicities of diseases. The sensation of detoxification one experiences at these doses is unmistakable. The effect is so reliable and dramatic in the tolerant patient as to make obvious the fact that something very important, that has not been widely appreciated before, is going on.

The Three Faces

Vitamin C probably always functions by being an electron donor. At the lowest dose level (up to 65 mg per day), it is necessary as a vitamin to prevent scurvy. It is essential for certain metabolic functions which are well described and mostly noncontroversial.

At the second level (the second face) vitamin C is still used as a vitamin, but larger doses are necessary to maintain its basic functions because the vitamin is destroyed rapidly in diseased or injured tissues where there is an overabundance of free radicals. When an ascorbate molecule gives up two reducing equivalents (available electrons) to neutralize free radicals, it becomes dehydroascorbate (DHA). If DHA (a relatively unstable form of ascorbate) is not rapidly rereduced by reducing equivalents from the mitochondria (site of energy production within the cell), the DHA is irreversibly lost. I describe the resulting state of deficiency, if the vitamin C is not replaced, as "acute induced scurvy."[12] There is ample evidence of this depletion of vitamin C by stress and disease, as recently reviewed in the literature.[20]

Additionally, the recent extensive research on vitamin C has concerned itself with certain functions that may be augmented by higher than minimal doses of vitamin C.[20] Strangely, any usefulness of these larger than minimal doses of vitamin C remain mostly neglected by clinicians. This level is from about 1,000 to 20,000 mg a day. Benefits vary from person to person.

At this second level, as in studies reviewed by Pauling[11] and more recently by

Harri Hemilä, MD, PhD,[20] there may be expected a slight decrease in the incidence of colds but a more significant reduction in the complications and the duration of colds. Personally, I am impressed by the number of patients (but certainly not all) who tell me that they have not had a cold for years since reading Pauling's book *Vitamin C and the Common Cold and Flu* (1976) and beginning to take vitamin C. Patients with chronic infections frequently have their infections cured for the first time. Antibiotics work synergistically with these doses. A surprising number of elderly persons benefit from doses of this magnitude and may indeed have what Irwin Stone described as chronic subclinical scurvy.[10]

The highest dose level (the third face) is virtually undiscussed in the literature but is the most interesting. These doses range usually from 30,000 to 200,000 mg or more per 24 hours. The most important concept to understand is that while incidentally at these dose levels the vitamin C performs all the functions of levels one and two, it is mostly thrown away for the reducing equivalents it carries.[3] With these doses it is possible to saturate the body with reducing equivalents, neutralize the excessive free radicals, and drive a reducing redox potential into involved tissues. Inflammations mediated by free radicals can be eliminated or markedly reduced. In many instances patients with allergies or autoimmune diseases have their humoral immunity (antibody meditated) controlled while their cellular immunity is augmented.[19] To the extent that free radicals are either essential to the perpetuation of a disease or just part of the cause of symptoms, the disease will be cured or just ameliorated. The list of diseases involving free radicals continues to grow. Infections, cardiovascular diseases, cancer, trauma, burns both thermal and radiation, surgeries, allergies, autoimmune diseases, and aging are now included. It is more difficult to think of a disease that does not involve free radicals.

> *"With vitamin C, research has shown that the more that is taken into the body, the greater is the amount retained and used by the body."*
>
> —ABRAM HOFFER, MD, PHD, AND JONATHAN PROUSKY, ND, *NATUROPATHIC NUTRITION*

Progressive nutritionists routinely give vitamin C, vitamin E, beta-carotene, selenium, N-acetylcysteine (NAC), and other antioxidant compounds to counter free radicals. I certainly agree with this practice. However, there is one important concept being neglected which results in these nutrients not being as effective as described.

In the spirit that if you throw a bucket of water on a fire, it is the water that puts the fire out, not the bucket, it is the reducing equivalents carried by the free-radical scavengers that quench the free radicals, not the free-radical scavenger itself.

Dietary free-radical scavengers carry in on ingestion only a small percentage of the total reducing equivalents carried by those scavengers during their lifetime in the body. After their first pass neutralizing free radicals, the free-radical scavenger must be recharged with reducing equivalents made available in the mitochondria.

The problem in inflamed tissues or in patients with severe illnesses is not so much that all the free-radical scavengers have been lost (although they may be lost); the problem is more that the mitochondria cannot furnish the reducing equivalents fast enough to rereduce adequate amounts of free-radical scavengers. The dynamic nature of this process must be emphasized. When free radicals injure cells, particularly their mitochondria, more free radicals are formed, and some injure adjacent cells. An inflammatory cascade results. Without enough reducing equivalents being provided by glycolysis in the mitochondria and the continuing rereduction of free-radical scavengers, the inflammatory cascade cannot be properly contained.

Early in this study a 23-year-old, 98-pound librarian with severe mononucleosis claimed to have taken 2 heaping tablespoons every two hours, consuming a full pound of ascorbic acid in two days without it producing diarrhea. She felt mostly well in three to four days, although she had to continue about 20,000 to 30,000 mg a day for about two months. Subsequently, all my young mononucleosis patients with excellent GI tracts have responded similarly and have had equivalent increases in bowel tolerance during the acute state of the disease. What is important here is the magnitude of this increased bowel tolerance.

I believe that the loose stools caused by excessive doses of ascorbic acid orally ingested are due to a resulting hypertonicity of ascorbate in the rectum. Water is attracted into the rectum by the increased osmotic pressure and results in a loosening of the stools. With toxic illnesses, the ascorbate is destroyed rapidly in the involved tissues, and this results in a rapid absorption of ascorbate from the gut. Of the ascorbate, what does not reach the rectum, does not cause diarrhea. Intravenous sodium ascorbate does not cause diarrhea and, in fact, increases bowel tolerance to orally ingested ascorbic acid while the IV is running. With hypertonicity of the ascorbate both in the blood and in the rectum, the osmotic pressure of the ascorbate is closer to equal on both sides of the bowel wall, so no diarrhea results. If the diarrhea was caused by other metabolic processes, diarrhea would be caused by intravenous ascorbate.

"Since I've learned to use vitamin C, I found that not only has my own health become extraordinarily better, but my prescription writing has gone down significantly, and the health of my patients has also improved greatly."

—SUZANNE HUMPHRIES, MD, Sweden Society for Orthomolecular Medicine, ABF Stockholm, 2014

It should be noted that in some cases of pathological diarrhea, ascorbic acid *stops* the diarrhea. Presumably in these cases some of the increased destruction of ascorbate is from free radicals in the bowel. However, in most toxic systemic diseases there is no reason to believe that the destruction of the additional ascorbate tolerated occurs directly in the bowel, so it is a safe hypothesis that this increased destruction occurs in the interior of the body. The increased tolerance to ascorbic acid orally provides an interesting and somewhat useful measure of the toxicity of a disease. Probably it is somewhat a measure of the free radicals involved in a disease. I have a term for a cold that at its maximum makes it possible for a patient to just tolerate per 24 hours 100 grams (100,000 mg) of ascorbic acid orally without diarrhea; I call it a "100 gram cold." Patients, appearing to be well, who have a tolerance over 20 to 25 grams (20,000–25,000 mg) per 24 hours probably have some subclinical condition which is being hidden by their own free-radical scavenging system. Patients with chronic infections (and a normally strong stomach) can ingest enormous amounts of ascorbic acid. One of my chronic fatigue patients is functional only because of his ingestion of 65 pounds of ascorbic acid in the past 12 months. In 22 years, I, personally, have ingested approximately 361 kilos (about 797 lbs., about 4.3 times my body weight) of ascorbic acid because of chronic allergies and perhaps chronic Epstein-Barr virus.

Considering the reducing equivalents carried by such amounts of ascorbic acid, one can only guess at the turnover rate of the nonenzymatic free-radical scavengers in a patient acutely ill with a 200 gram (200,000 mg) mononucleosis. However, one gains the impression that all the nonenzymatic free-radical scavengers would have to be rereduced many times a day.

An Analogy

Suppose you owned a farm and on one end of the property there was a barn and on the other end of the property there was a water well. One day the barn catches fire, and neighbors come with buckets to set up a bucket brigade between the water well and the barn and are putting out the fire when the well goes dry. My use of ascorbate is like thousands of neighbors coming from miles around, each with a bucketful of their own water, throwing their own water on your fire once, and then leaving.

Conclusion

Because of the invariable (in patients tolerant to ascorbic acid) increasing bowel tolerance to ascorbic acid in patients roughly in proportion to the toxicity of their disease, there has to be something happening to ascorbate in the sick patient other than its being used as vitamin C in the classic sense. The amelioration or sometimes cure of different diseases appears related to the importance of free radicals in the perpetuation of the particular disease.

The sudden marked benefit in many disease processes, which is achieved at doses near to the bowel tolerance level, suggests that a reducing redox potential is forced into the affected tissues only at those dose levels. This ascorbate effect only at the high-dose levels is also suggestive that something other than classic functions of vitamin C is involved. This ascorbate effect is more compatible with principles of redox chemistry.

Only a small percentage of the total reducing equivalents donated by non-enzymatic free-radical scavengers to neutralize free radicals come in on the ingested nutritional free-radical scavengers. Ascorbate is unique in that the body can tolerate doses adequate to supply the necessary reducing equivalents to quench the free radicals generated by severely toxic disease processes. The vitamin C is thrown away for the reducing equivalents it carries. Only in this way can the large amounts of free radicals generated by the most toxic disease processes be rapidly quenched.

REFERENCES FOR "THE THIRD FACE OF VITAMIN C"

1. Cathcart RF. The method of determining proper doses of vitamin C for the treatment of disease by titrating to bowel tolerance. *J Orthomolecular Psych* 1981; 10:125–132.

2. Cathcart RF. Vitamin C: Titrating to bowel tolerance, anascorbemia, and acute induced scurvy. *Med Hypotheses* 1981; 7:1359–1376.

3. Cathcart RF. A unique function for ascorbate. *Med Hypotheses* 1991; 35:32–37.

4. Klenner FR. Virus pneumonia and its treatment with vitamin C. *J South Med and Surg* 1948;110: 60–63.

5. Klenner FR. The treatment of poliomyelitis and other virus diseases with vitamin C. *J South Med and Surg* 1949; 111:210–214.

6. Klenner FR. Observations on the dose and administration of ascorbic acid when employed beyond the range of a vitamin in human pathology. *J App Nutr* 1971; 23:61–88.

7. Klenner FR. Significance of high daily intake of ascorbic acid in preventive medicine. *J Int Acad Prev Med* 1974; 1:45–49.

8. Stone I. Studies of a mammalian enzyme system for producing evolutionary evidence on man. *Am J Phys Anthro* 1965; 23:83–86.

9. Stone I. Hypoascorbemia: The genetic disease causing the human requirement for exogenous ascorbic acid. *Perspect Biol Med* l966; 10:133–134.

10. Stone I. *The Healing Factor: Vitamin C Against Disease.* New York: Grosset & Dunlapp, 1972.

11. Pauling L. *Vitamin C and the Common Cold.* San Francisco: W.H. Freeman & Co, 1970.

12. Pauling L. *Vitamin C, the Common Cold, and the Flu.* San Francisco: W.H. Freeman & Co, 1976.

13. Pauling L. *How to Live Longer and Feel Better.* New York: W.H. Freeman & Co, 1986.

14. Kalokerinos A. *Every Second Child.* New Canaan, CT: Keats Publishing, 1981.

15. Cathcart RF. Clinical trial of vitamin C. Letter to the Editor. *Medical Tribune,* June 25, 1975.

16. Cathcart RF. Vitamin C in the treatment of acquired immune deficiency syndrome (AIDS). *Med Hypothesis* 1984; 14(4): 423–433.

17. Cathcart RF. Vitamin C: The non-toxic, non-rate-limited, antioxidant free-radical scavenger. *Med Hypotheses* 1985; 18:61–77.

18. Cathcart RF. HIV infection and glutathione. Letter. *Lancet* 1990; 335(8683):235.

19. Cathcart RF. The vitamin C treatment of allergy and the normally unprimed state of antibodies. *Med Hypotheses* 1986; 21(3):307–321.

20. Hemila H. Vitamin C and the common cold. *Br J Nutr* 1992; 67:3–16.

THE METHOD OF DETERMINING PROPER DOSES OF VITAMIN C FOR THE TREATMENT OF DISEASE BY TITRATING TO BOWEL TOLERANCE

by Robert F. Cathcart, MD

From *J Orthomolecular Psych* 1981; 10(2): 125–132.

My experience in utilizing vitamin C in large doses has extended over a nine-year period and has involved over 9,000 patients.[4–7] Much of the original work with large amounts of vitamin C was done by Fred R. Klenner, MD, of Reidsville, North Carolina.[11–14] Klenner found that viral diseases could be detoxified and subsequently cured by intravenous sodium ascorbate in amounts up to 200,000 milligrams (mg) per 24 hours. Irwin Stone pointed out the potential of vitamin C in the treatment of many diseases, the inability of humans to synthesize ascorbate, and the resultant condition, hypoascorbemia.[18–20] Linus Pauling reviewed the literature on vitamin C and has led the crusade to make known its medical uses to the public and the medical profession.[16–17] Ewan Cameron, in association with Pauling, has shown the usefulness of ascorbic acid in the treatment of cancer.[2–3]

The purpose of this paper is to describe a method which maximizes the effectiveness of ascorbic acid (vitamin C) taken orally for various diseases and stress processes. Much of the controversy about ascorbic acid has been due to studies utilizing totally inadequate doses of vitamin C. It seems incredible to the growing number of physicians familiar with the proper doses of ascorbic acid that recent papers would describe studies utilizing only up to 4,000 mg per 24 hours. Also, the hypothesis that not only do humans suffer from chronic hypoascorbemia, but that stress and disease can induce localized and systemic aascorbemia (a type of scurvy) will be presented.

Bowel Tolerance Method

In 1970, I discovered the sicker a patient was, the more ascorbic acid he would tolerate by mouth before diarrhea was produced. At least 80 percent of adult patients will tolerate 10,000 to 15,000 mg of ascorbic acid fine crystals in one-half cup water in four divided doses per 24 hours without having diarrhea. The astonishing finding was that almost all patients will absorb far greater amounts without having diarrhea when ill. This increased tolerance is somewhat proportional to the toxicity of the disease being treated. Tolerance is increased some by stress (e.g., anxiety, exercise, heat, cold, etc.). Admittedly, increasing the frequency of doses increases tolerance perhaps to half again as much; but the tolerance exceeding sometimes 200,000 mg per 24 hours was totally unexpected. Representative doses taken by patients titrating their ascorbic acid intake between the relief of most symptoms and the production of diarrhea are shown in Table 1:

Table 1. Usual Bowel Tolerance Doses

Condition	Milligrams (Mg) Per 24 Hours	Number of Doses Per 24 Hours
Normal, well	4,000–15,000	4–6
Mild cold	30,000–60,000	6–10
Severe cold	60,000–100,000 or more	8–15
Influenza	100,000–150,000	8–20
Echovirus, coxsackievirus	100,000–150,000	8–20
Mononucleosis	150,000–200,000 or more	12–25
Viral pneumonia	100,000–200,000 or more	12–25
Hay fever, asthma	15,000–50,000	4–8
Environmental and food allergy	500–50,000	4–8
Burn, injury, surgery	25,000–150,000	6–20
Anxiety, exercise, and other mild stresses	15,000–25,000	4–6
Cancer	15,000–100,000	4–15
Ankylosing spondylitis	15,000–100,000	4–15
Reiter's syndrome	15,000–60,000	4–10
Acute anterior uveitis	30,000–100,000	4–15
Rheumatoid arthritis	15,000–100,000	4–15
Bacterial infections	30,000–200,000 or more	10–25
Infectious hepatitis	30,000–100,000	6–15
Candidiasis	15,000–200,000 or more	6–25

It was found that maximum relief of symptoms, the most shortening of the course of the disease, and the greatest reduction in complications could be obtained by the oral doses just below the point causing diarrhea. This titration to bowel tolerance (the amount and timing of doses) is usually easily sensed by the patient. In many conditions, symptoms are markedly suppressed but will return rapidly if the dose levels are not maintained long enough. In the case of very toxic diseases, doses may have to be taken every half hour. Even short delays in taking these doses may prolong the disease. The necessary duration of treatment is usually also easily sensed by patients.

Aascorbemia

The term "aascorbemia" is coined to mean complete absence of ascorbate from the blood. It accompanies the acutely and chronically induced scurvy.

The object of this titration to bowel tolerance is to eliminate the toxicity of the disease and to maintain a high level of ascorbate in all tissues of the body, especially the tissues directly involved by the disease process. Bearing in mind that almost continuous sipping of ascorbic acid would be optimum (especially with the more toxic diseases), for practical purposes compromising to the number of doses listed in Table 1 often suffices. Apparently, there is an almost unbelievable and unappreciated potential draw by diseased tissues on ascorbic acid. Only by fully satisfying this need of stressed tissues can the condition of aascorbemia and localized scurvy be absolutely prevented. Fully satisfying this need probably accounts for the striking amelioration of symptoms just before bowel tolerance is reached. This need for ascorbate is probably the reason many toxic diseases or stressful situations produce complications or even secondary diseases later on. The induced aascorbemia may predispose a patient to pneumonia, heart attacks, phlebitis, Guillian-Barre syndrome, and perhaps rheumatoid arthritis and cancer.

It is my custom to speak of 20- to 100-gram colds, etc. A 100-gram cold would mean that the patient is capable of ingesting 100 grams (100,000 mg) of ascorbic acid per 24 hours at the peak of the disease. In the case of systemic viral infections, it is often more important to properly estimate what gram disease it is and persuade the patient to take adequate doses than to know what virus is being treated. A patient who learns to start titrating at the earliest symptoms of a disease will have the best results. Nevertheless, adequate doses will usually reduce symptoms even late in the disease.

By this method large amounts of ascorbate are spilled into the urine, but this is necessary to push adequate amounts of ascorbate into the tissues of the very seat of the disease and maintain full vitamin C functions. One who argues that ascorbate can have no effect above renal (kidney) threshold misses the point entirely and would, I suppose, maintain that one could not become more intoxicated on ethyl alcohol above renal threshold. Also, large amounts of ascorbate in the urine will prevent many kidney and bladder infections.

In the case of the more toxic conditions, half-hourly doses may be necessary. Absorption and presumably destruction of ascorbate occur so rapidly as to require this frequency of doses for adequate amounts of ascorbic acid to keep the diseased tissues saturated without requiring too-large doses that produce diarrhea. Even short delays in taking these doses may prolong the disease and reduce the effectiveness of ascorbic acid in blocking symptoms.

Infants and children tolerate ascorbic acid remarkably. I encourage the use of water rather than juice because the unsweetened taste aids in helping the patient select the proper dose. Juice is allowed only if the child refuses doses otherwise. Children ten years old take adult doses; most teenagers take half again as much as adults. Older adults often tolerate ascorbic acid less well and more frequently require intravenous (IV) ascorbate. Young children refusing to take oral ascorbic acid often will subsequently take oral doses after intramuscular (IM) injections of ascorbate. Although this method of persuasion seems cruel, it is better than the complications of serious diseases and probably hurts no more than a penicillin shot.

> *"I have never seen a serious reaction to vitamin supplements. Since 1969 I have taken over two tons of ascorbic acid myself. I have put over 20,000 patients on bowel tolerance doses of ascorbic acid without any serious problems, and with great benefit."*
>
> —ROBERT F. CATHCART, MD

IM and IV Injections

Per milligram intravenous and intramuscular sodium ascorbate is more effective than oral ascorbic acid.[11,14] Solutions of sodium ascorbate, at 250 mg per cubic centimeter (cc) with no preservative except for ethylenediaminetetraacetic acid (EDTA) must be used. The volume of a single IM injection can be as much as one could give as a saline shot. Usually 2 cc are used; sometimes a little more, sometimes in two sites. The object of the intramuscular injection is to avert a crisis, break the fever, etc. Usually very rapid conversion to oral doses is possible.

In adults, intravenous injections can be made with the same 250 mg per cc solutions in pushes of 10 cc or very slowly up to 50 cc. Care is necessary here to make sure that the vein does not hurt as the injection is made and that the patient does not dehydrate or have tetany (muscle spasm). IV bottles can be prepared by using lactated Ringer's, one half normal saline, or normal saline, and diluting solutions to 60,000 mg sodium ascorbate per liter. At this concentration, sterile water can be used but care must be taken to make absolutely sure straight sterile water is never given.

These solutions can be run in two to eight hours for a liter. It is my experience that sodium ascorbate intravenously in an edematous patient will usually act as a diuretic. However, one should think about the sodium and examine the patient frequently. The most frequent difficulty is dehydration or tetany from running solutions too rapidly. Oral water will prevent dehydration. A 10 cc vial of calcium gluconate (1,000 mg) should be added to one bottle per day if solutions are run for longer than one day. Remember that most patients will convert to oral doses of ascorbic acid rapidly. In some cases, such as severe viral or bacterial pneumonias, one may want to give IV solutions of ascorbate at the same time that oral doses are being given.

Mononucleosis

Mononucleosis, an infectious viral disease, responds dramatically to ascorbic acid although the doses required can be very high. Early in this study a 23-year-old, 98-pound-female librarian with severe mononucleosis claimed to have taken two heaping tablespoons every two hours, consuming a full pound of ascorbic acid in two days. She felt mostly well in three to four days, although she had to continue about 20,000 to 30,000 mg a day for about two months. Most cases do not require maintenance doses for more than two to three weeks. The duration of need can be sensed by the patient. Professional ski patrol patients can be back on the slopes in a week. I care mostly that they carry their bota bags full of ascorbic acid in solution on the hills with them so as to keep the disease detoxified almost completely while the infection persists. Lymph nodes and the spleen return to normal rapidly.

Viral Hepatitis

Viral hepatitis (inflammation of the liver) of all types (A, B, and C), in my experience, is one of the easiest diseases for ascorbic acid to cure. A difficulty is that hepatitis often causes diarrhea; so titrating to bowel tolerance is more difficult. However, with experience one judges what milligram disease it is and gives this amount regardless of diarrhea. This amount could be from 40,000 to 100,000 mg. It soon becomes obvious whether it is the disease or the ascorbic acid causing the diarrhea. There is usually a paradoxical stopping of the diarrhea within a day or two. If too much difficulty is experienced in judging the dosages, intravenous ascorbate is extremely effective. Stools and urine return to normal color within two to three days in acute cases. Chronic cases take longer but in my experience respond rapidly. In acute cases the patient will usually feel fairly well in two to four days, but it usually takes the jaundice about six days to clear. There would appear to be a staining of the skin that persists even though physical findings and laboratory results return rapidly to normal. Liver function test values that are so high as to be unmeasurable, rapidly fall and reflect objectively the subjective feelings of the patient.

Gastroenteritis

Gastroenteritis of viral origin (stomach flu) responds very rapidly, but one must titrate boldly and anticipate paradoxical stopping of the diarrhea. If titration starts in the first hour of the disease, experienced ascorbic acid takers may never develop the diarrhea and only suspect what they have avoided because of the disease being epidemic. These diseases may require 60,000 to 150,000 mg of ascorbic acid to almost totally block symptoms. If a patient overtitrates and develops diarrhea from the ascorbic acid, the change in character of the diarrhea to a relatively painless, less foul, more watery diarrhea, and a generalized relief of malaise signals that the doses should be lowered.

Other acute self-limiting viral diseases respond similarly when the patient titrates properly. Antihistamines and decongestants should be used when appropriate.

Belfield and Stone have observed similar results in veterinary medicine with usually fatal viral diseases when intravenous ascorbate is utilized.[1]

Bacterial Infections

Ascorbic acid should be used in conjunction with the appropriate antibiotic. The effect of ascorbic acid is synergistic with antibiotics and would appear to broaden the spectrum of antibiotics considerably. The incidence of allergic reaction to penicillin in patients "saturated" with ascorbate is almost zero. One must understand that ascorbate does not always effectively protect against allergic reactions until the patient has titrated up to bowel tolerance. If a patient has an allergic reaction to penicillin before bowel tolerance is reached, subsequent saturation with ascorbate in conjunction with usual medications will more rapidly than expected resolve the reaction. It is especially interesting that mononucleosis would appear to cause more rapid destruction of ascorbate than other commonly encountered viral diseases. The high incidence of allergic reaction to penicillin in patients mistakenly given penicillin when they have mononucleosis is usually prevented by saturation with ascorbic acid. It is probable that this high incidence of allergic reaction to penicillin in mononucleosis patients is due to the tremendous draw on ascorbate by the disease. It has been my experience the indications for ampicillin are markedly reduced by ascorbic acid.

Candida Albicans

Candida (yeast) infections occur less frequently in patients being treated with antibiotics if bowel tolerance doses of ascorbic acid are simultaneously used. Antibiotics, which kill beneficial bacteria along with harmful ones, allow *Candida albicans* overgrowth. Ascorbic acid seems to have little effect on established candida infections. It should be used, nevertheless, to help the patient with the stress of the disease.

Fungus Infections

Although ascorbic acid should be given in some form in some way to all sick patients to help them meet the stress of the disease, it is my experience that ascorbate has little effect on the primary fungal infection. It will probably be found that certain complications can be reduced in incidence. It may be found that appropriate antifungal agents will better penetrate tissues that have been saturated in ascorbate.

Trauma, Surgery

Swelling and pain from trauma and surgery are markedly reduced by bowel tolerance doses of ascorbic acid. Doses should be given a minimum of six times a day. More major surgeries should require IV sodium ascorbate postoperatively. The effect of ascorbate on anesthetics should be studied. Barbiturates and many narcotics are blocked. Refer to the work of Libby and Stone.[15] The need for these substances postoperatively is greatly reduced.

Cancer

I have avoided the treatment of cancer patients for legal reasons; however, I have given nutritional consults to a number of cancer patients and have observed an increased bowel tolerance to ascorbic acid. Were I treating cancer patients, I would not limit their ascorbic acid ingestion to a set amount but would titrate them to bowel tolerance. Dr. Cameron's advice against giving cancer patients with widespread metastasis large amounts of ascorbate too rapidly at first should be heeded. He found that sometimes extensive necrosis or hemorrhage of the cancer could kill the patient if the vitamin was started too rapidly in patients with widespread metastasis. Hopefully, ascorbic acid will become the first treatment given cancer patients and not the last. The nutritional treatment of cancer should not be limited to ascorbic acid.

Stress and Disease in General

After considerable experience with patients in stressful situations and with diseases producing stress, it is my opinion that saturation with ascorbate continuously has markedly reduced the incidence of secondary complications.[7] It is difficult to prove, but it is my definite impression that the incidence of disease months following stress is reduced.

Allergies

Hay fever and asthma are most frequently benefited. Sometimes, pantothenic acid and/or pyridoxine (vitamin B_6) are helpful in acting synergistically with ascorbic acid. Frequently, hay fever and asthma are benefited at dose levels lower and more comfortable than bowel tolerance doses. However, treatment should be begun with bowel tolerance doses at least six times a day so that the response of some more difficult cases will not be missed.

Back Pain from Disc Disease

Greenwood observed that 1,000 mg a day would reduce the incidence of necessary surgery on discs.[8] At bowel tolerance levels, ascorbic acid more markedly reduces pain by about 50 percent and lessens the difficulties with narcotics and muscle relaxants. It is not the total answer for back pain patients, however.

Rheumatoid Arthritis and Ankylosing Spondylitis

Bowel tolerance is increased by rheumatoid arthritis and ankylosing spondylitis (a type of arthritis that affects the base of the spine). Clinical response varies. Sometimes, these diseases are put into remission; sometimes not. I would advise that the patient's increased needs for ascorbate be met regardless.

Scarlet Fever

Three cases with typical sandpaper-like rash, peeling skin, and diagnostic laboratory findings of scarlet fever have responded within an hour or overnight. It is thought this immediate response is due to the neutralization of the small amount of residual streptococcus toxin causing the disease.

Herpes: Cold Sores, Genital Lesions, and Shingles

Acute herpes infections are usually ameliorated with bowel tolerance doses of ascorbic acid. However, recurrences are common especially if the disease has already become chronic. Zinc in combination with ascorbic acid is more effective for herpes infections.

Crib Deaths (Sudden Infant Death Syndrome)

I would agree with Kalokerinos and Klenner that crib deaths are caused by sudden ascorbate depletions.[10,13] The induced aascorbemia in some vital regulatory center kills the child. This induced deficiency is more likely to occur when the diet is poor in vitamin C. All of the epidemologic factors predisposing infants to crib death are associated with low vitamin C intake or high vitamin C destruction. I have never heard of a crib death in an infant saturated with ascorbate.

Maintenance Doses

I advise patients to take bowel tolerance doses of ascorbic acid for about a week and observe if anything beneficial happens. Some patients clear sinuses, or get a lift from it, and so forth. In these cases, doses are reduced to a comfortable effective level. If a patient feels nothing then the amount is lowered to about 4,000 mg a day divided in about three to four doses for a good day. During a stressful day, doses are raised to a total of perhaps 10,000 mg or more. When ascorbic acid crystals are dissolved in a small amount of plain water, the patient usually develops a taste for the substance that tells him how much to take. At the slightest hint of a threatening viral disease, doses are increased in frequency and to bowel tolerance.

In many patients viral infections still occur despite high ascorbic acid intake, although the symptoms of the disease will be mostly ameliorated. Vitamin A in dosages from 25,000 to 50,000 international units (IU) per day should be taken if high doses of ascorbic acid are maintained for more than several months. Supplements of all essential minerals should also be taken along with long-run maintenance doses of vitamin C.

Avoidance of sugar and processed foods will prove valuable if a patient's goal is almost complete prevention of viral diseases.

Complications

It is my experience that ascorbic acid never causes kidney stones, but, in fact, probably prevents them. Acute and chronic urinary tract infections are usually eliminated. One patient in a thousand will experience some discomfort while urinating. A small number will have a light rash, usually clearing with subsequent doses. Patients with hidden peptic ulcers may have pain, but some are benefited. The few patients complaining of canker sores with small doses of vitamin C do not usually have problems with large bowel tolerance closes. Patients with canker sores should be given large doses of vitamin E.

Some patients complaining of acid conditions do not tolerate ascorbic acid. These cases are very few. Older patients will have more nuisance problems with ascorbic acid and have more difficulty reaching bowel tolerance.

Patients started on maintenance doses of ascorbic acid when well will have a moderately high incidence of nuisance complaints. Patients treated with bowel tolerance doses for acute diseases have very few complaints because of the increased tolerance and the marked relief of symptoms. It is my experience that high maintenance doses of ascorbic acid reduce the incidence of gouty arthritis. Since that discovery, I have not had difficulties giving large amounts of ascorbic acid to patients with gout.

There has been no evidence as Herbert and Jacob suspected that ascorbic acid destroys vitamin B_{12}.[9]

The major problem, if one wishes to call it a problem, is a certain dependency on ascorbic acid that a patient acquires over a long period of time when he takes large maintenance doses. Apparently, certain metabolic reactions are encouraged by large amounts of ascorbate, and if the substance is suddenly withdrawn, certain problems result, such as a cold, return of allergy, fatigue, etc. Mostly, these problems are a return of problems the patient had before taking the ascorbic acid. Patients have, by this time, become so adjusted to feeling better that they refuse to go without vitamin C. Patients do not seem to acquire this dependency in the short time they take doses to bowel tolerance to treat an acute disease. Maintenance doses of 4,000 mg per day do not seem to create a noticeable dependency. The majority of patients who take 10,000 to 15,000 mg of ascorbic acid per day probably have a certain metabolic need for ascorbate which exceeds the universal human species need.

"Except in individuals with established, significant renal insufficiency, vitamin C is arguably the safest of all nutrients that can be given."
—THOMAS LEVY, MD

The major problem feared by patients benefiting from these large maintenance doses of ascorbic acid is that they may be forced into a position where their body is deprived of ascorbate during a period of great stress such as emergency hospitalization. Physicians should recognize the consequences of suddenly withdrawing vitamin C under these circumstances and be prepared to meet these increased metabolic needs for ascorbate in even an unconscious patient. These consequences, which may include shock, heart attack, phlebitis, pneumonia, allergic reactions, and more, can be averted only by intravenous ascorbate. All hospitals should have supplies of large amounts of ascorbate for intravenous use to meet this need. The millions of people taking ascorbic acid makes this an urgent priority. Patients should carry warning of these needs in a card prominently displayed in their wallets or should have a medic alert type bracelet or necklace engraved with this warning. Physicians should, in addition, carefully ask patients' families about the patients' ascorbic acid maintenance doses. Regardless of a physician's philosophical feelings about the usefulness of vitamin C, the physician should not withhold this essential nutrient from patients who have previously adjusted their body's metabolism to their increased needs. It would be like withholding vitamin B_{12} from a patient with pernicious anemia just because he was hospitalized. In the case of ascorbic acid, the effect would be much more rapid, however.

Conclusion

The method of titrating a patient's dosage of ascorbic acid between the relief of most symptoms and bowel tolerance has been described. This titration method is absolutely necessary to obtain excellent results. Studies of lesser amounts are almost useless. This method cannot by its nature be studied by double-blind methods because no placebo will mimic this bowel tolerance phenomenon. The method produces such spectacular effects in all patients capable of tolerating these doses, especially in the cases of acute self-limiting viral diseases, as to be undeniable. A placebo could not possibly work so reliably, work in infants and children, and have such a profound effect on critically ill patients. More stable patients will tolerate bowel tolerance doses of ascorbic acid and almost uniformly have excellent results. The more suggestable unstable patient is more likely to have difficulty with the taste.

REFERENCES FOR "THE METHOD OF DETERMINING PROPER DOSES OF VITAMIN C"

1. Belfield WO, Stone I. Megascorbic prophylaxis and megascorbic therapy: A new orthomolecular modality in veterinary medicine. *Journal of the International Academy of Preventive Medicine* 1975; 2:10–26.

2. Cameron E, Pauling L. Supplemental ascorbate in the supportive treatment of cancer: Prolongation of survival times in terminal human cancer. *Proc Natl Acad Sci USA* 1976; 73:3685–3689.

3. Cameron E, Pauling L. The orthomolecular treatment of cancer: Reevaluation of prolongation of survival times in terminal human cancer. *Proc Natl Acad Sci USA* 1978; 75:4538–4542.

4. Cathcart, RF. Clinical trial of vitamin C. *Medical Tribune,* June 25, 1975.

5. Cathcart, RF. Clinical use of large doses of ascorbic acid. Annual Meeting of the California Orthomolecular Medical Society, San Francisco, February 19,1976.

6. Cathcart RF. Vitamin C as a detoxifying agent. Annual Meeting of the Orthomolecular Medical Society, San Francisco, January 21,1978.

7. Cathcart RF. Vitamin C: The missing stress hormone. Annual Meeting of the Orthomolecular Medical Society, San Francisco, March 3,1979.

8. Greenwood J. Optimum vitamin C intake as a factor in the preservation of disc integrity. *Med Ann Dist Columbia* 1964; 33: 274–276.

9. Herbert V, Jacob E. Destruction of vitamin B_{12} by ascorbic acid. *JAMA* 1974; 230: 241–242.

10. Kalokerinos A. *Every Second Child.* New Canaan, CT: Keats Publishing, 1981.

11. Klenner FR. Virus pneumonia and its treatment with vitamin C. *J South Med and Surg* 1948; 110: 60–63.

12. Klenner FR. The treatment of poliomyelitis and other virus diseases with vitamin C. *J South Med and Surg* 1949;111: 210–214.

13. Klenner FR. Observations on the dose and administration of ascorbic acid when employed beyond the range of a vitamin in human pathology. *J App Nutr* 1971; 23:61–88.

14. Klenner FR. Significance of high daily intake of ascorbic acid in preventive medicine. *J Int Acad Prev Med* 1974; 1:45–49.

15. Libby AF, Stone I. The hypoascorbemia kwashiorkor approach to drug addiction therapy: A pilot study. *J Ortho Psychiat* 1977; 6:300–308.

16. Pauling L. *Vitamin C and the Common Cold.* San Francisco: W.H. Freeman & Co, 1970.

17. Pauling L. *Vitamin C, the Common Cold, and the Flu.* San Francisco: W.H. Freeman & Co, 1976.

18. Stone I. Studies of a mammalian enzyme system for producing evolutionary evidence on man. *Am J Phys Anthro* 1965; 23:83–86.

19. Stone I. Hypoascorbemia: The genetic disease causing the human requirement for exogenous ascorbic acid. *Perspect Biol Med* 1968; 10:133–134.

20. Stone I. *The Healing Factor: Vitamin C Against Disease.* New York: Grosset & Dunlap, 1972.

HIDDEN IN PLAIN SIGHT: THE PIONEERING WORK OF FREDERICK ROBERT KLENNER, MD

by Andrew W. Saul, PhD

From *J Orthomolecular Med* 2007; 22(1): 31–38.

"Some physicians would stand by and see their patient die rather than use ascorbic acid because in their finite minds it exists only as a vitamin."

—F. R. KLENNER, MD

Vitamin C Against Polio

The sound barrier was broken in 1947. The Korean War began in 1950. In between was the polio epidemic of 1948–1949, during which Frederick Robert Klenner, MD, cured every polio case he saw by using vitamin C.

Claus W. Jungeblut, MD,[1] had the initial idea; William J. McCormick, MD,[2] was an early proponent of frequent gram-sized doses. But it was Dr. Klenner who first gave polio patients tens of thousands of milligrams of vitamin C per day. He had been doing so since before D-Day.

"From 1943 through 1947," writes Robert Landwehr,[3] "Dr. Klenner reported successful treatment of 41 more cases of viral pneumonia using massive doses of vitamin C. From these cases he learned what dosage and route of administration—intravenously, intramuscularly, or orally—was best for each patient. Dr. Klenner gave these details in a February 1948 paper published in the *Journal of Southern Medicine and Surgery* entitled 'Virus Pneumonia and Its Treatment with Vitamin C.'[4] This article was the first of Dr. Klenner's twenty-eight (through 1974) scientific publications."

"When I first came across Dr. Klenner's work on polio patients," writes Thomas Levy, MD, "I was absolutely amazed and even a bit overwhelmed at what I read. . . To know that polio had been easily cured and so many babies, children, and some adults still continued to die or survive to be permanently crippled by this virus was extremely difficult to accept. . . Even more incredibly, Dr. Klenner briefly presented a summarization of his work on polio at the Annual Session of the American Medical Association on June 10, 1949 in Atlantic City, New Jersey:

"It might be interesting to learn how poliomyelitis was treated in Reidsville, N.C., during the 1948 epidemic. In the past seven years, virus infections have been treated and cured in a period of seventy-two hours by the employment of massive frequent injections of ascorbic acid, or vitamin C. I believe that if vitamin C in these massive doses—6,000 to 20,000 milligrams (mg) in a twenty-four hour period—is given to these patients with poliomyelitis (polio) none will be paralyzed and there will be no further maiming or epidemics of poliomyelitis." Dr. Levy concludes: "The four doctors who commented after Dr. Klenner did not have anything to say about his assertions."[5]

"How then," asks Landwehr, "could a Dr. Fred R. Klenner, a virtually unknown general practitioner specializing in diseases of the chest, from a town no one ever heard of, with no national credentials, no research grants and no experimental laboratory, have the nerve to make his sweeping claim in front of that prestigious body of polio authorities?" Indeed, Dr. Klenner was hardly a man to mince words. "When proper amounts are used, it will destroy all virus organisms," he would say. "Don't expect control of a virus with 100 to 400 mg of C."[6] Dr. Klenner administered ascorbate by injection, and, as Lendon H. Smith, MD, describes in great detail in the *Clinical Guide to the Use of Vitamin C: The Clinical Experiences of Frederick R. Klenner, M.D.,* Dr. Klenner found that "the most effective route was intravenous, but the intramuscular route was satisfactory. He gave at least 350 mg per kilogram (kg) of body weight." That quantity per day is a dose of 25,000–30,000 mg or so for an adult. Yet, Dr. Smith adds, "With 350 mg per kilogram of body weight every two hours, he could stop measles and dry up chicken pox."

This is indeed a large amount of vitamin C. Such use exemplifies the modern orthomolecular physician. Dr. Klenner's doses were enormous, flexible, and symptom-driven. The sicker the patient, the higher the dose. Massive ascorbate treatment cured every one of 60 polio cases Dr. Klenner saw. He published his report in *Southern Medicine and Surgery* in July of 1949.[7] All patients were well in three days. None had any paralysis.

In a 1950 letter, Dr. Klenner wrote: "Since my last communication, I have seen four new cases of poliomyelitis. All of these have completely recovered. Three cases were seen in the acute febrile stage and in each instance, using 65 mg per kg body weight (by injection) every two (to) four hours, recovery was spontaneous in 48 hours."[8]

In 1951, "In an especially incredible case," Dr. Levy says, "Dr. Klenner[9] described a five-year-old girl stricken with polio. This child had already been paralyzed in both her lower legs for over four days. The right leg was completely limp, and the left leg was determined to be 85 percent flaccid. Pain was noticed especially in the knee and lumbar areas. Four consulting physicians confirmed the diagnosis of polio. Other than massage, vitamin C was the only therapy initiated. After four days of vitamin C injections, the child was again moving both legs, but with only very slow and deliberate movement. Dr. Klenner also noted that there was a 'definite response' after only the first injection of vitamin C. The child was discharged from the hospital after four days, and 1,000 mg of oral vitamin C was continued every two hours with fruit juice for seven days. The child was walking about, although slowly, on the 11th day of treatment. By the 19th day of treatment there was a 'complete return of sensory and motor function,' and no long-term impairment ever resulted. Vitamin C not only completely cured this case of polio, it completely reversed what would undoubtedly have been a devastating, crippling result for the remainder of this girl's life."[4] For such elegant results, in the days before widespread use of either antibiotics or vaccination, one may wonder why Dr. Klenner was not awarded the Nobel Prize for Medicine.

Orthomolecular Originator

Born 22 October 1907 in Johnstown, Pennsylvania, Frederick Robert Klenner earned his undergraduate and graduate degrees in biology, magna cum laude, from St. Vincent and St. Francis Colleges. After two teaching fellowships, he entered Duke University School of Medicine. There, while he was ill, he met his future wife, Annie Hill Sharp (b. 19 Feb 1914), then a senior nursing student who "helped nurse him back to health, and romance blossomed."[10] At the time, Annie would be only the second woman in the school's history to graduate with a Bachelor of Science degree. Klenner received his MD in 1936, and "the couple settled in Winston-Salem, where Dr. Klenner was completing his residency at the North Carolina Tuberculosis Sanitarium."[10] There, according to a short biography published in the *Journal of Applied Nutrition,* he "served three years in post-graduate hospital training before embarking on a private practice. Although specializing in diseases of the chest, he continued to do general practice because of the opportunities it afforded for observations in medicine. His patients were as enthusiastic as he in playing 'guinea pigs' to study the action of ascorbic acid."[11]

Dr. Klenner had hospital privileges at Reidsville's Annie Penn Memorial Hospital where, among other things, he delivered hundreds of babies. Given supplemental ascorbate, not merely from birth but also all throughout gestation, Dr. Klenner's uniformly healthy, trouble-free infants were known by the staff as the "Vitamin C Babies."[12]

In a 1978 letter to Dr. Klenner, biochemist Irwin Stone writes that he thinks that "giving levels of ascorbate for long periods of time at the daily levels you recommend. . . is equivalent to creating a new human subspecies, 'Homo sapiens ascorbicus' . . . with unusual resistance to disease and stress and with a prolonged life span." Stone adds, "I was sorry to hear that the book you intend to write is still only a gleam in your eye."[13]

Although he never would publish a book on vitamin therapy, Dr. Klenner was a Fellow of the American College of Chest Physicians, the American College of Angiology, the American Association for the Advancement of Science, and one of the founders of the American Geriatrics Society. He was inducted into the Orthomolecular Medicine Hall of Fame in 2005.[14]

Greensboro Daily News reporter Flontina Miller has colorfully described Dr. Klenner's office, above a drugstore in Reidsville. "Up a creaking stairway is a dimly-lighted hallway. . . On one side of the hall is a stark waiting room nearly filled with patients. . .

A hand-printed sign tacked by the door reads, 'Limited General Practice'. . . Two walls (are) covered with framed certificates and honors awarded by medical schools and organizations. A crude hand-scrawled cardboard sign on a window air-conditioning unit reads, 'Snake Inside.' No snake actually lives inside the air conditioner, but Mrs. Klenner declares the sign has worked miracles to keep visitors' hands off. She said patients, waiting to talk with the doctor, often would tamper with the unit, causing continual need for repairs. . . For the past 12 years, Mrs. Klenner has been her husband's fulltime nurse, and they manage the office with no other help. 'I'd never see my husband if I didn't work with him,' said Mrs. Klenner. . . 'Sometimes he overworks and feels kind of tired.'"[15] He was also subject to severe headaches, including migraines. Still, according to journalist Jerry Bledsoe, Dr. Klenner never sent bills to his patients. "If a patient couldn't pay when treated, then he could pay when he could. And even if he couldn't pay and still needed a doctor, Dr. Klenner would be there, making house calls no matter the hour."[16]

Another *Greensboro Daily News* article written by Miller recounts how Dr. Klenner first used injections of vitamin C: "Dr. Klenner remembers using (ascorbate) for a man, who was lying near death from severe virus pneumonia, but refused to be hospitalized. 'I went to his house and gave him one big shot with five grams or 5,000 milligrams of vitamin C,' he recalled. 'When I went back later in the day, his temperature was down three degrees and he was sitting on the edge of the bed eating. I gave him another shot of C, 5,000 milligrams and kept up that dosage for three days, four times a day. And he was well. I said then, well, my gosh! This is doing something.'"[17]

Dr. Klenner devised an early office test for vitamin C.[18] He would go on to administer massive amounts of ascorbate against any and all viral diseases. And, in the course of some forty years of general practice, Dr. Klenner used vitamin C, often accompanied with high doses of other nutrients, to fight a striking variety of other illnesses. Dr. Smith[6] itemizes a list that includes Rocky Mountain Spotted Fever, bladder infections, alcoholism, arthritis, leukemia, atherosclerosis, ruptured intervertebral discs, high cholesterol, corneal ulcer, diabetes, glaucoma, burns and secondary infections, heat stroke, radiation burns, heavy metal poisoning, chronic fatigue, and complications resulting from surgery. Additionally, Dr. Klenner also reported meganutrient cures of tetanus,[19,20] trichinosis,[21] venomous bites from spiders or snakes,[22,23] and, perhaps most controversially, multiple sclerosis.

Vitamins against Multiple Sclerosis

Nearly every person with multiple sclerosis I've met has had two things in common: a lack of hope, and a lack of vitamins. Dr. Klenner's patients lacked neither, with a treatment schedule calling for massive quantities of B vitamins to, said Dr. Klenner, "effect nerve repair." He based his protocol in part on work, in the late 1930s, by "Stern from Columbia University, (who) was employing thiamine hydrochloride intraspinally with astonishing results in multiple sclerosis. He reported taking patients to the operating room on a stretcher, and following 30 mg thiamine given intraspinally, they would walk back to their room."[24] While, Dr. Klenner commented, "the response was relatively transient," it indicated that multiple sclerosis might be a severe form of avitaminosis.

If one vitamin helped, two seemed likely to work better. Dr. Klenner writes: "Moore,[25] in 1940, published a monograph on the use of high intravenous doses of nicotinic acid for the cure of multiple sclerosis. Moore employed a drug combination called 'Nicobee.' This preparation contained 100 mg nicotinic acid and 60 mg of thiamine in each 10 cc solution." Moore, like Dr. Klenner, was influenced by earlier work showing that nerve degeneration results from multiple nutritional deficiencies.[26] Subsequently, Dr. Klenner would employ what may only be described as a wide-ranging nutritional approach. His protocol for multiple sclerosis and myasthenia gravis follows, as described in his paper, "Response of Peripheral and Central Nerve Pathology to Mega-Doses of the Vitamin B-Complex and Other Metabolites":[27]

Thiamine hydrochloride (B_1): "300 mg to 500 mg, 30 minutes before meals and bed hour, and during the night if awake" plus "400 mg daily by needle, given intramuscularly."

Niacin (B_3): "100 mg to 3,000 mg, thirty minutes before meals and at bed hour, and also during the night if awake—whichever dose will produce a strong body flush."

Pyridoxine (B_6): "100 mg to 200 mg is given before meals and bed hour. At least 100 mg daily is given intramuscularly."

Cobalamin (B_{12}): "1,000 micrograms (mcg) three times each week by needle."

Ascorbic acid (vitamin C): "10,000 to 20,000 mg should be taken daily by mouth in divided doses."

Riboflavin (Vitamin B_2): "40 mg to 80 mg given daily by needle intramuscularly; 25 mg before meals and bed time."

Choline: "700 mg to 1,400 mg after each meal and at bed hour."

Lecithin: "1,200 mg soybean lecithin after each meal."

Magnesium: "100 mg after each meal."

Pantothenic acid (B_5): 200 mg "after each meal and at bed hour."

Aminoacetic acid (glycine): "1 heaping tablespoon of the powder in a glass of milk four times each day."

Zinc gluconate: "10 mg three times each day has some value in myasthenia gravis. Take several hours after vitamin B_2."

Additionally, Dr. Klenner gave vitamin E (800 to 1,600 international units [IU] per day), crude liver extract, adenosine-5-monophosphoric acid, and a multi-vitamin/

multi-trace-mineral tablet, which would have included some vitamin D, and a calcium supplement. Dr. Klenner prescribed a high-protein diet, and used available drugs to relieve tremor and stiffness. He might also specify linolenic acid, thyroid, fresh green vegetables, fresh fruits, a considerable quantity of milk (1 quart per day) and eggs (up to six per day). Dr. Klenner required patients to limit fats, eat only whole-grain bread, and specified "no junk foods, especially sweets."[28]

Dr. Klenner also offered what he considered to be an abbreviated, compromise program. "Should a given patient's physician refuse to administer this schedule, I have this recommendation: 1 gram thiamin hydrochloride one hour before meals and at bed hour, and during the night if awake. Niacin taken at the same time, and in amounts sufficient to produce a good body flush. Two hundred mg calcium pantothenate (B_5) and 100 mg pyridoxine (B_6) before meals and at bed hour. Ten grams (10,000 mg) ascorbic acid, taken in divided doses. Amino acetic acid: 1 heaping tablespoon in a glass of milk, four times each day. Naturally, the full schedule will afford more dramatic response." He declares, "We categorically make this statement: Any victim of multiple sclerosis who will dramatically flush with the use of nicotinic acid (B_3), and who has not yet progressed to the stage of myelin degeneration, as witnessed by sustained ankle clonus elicited in the orthodox manner, can be *cured* with the adequate employment of thiamine hydrochloride and other factors of the vitamin B complex in conjunction with essential proteins, lipids, carbohydrates, and injectable crude liver."[27]

Media Muckraking

Perhaps it is not a complete surprise that the print and broadcast media have been obsessively interested in the scandal that rocked Dr. Klenner's family following the doctor's death from heart disease in 1984. Fred Klenner Jr., known as Fritz, implicated in the murders of at least five people, died by his own hand in 1985.[29] The tragedy was the subject of a best-selling 1988 tell-all book,[30] in which Dr. Klenner is mentioned over 50 times, and then, in 1994, a two hundred–minute made-for-TV movie.[31] It is instructive to note that the news media reported on the son's crimes far more than it reported on the father's cures. There have been countless television programs and Hollywood films about crime, but not one ever made about the lifesaving achievements of megavitamin therapy. Perhaps that is an even greater tragedy. "We've used massive doses of vitamins on over 10,000 people over a period of 30 years," said Dr. Klenner, "and we've never seen any ill effects from them. The only effects we've seen have been beneficial."

Dr. Klenner's immensely valuable work is his legacy. Chemist and double Nobel Laureate Linus Pauling said, "The early papers by Dr. Fred R. Klenner provide much information about the use of large doses of vitamin C in preventing and treating many diseases. These papers are still important."[32] Dr. Klenner is justly remembered as the doctor who was first to boldly assert that "Ascorbic acid is the safest and most valuable substance available to the physician" and that patients should be given "large doses of vitamin C in all pathological conditions while the physician ponders the diagnosis." Whether overshadowed by scandal or stubbornly ignored by the medical profession, high-dose ascorbate therapy is here to stay. "I have used Dr. Klenner's methods on hundreds of patients," said Lendon H. Smith, MD. "He is right."

Editor's note: Dr. Klenner's "Observations on the Dose and Administration of Ascorbic Acid When Employed Beyond the Range of a Vitamin in Human Pathology" immediately follows this article.

REFERENCES FOR "HIDDEN IN PLAIN SIGHT"

1. Saul AW. Claus Washington Jungeblut, M.D.: Polio pioneer; ascorbate advocate. *J Orthomolecular Med* 2006;. 21(2):102–106.

2. Saul AW. The pioneering work of William J. McCormick, M.D. *J Orthomolecular Med* 2003; 18(2):93–96.

3. Landwehr R. The origin of the 42-year stonewall of vitamin C. *J Orthomolecular Med* 1991; 6(2):99–103.

4. Klenner FR. Virus pneumonia and its treatment with vitamin C. *Southern Medicine and Surgery* 1948; 110(2):36–38, 46.

5. Levy TE. *Vitamin C, Infectious Diseases, and Toxins: Curing the Incurable.* Philadelphia, PA: Xlibris Corporation, 2002.

6. Smith, LH. *Clinical Guide to the Use of Vitamin C: The Clinical Experiences of Frederick R. Klenner, M.D.* Portland, OR: Life Sciences Press, 1988. Originally titled: *Vitamin C as a fundamental medicine: Abstracts of Dr. Frederick R. Klenner, M.D.'s published and unpublished work.*

7. Klenner FR. The treatment of poliomyelitis and other virus diseases with vitamin C. *South Med J* 1949; 3(7):209–214.

8. Klenner FR. Letter to M.G. Farnsworth, Farnsworth Laboratories, Inc., Chicago, dated October 14, 1950.

9. Klenner FR. Massive doses of vitamin C and the virus diseases. *South Med J* 1951; 113(4):101–107.

10. Bledsoe J. *Bitter Blood: A True Story of Southern Family Pride, Madness, and Multiple Murder.* NY: Dutton, 1988. Also: NY: New American Library, 1989.

11. Klenner FR. Observations on the dose of administration of ascorbic acid when employed beyond the range of a vitamin in human pathology. *J Applied Nutrition* 1971; 23(3 & 4): 61–68.

12. Stone I. *The Healing Factor: Vitamin C Against Disease.* NY: Grosset and Dunlap, 1972.

13. Letter from Irwin Stone to Dr. & Mrs. Frederick R. Klenner, Gilmer Street, Reidsville, North Carolina, dated 3 June 1978.

14. Saul AW. The 2005 Orthomolecular Medicine Hall of Fame. *J Orthomolecular Med* 2005; 20(2):113–117.

15. Miller F. Klenner's office recalls old-fashioned practitioner. *Greensboro Daily News,* undated reprint. This medium-circulation newspaper, founded in 1909, has been known since 1982 as the *News-Record.*

16. Bledsoe J. *Bitter Blood: A True Story of Southern Family Pride, Madness, and Multiple Murder.* NY: Dutton, 1988. Also: NY: New American Library, 1989.

17. Miller F. Dr. Klenner urges taking vitamins in huge doses. *Greensboro Daily News,* Tuesday, Dec 13, 1977, A8-A10.

18. Klenner FR. A new office procedure for the determination of plasma levels for ascorbic acid. *Tri-State Medical J* 1956; 26–28.

19. Klenner FR. The history of lockjaw. *Tri-State Med J* 1954, June.

20. Klenner FR. Recent discoveries in the treatment of lockjaw with vitamin C and tolserol. *Tri-State Med J* 1954, July.

21. Klenner FR. A treatment of trichinosis with massive doses of vitamin C and para-aminobenzoic acid. *Tri-State Medical J* 1954, April.

22. Klenner FR. Case history: The black widow spider. *Tri-State Med J* 1957, December.

23. Klenner FR. Case history: Cure of a 4-year old child bitten by a mature Highland Moccasin with vitamin C. *Tri-State Med J* 1954, July.

24. Sern EL. The intraspinal injection of vitamin B-1 for the relief of intractable pain, and for inflammatory and degenerative diseases of the central nervous system. *Amer J Surg* 1938; 34:495.

25. Moore MT. Treatment of multiple sclerosis with nicotinic acid and vitamin B-1. *Archives Int Med* 1940;65:18.

26. Zimmerman HH, Burack F. Lesions of the nervous system resulting from a deficiency of the vitamin B complex. *Arch Pathology* 1932;13:207.

27. Klenner FR. Response of peripheral and central nerve pathology to mega-doses of the vitamin B-complex and other metabolites. Parts 1 and 2. *J Applied Nutrition* 1973; 25:16–40. Klenner, FR. Treating multiple sclerosis nutritionally. *Cancer Control J* 2(3):16–20. And, a similar, comprehensive MS/MG protocol is to be found in the *Clinical Guide to the Use of Vitamin C: The Clinical Experiences of Frederick R. Klenner, M.D.,* reference 6.

28. Program prescribed by Dr. Fred R. Klenner, a two-page itemized check-off list of nutritional recommendations for patients. Hand-dated January 25, 1979, by Irwin Stone, who added a notation that it had been "Rec'd from L. P. Institute." (Linus Pauling Institute of Science and Medicine). Provided by Steve Stone.

29. While it has sometimes been assumed that son Fritz Klenner (Fred Klenner Jr.) was a physician, he was not. He never attended medical school.

30. Bledsoe J. *Bitter Blood: A True Story of Southern Family Pride, Madness, and Multiple Murder.* NY: Dutton, 1988. Also: NY: New American Library, 1989.The book contains three black-and-white photos of Dr. Klenner. Chapter 22 focuses on his work. That chapter, and the balance of the book, is less than flattering. Publisher's notes say that Jerry "Bledsoe wrote an award-winning series about the (Fritz Klenner) case in 1985 in the Greensboro (NC) News & Record," where he is a senior writer and columnist. http://company.news-record.com/library.htm. Bledsoe is a *New York Times*–bestselling author.

31. *In the Best of Families: Marriage, Pride & Madness* stars Kelly McGillis as Susie Lynch and Harry Hamlin as Fritz Klenner (Fred Klenner Jr.). Produced by Ambroco Media Group and Dan Wigutow Productions. Directed by Jeff Bleckneritz. Originally telecast in the USA by CBS in two parts, on 16 and 18 January, 1994. Later shown in Britain by BBC 1 on 19 and 20 April, 1997. The film is not known to have won any awards.

32. Pauling L. Foreword to: Smith LH. Clinical guide to the use of vitamin C: The clinical experiences of Frederick R. Klenner, M.D. Portland, OR: Life Sciences Press, 1988.

OBSERVATIONS ON THE DOSE AND ADMINISTRATION OF ASCORBIC ACID WHEN EMPLOYED BEYOND THE RANGE OF A VITAMIN IN HUMAN PATHOLOGY

by Frederick R. Klenner, MD

From *J Orthomolecular Med* 1998; 13(4):198–210.

"Recently in browsing the Net I ran across Dr. Robert F. Cathcart III's reprint of Dr. Frederick R. Klenner's pioneering report on ascorbic acid. Dr. Cathcart probably has more experience using ascorbic acid than any other living physician. He discovered how to determine the optimum dose by increasing the amount until the stools become too soft and too much gas developed. He pointed out that the optimum amount varied tremendously depending upon the nature of the disease, the nature of the stress and many other factors. I agree with Dr. Cathcart that the report by Klenner deserves wide exposure as an honor to one of our many pioneers, perhaps the first to use huge dosages of vitamin C with safety, and to remind modern physicians that the history of mega ascorbic acid goes back at least forty-five years."

–ABRAM HOFFER, MD, PHD

Ancient History and Homespun Vitamin C Therapies

Folklore of past civilizations reports that for every disease afflicting man there is an herb or its equivalent that will effect a cure. In Puerto Rico the story has long been told that to have the health tree acerola in one's backyard would keep colds out of the front door.[1] The ascorbic acid content of this cherry-like fruit is thirty times that found in oranges. Boneset, scientifically called *Eupatorium perfoliatum*,[2] is now rarely prescribed by physicians, but was once the most commonly used medicinal plant of the eastern United States. Most farmsteads had a bundle of dried boneset in the attic or woodshed from which a most bitter tea would be meted out to the unfortunate victim of a cold or fever. Having lived in that section of the country, we qualified many times for this particular drink.

The flu pandemic of 1918 stands out very forcefully in that the Klenners survived when scores about us were dying. Although bitter, it was curative, and most of the time the cure was overnight. Several years ago my curiosity led me to assay this "herbal medicine," and to my surprise and delight I found that we had been taking from 10,000 to 30,000 milligrams (mg) of natural vitamin C at one time. Even then it was given by body weight. Children one cupful; adults two to three cupfuls. Cups those days held 8 ounces. Twentieth-century man seemingly forgets that his ancestors made crude drugs from various plants and roots, and that these decoctions served his purpose. Elegant pharmacy has only made the forms and shapes more acceptable.

Early Specifications, Action, and Dosages for Administration

To understand the chemical behavior of ascorbic acid in human pathology, one must go beyond its present academic status either as a factor essential for life or as a substance necessary to prevent scurvy. This knowledge is elementary. Listen to what appeared in *Food and Life Yearbook 1939,* US Department of Agriculture: "In fact even when there is not a single outward symptom of trouble, a person may be in a state of vitamin C deficiency more dangerous than scurvy itself. When such a condition is not detected, and continues uncorrected, the teeth and bones will be damaged, and what may be even more serious, the blood stream is weakened to the point where it can no longer resist or fight infections not so easily cured as scurvy."[3] It is true that without these infinitesimal amounts myriads of body processes would deteriorate and even come to a fatal halt.

Ascorbic acid has many important functions. It is a powerful oxidizer, and when given in massive amounts—that is, 50,000 mg to 150,000 mg, intravenously, for certain pathological conditions, and "run in" as fast as a 20-gauge needle will allow—it acts as a "flash oxidizer,"[4] often correcting the pathology within minutes. Ascorbic acid is also a powerful reducing agent. Its neutralizing action on certain toxins, exotoxins (external toxins), virus infections, endotoxins (internal toxins), and histamine is in direct proportion to the amount of the lethal factor involved *and the amount of ascorbic acid given.* At times it is necessary to use ascorbic acid intramuscularly. It should always be used orally, when possible, along with the needle.

If one is to employ ascorbic acid intelligently, some index for requirements must be realized. Unfortunately, there exists today a sort of "brand" called "minimum daily requirements." This illegitimate "child" has been co-fathered by the National Academy of Science and the National Research Council and represents a tragic error in judgment. There are many factors which increase the demand by the body for ascorbic acid, and unless these are appreciated, at least by physicians, there can be no real progress. It is vitally important that cognizance be taken of the demand by the body for ascorbic acid far beyond so-called scorbutic levels. Briefly these demands can be summarized as:

- The age of the individual
- Body chemistry
- Body weight
- Drugs
- Habits such as smoking, alcohol use, and lifestyle

- Inadequate storage
- Kidney threshold
- Loss in the stool
- Physiological stress
- Season of the year
- Sleep, especially when induced artificially
- Trauma caused by a pathogen, work, surgery, or accident
- Exposure to pesticides
- Environment
- Variations in binders in commercial tablets
- Variations in individual absorption

With such knowledge it is no longer possible to accept a set numerical unit in terms of minimal daily requirements. This is true because of the simple fact that people are different, and these same people experience different situations at various times. With ascorbic acid, today's adequate supply means little or nothing in terms of the needs for tomorrow. Let us start thinking in terms of maximum requirements. For too long a time we have undersupplied our children and ourselves by accepting through negative ignorance and acquiescence so-called standards. Based on scant data on mammalian synthesis, available for the rat, a 70 kg (154 lbs.) individual would produce 1.8 grams (1,800 mg)[5] to 4.0 grams (4,000 mg)[6] of ascorbic acid per day in the unstressed condition; under stress, up to 15.2 grams (15,200 mg).[7] Compare this to the 70 mg recommended for daily requirements without stress and 200 mg for the simple stress of the obstetrical patient, and you will recognize the disparity and understand why we have been waging a one-man war against the establishment in Washington for 23 years.

Ascorbic Acid Not Synthesized by Man

Work on mammalian biosynthesis of ascorbic acid indicates that the vitamin C story, as is generally accepted, represents an oversimplification of available evidence.[6–8] This often leads to misinterpretations and false impressions. It has been proposed that the biochemical lesion which produces the human need for exogenous sources of ascorbic acid is the absence of the active enzyme gulonolactone oxidase from the human liver.[9] A defect or loss of the gene controlling the synthesis of this enzyme in humans blocks the final phase in the series for converting glucose to ascorbic acid. Such a mutation could have happened by a virus, by radiation, or simply by chance, thus denying all progenies of this mutated animal the ability to produce ascorbic acid. Survival demanded ascorbic acid from an exogenous source. This is not remarkable. Other recognized genetic diseases in which a missing enzyme causes a pathological syndrome in man are phenylketonuria, galactosemia, and alkaptonuria. The inability of humans to manufacture their own ascorbic acid, due to genetic fault, has been called hypoascorbemia by Irwin Stone, PhD.[10] This is another reason for abolishing the present concept of daily minimal requirements. The physiological requirements in man are no different from other mammals capable of carrying out this synthesis.

Various Procedures for Testing Vitamin C Levels and Body Requirements

Various tests have been employed to determine the degree of body saturation of vitamin C, but for the most part they have been misleading. Blood and urine samples analyzed with 2,6-dichlorophenol-indophenol will give values roughly 7 percent less than when testing with dinitrophenol-hydrazine (a sensitive compound). The capillary fragility test is similar to the tourniquet test in results. Both can be used to estimate the quantity of vitamin C necessary to maintain capillary integrity. The intradermal test as modified by Lawrence Slobody[11] is again gaining new recruits. In principle it is the same as the lingual test of William Ringdorf and Emanuel Cheraskin,[12] since both are based on the time required to decolorize dye. The lingual test is rapid and simple to perform, but it requires a syringe with a 25-gauge needle and a stop watch. This test was helpful in gauging requirements for simple stress, but not accurate enough when using needle therapy. Fifteen years ago, I helped to develop the silver nitrate-urine test.[13] This test employs ten drops of 5 percent silver nitrate and ten drops urine which are placed in a test tube. When read in two minutes, it will give a color pattern showing white, beige, smoke gray, or charcoal or various combinations of any two depending upon the degree of saturation. We have found that this color index test is all one will need for establishing the correct amount of ascorbic acid to use by mouth, by muscle, or by vein in the handling of all types of human pathology, either as the specific drug or as an adjuvant with other antibiotics or neutralizing chemicals. In severe pathological conditions, the urine sample, taken every four hours, must show a fine charcoal-like precipitation.

Role of Ascorbic Acid in Intercellular Reactions and in Neutralizing and Possibly Controlling Virus Production

In 1935, chemist Wendell Stanley isolated a crystalline protein possessing the properties of tobacco mosaic virus (the first virus to be discovered). It contained two substances: ribonucleic acid (RNA) and protein. The simple structure characteristic of tobacco mosaic virus was soon found to be a basic property of many human viruses, such as Coxsackie virus (which I believe to be the cause of multiple sclerosis), the echovirus (one of several viruses that affect the gastrointestinal tract), and the poliovirus. They all contain only RNA and protein. There exist minor variations. The adenovirus, which causes most repiratory illnesses, contains deoxyribonucleic acid (DNA) and protein. Other viruses such as those causing influenza contain added lipids and polysaccharides. DNA is used to program the large viruses like mumps; RNA is used to program the small viruses like measles. The role of the protein coat is to protect the parasitic but unstable nucleic acid as it rides the "blood highway" or "lymphatic system" to gain specific cell entry. Pure viral nucleic acid without its protein coat can be inactivated by constituents of normal blood. There are several theories as to what happens after cell entry:

- Once inside a given cell, the virus nucleic acid sheds its protein coat and proceeds to modify the host cell by either creating mutations or by directly substituting its own nucleic acid.
- The infectious nucleic acid, after entering a human cell, retains its protein coat and starts to produce its own type of protein coat[14] and viral nucleic acid, so that new units can either depart to enter other cells or destroy the cell, thus making the infection more severe.
- The introduction of a foreign fragment of nucleic acid in the cell-virus interaction approach as postulated by virologist T. J. Starr[15] suggests that there can exist cells with partial chromosome makeup and cells with multi-nuclei. Hiliary Kropowski, also a virologist, holds that these partial cells are "pseudo-virons"[16] and are found in some tumor-virus infections. A key factor in the Starr-Kropowski thinking is that the cell maintains its biological integrity to support virus development despite the abnormal morphology and genetic deficiency. If these invaded cells could be destroyed or the invader neutralized, the illness would suddenly terminate. Ascorbic acid has the capability of entering all cells. Under normal circumstances its presence is beneficial to the cell. However, when the cell has been invaded by a foreign substance, like virus nucleic acid, enzymatic action by ascorbic acid contributes to the breakdown of virus nucleic acid. Ascorbic acid also joins with the available virus protein, making a new macromolecule, which acts as the repressor factor. It has been demonstrated that when combined with the repressor (the operator gene), virus nucleic acid cannot react with any other substance and cannot induce activity in the structural gene, therefore inhibiting the multiplication of new virus bodies. The strength of the cell membrane is exceeded by these macromolecules with rupture and destruction.

Promptness of Massive Ascorbic Acid in Avoiding Fatal Encephalitis Related to Stubborn Head and Chest Colds

In 1953,[17] my colleagues and I presented a case history and films of a patient with virus pneumonia. This patient was unconscious, with a fever of 106.8°F when admitted to the hospital. She was given 140,000 mg of ascorbic acid intravenously over a period of 72 hours, at which time she was awake, sitting up in bed, and taking fluids freely by mouth. Her temperature was normal. Since that time we have observed a more deadly syndrome associated with a virus causing head and chest colds. This is one of the adenoviruses, which strikes in the area of the upper respiratory tract with resulting fever, sore throat, and watery eyes, and when appearing in children can cause fatal pneumonia. More often death is indirect by way of incipient encephalitis (inflammation of the brain) the child can be dead in 30 minutes. These are the babies and children found dead in bed whose deaths are attributed to sudden infant death syndrome (SIDS). It is suffocation but by way of a syndrome we observed and reported in 1957,[18] which is similar to that found in cephalic tetanus-toxemia, culminating in diaphragmatic spasm, with dyspnea (shortness of breath) and finally asphyxia.[19] By 1958, we had collected sufficient information from our office and hospital patients to catalog this deadly syndrome into two important stages:[20]

- **Stage 1:** There is always a history of having had the flu, which lasts 48 to 96 hours, complicated with extreme physical or mental distress, or a mild cold, similar to an allergic rhinitis, which lingers on for several weeks but does not incapacitate the individual.
- **Stage 2:** This stage, which is always sudden, presents itself in at least several forms, including convulsive seizures; extreme excitability, resembling delirium tremens if an adult and with dancing of the eyeballs if a child; severe chill; strangling in the course of eating or drinking; collapse; and stupor and hemiplegia. Other findings of this dramatic second stage are rapid pulse; respiration, two to three times normal, that in some cases will be suggestive of air hunger; moderately dilated pupils; and a high white blood cell count.

The second stage of this syndrome is triggered by a breakthrough at the site of the blood-brain barrier. The time required for neurological changes to become evident is roughly comparable to the time necessary for similar neuropathology to be demonstrated following a severe head injury. Cerebral edema (severe brain swelling) exists in both severe head injury and viral encephalitis. In my practice, I start massive ascorbic acid therapy immediately. Physicians must realize the inherent danger of a lingering head or chest cold and appreciate the importance of early massive vitamin C therapy. I have seen children dead in two hours because their attending physician was not impressed with their illness upon hospital admission. An autopsy on one of these patients showed bilateral pneumonia (infection that affects both lungs)—all one needs to spark a deadly encephalitis.

How does the brain become involved in encephalitis? Some speculate on the pathways in which the virus gains entrance into the brain, summarized as follows:

- Through the olfactory nerves;
- Through the portals of the stomach from material swallowed, either pulmonary or upper respiratory drainage;
- Through direct extension from otitis media or from mastoid cells;
- Through the bloodstream; arriving in the brain, the virus goes through the blood–

cerebrospinal fluid barrier and/or the blood-brain barrier by one of three ways: electrical charge; chemical lysis of tissue; or osmosis. Louis Bakay[21] reported that the permeability of the blood-brain barrier can be changed by introducing various toxic agents into the blood circulation. Researchers R. Chambers and B. W. Zweifach[22] emphasized the importance of the intercellular cement of the capillary wall in regulating permeability of the blood vessels of the central nervous system. In this syndrome the toxic substance is an adenovirus. Ascorbic acid will repair and maintain the integrity of the capillary wall.

Burn Degrees Explained and Some Therapy Rationale

In the treatment of burns, ascorbic acid, in sufficient amounts, reflects itself as a truly miracle substance. In the early 1940s, when I was using ascorbic acid intramuscularly in treating bacillary dysentery (an acute infection of the intestines by shigella bacteria) with excellent results, Charles Lund and many others were using what they called massive doses of ascorbic acid in the treatment of burn-damaged skin. One or two grams (1,000 to 2,000 mg) each day, in fluids, was the recognized dose. Burns are at the beginning first degree and some remain as just an erythema. Many times the first-degree burn progresses rapidly to the second-degree stage and remains as "blisters." Still others go on to third degree, which usually is more pronounced on the third-plus post burn day. There is a fourth stage which results from lack of knowledge in treatment. It terminates with skin grafting and plastic surgery. I believe that ascorbic acid can eliminate the third and fourth stages.

The pathologic physiology of a burn wound from the moment of the accident is in a state of dynamic change until the wound heals or the patient dies. The primary consideration is the phenomenon of intravascular agglutination or blood sludging (clotting of red blood cells), originally recognized by Melvin Knisely in 1945.[23,24] Initially, there is intravascular agglutination of red blood cells into distinctly visible, smooth, hard, rigid, basic masses. Oxygen uptake by the tissues is greatly reduced because of the sludging and subsequent reduced rate of blood flow. Research in 1960[25] concluded that this phenomenon of sludging or agglutination results in capillary thrombosis in the area of the burn, extending proximally to involve the large arterioles (arteries) and venules (small veins), and thereby creating tissue destruction greater than that originally produced by the burn. Anoxia (a lack of oxygen in the tissues) produces added tissue destruction. Charles Lund and Stanley Levenson[26] found that after severe burns there is considerable alteration in the metabolism of ascorbic acid as shown by a low concentration of ascorbic acid in the plasma, either with the patient fasting or after saturation tests, and also low urinary excretion of vitamin C, either with the patient fasting or after the injection of test doses. The extent of the abnormality closely paralleled the severity of the burn. One study[27] reported an increased demand for ascorbic acid in burns, especially when epithelization and formation of granulation tissue (connective tissue and tiny blood vessel repair) are taking place. Another study[28] also reported in 1941 a marked decrease in the plasma ascorbic acid concentration in patients with severe burns. David Klasson,[29] although limiting the amount of ascorbic acid to a dose range of 300 mg to 2,000 mg daily, in divided doses, found that it hastened the healing of wounds by producing healthy granulation tissue and also that it reduced local edema. He rationalized that ascorbic acid used locally as a 2 percent dressing possessed astringent properties similar to hydrogen peroxide. He also reported that antibiotic therapy was rarely necessary.

Harlen Stone[30] suggested the use of gentamicin in major, severe burns to lower the sepsis (a severe, often system-wide infection) caused by pseudomonas, a bacteria often seen in burn patients that is very resistant to antibiotics. Absorption of its exotoxin (a poisonous substance) from the infected burn wound inhibits the body's bacterial defense mechanism. Death can result either from the toxemia alone or from an associated septicemia. My colleagues and I have found that the secret in treating burns can be summarized in five steps:

1. Make a covered wagon–type cradle over the burn and keep warm with three 25-watt bulbs. The patient can control the heat by turning on and off the first bulb as needed. No garments or dressings are allowed.
2. Spray a 3 percent ascorbic acid solution over the entire area of the burn, every two to four hours for about five days.
3. Apply a vitamin A and D ointment over the area of the burn and alternate with the 3 percent ascorbic acid solution.
4. Give massive doses of ascorbic acid intravenously and by mouth. By injection, use 500 mg per kg of body weight diluted to at least 18 cubic centimeters (cc) per gram of vitamin C using 5 percent dextrose or saline in water or Ringer's solution, repeated every eight hours for several days, then at twelve-hour intervals (include 1,000 mg of calcium gluconate daily). Ascorbic acid, by mouth, is given to tolerance.
5. Supportive treatment; that is, whole blood and maintaining electrolyte balance. If seen early after the burn, there will be no infections and no dead skin formations. This eliminates fluid formation, since the dead skin traps will not exist and there will be no edema in the extremities because the venous and lymphatic systems will remain open. There will be no arterial obstruction and no nerve compression. Pseudomonas will not be a problem, since ascorbic acid destroys the exotoxin systemically and locally. Even if the burn is seen late, when pseudomonas is a major problem, the gram-negative bacilli will be destroyed in a few days, leaving a clean, healthy surface. Ascorbic acid also eliminates pain so that opiates or their equivalent are not required. What has been overlooked in burns is that there are

many living epithelial cells in the area. With the use of ascorbic acid these cells are kept viable, will multiply, and will soon meet with other proliferating units in the establishment of new skin.

Primary and Lasting Benefits in Pregnancy

Observations made on more than 300 consecutive obstetrical cases using supplemental ascorbic acid, by mouth, convinced me that failure to use this agent in sufficient amounts in pregnancy borders on malpractice. The lowest amount of ascorbic acid used was 4,000 mg and the highest amount 15,000 mg each day. Requirements were roughly 4,000 mg the first trimester, 6,000 mg the second trimester, and 10,000 mg the third trimester. Approximately 20 percent of the pregnancies required 15,000 mg each day during the last trimester. Eighty percent of this group received a booster injection of 10,000 mg, intravenously, on admission to the hospital.

The simple stress of pregnancy demands supplemental vitamin C. During the pregnancy, hemoglobin levels were much easier to maintain; leg cramps developed in less than 3 percent of cases; and stretch marks seldom developed, and when they were present, they occurred due to an associated problem of too much eating and too little walking. The capacity of the skin to resist the pressure of an expanding uterus will also vary in different individuals. Labor was shorter and less painful; there were no postpartum hemorrhages; and the perineum was found to be remarkably elastic, and episiotomy was performed electively. Even 15 to 20 years following the birth of the last child, the firmness of the perineum was found to be similar to that of a woman pregnant for the first time in those who continued their daily supplemental vitamin C. No patient required catheterization. No toxic manifestations were demonstrated in this group. There was no cardiac stress, even though 22 patients in the group had rheumatic hearts. One patient, in particular, carried two pregnancies without complications. She had been warned by her previous obstetrician that a second pregnancy would terminate with a maternal death. She received no ascorbic acid with her first pregnancy. This woman has been back teaching school for the past ten years. She still takes 10,000 mg of ascorbic acid daily.

Infants born under massive ascorbic acid therapy were all robust. Not a single case required resuscitation. No feeding problems were experienced. The Fultz quadruplets (the first identical African-American quadruplets on record) were in this group. They took milk nourishment on the second day. These babies were started on 50 mg of ascorbic acid the first day and, of course, this dosage was increased as time went on. Our only nursery equipment was one hospital bed; an old, used single-unit hot plate; and an equally old ten-quart kettle. Humidity and ascorbic acid tells this story. They are the only quadruplets to have survived in the southeastern United States. Another case of which I am justly proud is one in which we delivered ten children to one couple. All are healthy and good looking. There were no miscarriages. All are living and well. They are frequently referred to as the "vitamin C kids." In fact, all of the babies from this group were called "vitamin C babies" by the nursing personnel.

In my own practice I was able to take women who had had as many as five abortions without a successful pregnancy and carry them through two and three uneventful pregnancies with the use of supplemental vitamin C. The German literature is "stacked" with articles recommending high doses of vitamin C during gestation because German doctors believe that this substance is of great benefit in influencing the health of the mother and in preventing infections. The vital contribution of ascorbic acid to the body tissues can be summed up in the formation and maintenance of normal intercellular material, especially in the connective tissue, bones, teeth, and blood vessels. Genetic errors might be prevented if prospective mothers were advised to take 10,000 mg or more of ascorbic acid daily. It is significant that we found in the simple stress of pregnancy, a normal physiological process, that equivalent requirements paralleled those found in the rat when under stress. Experiments by many researchers have shown that the need for supplemental vitamin C begins with the embryo.

Diabetes Mellitus Response to 10,000 Milligrams of Ascorbic Acid by Mouth

Over the past 17 years my coworkers and I have studied the effect of 10,000 mg of vitamin C taken by mouth in patients with diabetes mellitus. We found that every diabetic not taking supplemental vitamin C could be classified as having subclinical scurvy (long-term marginal deficiency). For this reason they find it difficult to heal wounds. The diabetic patient will use the supplemental vitamin C for better utilization of his insulin. It will assist the liver in the metabolism of carbohydrates and to reinstate his body to heal wounds like a normal individual. We found that 60 percent of all diabetics could be controlled with diet and 10,000 mg of ascorbic acid daily. The other 40 percent will need much less needle insulin and less oral medication.

Observations Following Postsurgery Cases on Blood Plasma Levels of Ascorbic Acid

Deduction is evident of the need for substantial amounts of ascorbic acid prior to surgery. Plasma levels, recorded before starting anesthesia and after completion of surgery, remained unchanged. This has led many to believe that surgery created little or no demand for supplemental C. We found, however, that samples of blood taken six hours after surgery showed drops of approximately one-quarter the starting amount of vitamin C, and at 12 hours the levels were down to one-half. Samples taken 24 hours later, without added ascorbic acid to fluids, showed levels three-quarters lower than the original samples. A Baylor University research team reported similar findings in 1965. Marshall Bartlett, Chester Jones,[31] and others reported that in spite of low blood levels of plasma ascorbic acid at time of surgery, normal wound healing may be produced by adequate vitamin C therapy during the postoperative period. Thomas Lanman and Theodore Ingalls[32] showed that the strength of healing wounds is decreased at low plasma levels of vitamin C. Schumacher and colleagues[33] reported that the preoperative use of as little as 500 mg of vitamin C given orally was remarkably successful in preventing shock and weakness following dental extractions. Many other investigators have shown in both laboratory and clinical studies that optimal primary wound healing is dependent to a large extent upon the vitamin C content of the tissues.

In 1949, it was my privilege to assist at an abdominal exploratory laparotomy. A mass of small viscera was found glued together. The area was so friable that every attempt at separation produced a torn intestine. After repairing some 20 tears the surgeon closed the cavity as a hopeless situation. Two grams (2,000 mg) ascorbic acid was given by syringe every two hours for 48 hours and then four times each day. In 36 hours, the patient was walking the halls and in seven days was discharged with normal elimination and no pain. She has outlived her surgeon by many years. We recommend that all patients take 10,000 mg ascorbic acid each day. At least 30,000 mg should be given, daily, in solutions, postoperatively, until oral medication is allowed and tolerated.

Could Ascorbic Acid Have Anticancer Features?

Jorgen Schlegel from Tulane University has been using 1,500 mg of ascorbic acid daily to prevent recurrences of cancer of the bladder.[34] He and other biochemists have been able to demonstrate that in the presence of ascorbic acid, carcinogenic metabolites will not develop in the urine. They suggest that spontaneous tumor formation is the result of faulty tryptophan metabolism while urine is retained in the bladder. Schlegel termed ascorbic acid "an anticancer vitamin." Research has also shown that the depletion of mast cells (initiators of inflammation) from guinea pigs' skin was due to ascorbic acid deficiency.[35] The possibilities indicated are that vitamin C is necessary either directly or indirectly for formation of mast cells, or for their maintenance once formed, or both. Ascorbic acid will control myelocytic leukemia (a cancer that affects white blood cells) provided 25,000 to 30,000 mg is taken orally each day.

One can only speculate on what massive therapy would do in all forms of cancer. Many pathologic conditions are cured by giving 5 million to 100,000 million units of penicillin as an intravenous drip over a period of four to six weeks. How long must we wait for someone to start continuous ascorbic acid drip for two to three months, giving 100,000 to 300,000 mg each day, for various malignant conditions?

Cholesterol Is Not a Problem When Daily Intake of Ascorbic Acid Is High

Mention should be made of the role played by vitamin C as a regulator of the rate at which cholesterol is formed in the body.[36] A deficiency of the vitamin speeds the formation of this substance. In experimental work, guinea pigs fed a diet free of ascorbic acid showed a 600 percent acceleration in cholesterol formation in the adrenal glands. Take 10,000 mg or more each day and then eat all the eggs you want—that is my schedule and my cholesterol remains normal. Russia has published many articles demonstrating these same benefits.

Infectious Hepatitis Relieved

Viral hepatitis needs brief mentioning. There are two types: infectious hepatitis and needle hepatitis. Physical activity has always been considered to increase the severity and prolong the course of the disease.[37] Researchers in Vietnam showed that pick-and-shovel details had no effects on the 199 controls as against 199 kept at bed rest.[38] One thing is certain: given massive intravenous ascorbic acid therapy, patients are well and back to work in three to seven days. In these cases, the vitamin is also employed by mouth as follow-up therapy. A study at the University Clinic of Switzerland in Basel reported that just 10,000 mg daily, intravenously, proved the best treatment available.

Various Maladies

We could continue indefinitely extolling the merits of ascorbic acid . . .

- Excellent results in the healing of corneal ulcers at a dose of 1,500 mg daily.[39]
- One single injection of ascorbic acid, calculated at 500 mg per kg of body weight, will reverse heat stroke.
- One to three injections of the vitamin in a dose range of 400 mg per kg of body weight will effect a dramatic cure in viral pancarditis (inflammation of the heart).
- Intravenous injections will quickly relieve the pain and erythema even of second-degree burns when precautions are not taken.
- One to three injections of 400 mg per kg of body weight given every eight hours will dry up chickenpox in 24 hours; if nausea is present, it will stop the nausea.
- A 5 percent ointment using a water soluble base will cure acute fever blisters if applied ten or more times a day, and a 30 percent ointment can remove several small basal cell epithelioma.
- Very promising results have been reported in glaucoma with a dose schedule of 100 mg per kg of body weight taken after meals and at bed hour.[40]

- Oral doses of 1,000 mg every one to two hours during exposure will prevent sunburn.
- In arthritis, those taking at least 10,000 mg daily, and those taking 15,000 to 25,000 mg daily, will experience commensurate benefit. Supportive treatment must also be given. Repair of collagenous tissue is dependent on adequate ascorbic acid.
- In herpes zoster, 2,000 mg of vitamin C given intramuscularly with 50 mg adenosine-5 monophosphoric acid, also intramuscularly, every 12 hours is beneficial.
- In massive shingles, ascorbic acid should be given by vein and always as much by mouth as can be tolerated.
- Heavy-metal intoxication is resolved with adequate vitamin C therapy.
- In the common cold, 1,000 mg each hour for 48 hours and then 10,000 mg each day by mouth can help reduce the cold's symptoms and duration. Regnier reported that the larger the dose of ascorbic acid, the better were the results.[41]

Note: Injections are usually given with a syringe dilution of 1,000 mg to 5 cc of fluid. This concentration will produce immediate thirst and can be prevented by having the patient drink a glass of juice just before giving the injection.

Severe Viral Diseases

Severe viral diseases can be deadly and must be treated heroically with intravenous and/or intramuscular injections of ascorbic acid. We recommend a dose schedule of 350 mg to 700 mg per kg of body weight diluted to at least 18 cc of 5 percent dextrose water to each 1,000 mg of vitamin C. Ten thousand milligrams of ascorbic acid daily in divided doses is also given by mouth. In small children, 2,000 and 3,000 mg can be given intramuscularly, every two hours. An ice cap to the buttock will prevent soreness and induration.

Ascorbic acid in amounts under 400 mg per kg of body weight can be administered intravenously with a syringe in dilutions of 5 cc to each 1,000 mg, provided the ampoule is buffered with sodium bicarbonate with sodium bisulfite added. As much as 12,000 mg can be given in this manner with a 50 cc syringe. Larger amounts must be diluted with bottle dextrose or saline solutions and run in by needle drip. This is true because amounts like 20,000 to 25,000 mg, which can be given with a 100 cc syringe, can suddenly dehydrate the cerebral cortex so as to produce convulsive movements of the legs. This represents a peculiar syndrome, symptomatic epilepsy, in which the patient is mentally clear and experiences no discomfort except that the lower extremities are in mild convulsion. This epileptiform-type seizure will continue for 20-plus minutes and then abruptly stop. Mild pressure on the knees will stop the seizure so long as pressure is maintained. If still within the time limit of the seizure, the spasm will reappear by simply withdrawing the hand pressure. I have seen this in two patients receiving 26,000 mg intravenously with a 100 cc syringe on the second injection. One patient had polio; the other malignant measles. Both were adults. I have duplicated this on myself to prove no aftereffects. Intramuscular injections are always 500 mg to 1 cc solution. With continuous intravenous injections of large amounts of ascorbic acid, one gram (1,000 mg) of calcium gluconate must be added to the fluids each day.

Multiple Uses

We have reviewed many other pathological conditions in which ascorbic acid plays an important part in recovery. To these might be added cardiovascular diseases, abnormally heavy or prolonged menstruation, peptic and duodenal ulcers, postoperative and radiation sickness, rheumatic fever, scarlet fever, polio, acute and chronic pancreatitis, tularemia (rabbit fever), whooping cough, and tuberculosis.

In one case of scarlet fever in which penicillin and the sulfa drugs were causing no improvement, 50,000 mg of ascorbic acid given intravenously resulted in a dramatic drop in the fever curve to normal. Here the action of ascorbic acid was not only direct but also synergistic.

A similar situation was observed in a case of lobar pneumonia. In another case of puerperal sepsis following a criminal abortion, the initial dose of ascorbic acid was 1,200 mg per kg body weight, and two subsequent injections were at the 600 mg level. These dosages were administered in conjunction with penicillin and sulfadiazine. An admission temperature of 105.4°F resolved to normal in nine hours. The patient made an uneventful recovery.

In one spectacular case of black widow[42] spider bite in a three-year-old child, in coma, 1,000 mg calcium gluconate and 4,000 mg of ascorbic acid were administered intravenously. Then 4,000 mg of ascorbic acid was given every six hours with a syringe. The child was awake and well in 24 hours. On physical examination, the child was comatose with a rigid abdomen. The area about the umbilicus was red and indurated, suggesting a strangulated hernia. With a 4x camera lens, fang marks were in evidence. Thirty hours after starting the vitamin C therapy, the child expelled a large amount of dark, clotted blood; there was no other residual. A review of the literature confirmed that this individual has been the only one to survive with such findings—the others were reported at autopsy.

As for other bites, 10,000 mg daily of vitamin C with 200 mg to 400 mg vitamin B_6, by mouth, will shield one from mosquito bites. Twenty percent of these patients will also require 100 mg vitamin B_6 intramuscularly each week.

General All-Around Benefit

Vitamin C plays a very important role in general health. A deficiency of this substance in sufficient amounts can be a factor in loss of appetite, loss of weight or failure to grow, muscular weakness, anemia, and various skin lesions. The relationship between vitamin C and the health of the gums and teeth has long been recognized. Laboratory studies on gum-teeth connective tissue have reaffirmed this relationship.[43] Our son, who will be 19 in July, has never developed a tooth cavity. Since age ten he has received at least 10,000 mg of ascorbic acid, daily, by mouth. Before age 10, the amount given was on a sliding scale.[44]

In general, vitamin C is beneficial for all-around good health, and its benefits accrue with daily use. Adults taking at least 10,000 mg of ascorbic acid daily, and children under ten at least 1,000 mg for each year of life, will find that the brain will be clearer, the mind more active, the body less wearied, and the memory more retentive.

Conclusion

The types of pathology treated with massive doses of ascorbic acid run the entire gamut of medical knowledge. Body needs are so great that so-called minimal daily requirements must be ignored. A genetic error is the probable cause for our inability to manufacture ascorbic acid, thus requiring exogenous sources of vitamin C. Simple dye or chemical tests are available for checking individual needs. Ascorbic acid destroys virus bodies by taking up the protein coat so that new units cannot be made, by contributing to the breakdown of virus nucleic acid with the result of controlled purine metabolism. Its action in dealing with virus pneumonia and virus encephalitis has been outlined. The clinical use of vitamin C in pneumonia has a very sound foundation. In experimental tests, monkeys kept on a vitamin C–free diet all died of pneumonia, while those with adequate diets remained healthy.[45] Many investigators have shown an increased need for ascorbic acid in this condition,[46,47] as well as for burns, cancer, high cholesterol, diabetes, pregnancy, healing from surgery, and many more conditions.

It must be remembered when using ascorbic acid that experiments on man are the only experiments which can give positive evidence of therapeutic action in man. Likewise, the use of ascorbic acid in human pathology must follow the law of mass action: in reversible reactions, the extent of chemical change is proportional to the active masses of the interacting substance. I am in full agreement with statistician Lancelot Hogben, who said, "A scientific idea must live dangerously or die of inanition. Science thrives on daring generalizations. There is nothing particularly scientific about excessive caution. Cautious explorers do not cross the Atlantic of truth."

REFERENCES FOR "OBSERVATIONS ON THE DOSE AND ADMINISTRATION OF ASCORBIC ACID"

1. Correspondence with colleague from Puerto Rico.

2. Jennings OE, Avinoff A. *Wild Flowers of Western Penna. & Upper Ohio Basin.* University of Pittsburgh Press, Vol. 2, Plate 156.

3. Food and Life. 1939 Yearbook, U.S. Dept. Agriculture, U.S. Printing Office, Washington, DC:236.

4. Klenner, FR. Correspondence with Dr. Bauer, University of Switzerland.

5. Salomon LL, et al. *NY Acad Science* 1961; 93: 115.

6. Grollman AP, Lehninger AL. *Arch Biochem* 1957;69:458.

7. Chattejee IB, Kar NC, Guha BC. *NY Acad Science* 1961;92:36.

8. Isherwood FA, Mapson LW. *NY Acad Science* 1961;92:6.

9. Burns JJ. *Am J Med* 1959;26:740.

10. Stone I. Brief Proposal Per. *Biology & Medicine,* Autumn 1966.

11. Slobody, LB. *J Lab & Clinical Med* 1944;29(5):464–472.

12. Ringsdorf WM, Cheraskin E. Sec., Oral Med., U. of Ala. Med. Center, Birmingham, Ala.

13. Klenner FR. *Tri-State Med J* Feb 1956.

14. Larson C. *Ordnance* Jan-Feb 1967:359–360.

15. Starr TJ. *Hospital Practice,* Nov 1968: 52.

16. Kropowski H. *Med World News,* June 1970: 24.

17. Klenner FR. *J Applied Nutr,* 1953.

18. Klenner FR. *Tri-State Med. J,* June 1957.

19. Klenner FR. *Tri-State Med. J,* Oct. 1958.

20. Klenner FR. *Tri-State Med. J,* Feb. 1960.

21. Bakay L. *The Blood-Brain Barrier.* Springfield, IL: C. Thomas, 1956.

22. Chambers R, et al. *Physiol Rev* 1947;27: 436–463.

23. Knisely MH, et al. *Arch Surg* 1945; 51–220.

24. Knisely MH. *Science* 1947;106: 431.

25. Berkeley WT. Jr. *Southern Med J* 58:1182–1184.

26. Lund C., Levenson SM. *Arch Surg* 1947;55: 557.

27. Bergman HC, et al. *Am Heart J* 1945;29: 506–512.

28. Lam CR. *Col Rev Surg Gyn & Obst* 1941;72: 390–400.

29. Klasson DH. *NY J Med* 1951:51: 2388–2392.

30. Stone HH. *Med J* Aug. 1970;1: 6–10.

31. Bartlett MK, et al. *New Eng J of Med* 1942;226: 474.

32. Lanman TH, Ingalls TH. *Am Surgery* 1937;105: 616.

33. Schumacher. *Ohio State Med J* 1946;42: 1248.

34. Schlegal GE, et al. *Trans Am Ass Genito Urinary Surgery* 1989; 61.

35. Glick D, Hosoda T. *Proc Sec Exp Biology and Med* 1965;119.

36. Becker RR, et al. *J Am Chem Sec* 1953;75: 2020.

37. Capps RB. *Modern Med* Jan. 11, 1971.

38. Freeben RK, Repsher LR. *Mod World News* Jan. 23, 1970.

39. Boyd TA, Campbell FW. *B Med J* 1950; 2: 1145.

40. Virno M. *Eye, Ear, Nose & Throat Monthly* 1967; 46:1502.

41. Regnier E. *Review of Allergy* Oct 1968; 22: 948.

42. Klenner FR. *Tri-State Med J* Dec 1957.

43. Baume LJ. *Science News Letter* 1953;64: 103.

44. Klenner FR. *Tri-State Med J* Nov 1955.

45. Sabin J. *Exp Med* 1939; 89: 507–515.

46. Wright. *Ann Int Med* 1938;12(4): 518–528.

47. Brody HD. *J Am Diet Assoc* 1953;29: 588.

ASCORBIC ACID VITAMIN C: WHAT'S THE REAL STORY?

by Andrew W. Saul, PhD

From the *Orthomolecular Medicine News Service,* December 6, 2013.

Heard anything bad lately about ascorbic acid vitamin C? If you haven't, you may have been away visiting Neptune for too long. For nearly four decades, I have seen that, like all other fashions, vitamin-bashing goes "in" and "out" of style. Lately it has (again) been open season on vitamin C, especially if taken as cheap ascorbic acid. Linus Pauling, PhD, the world's most qualified advocate of vitamin C, urged people to take pure ascorbic acid powder or crystals.

Without having met Dr. Pauling, I know they are also what great-grandma used when she home-canned peaches. Vitamin C powder remains cheap and readily available on the internet. One-quarter teaspoon is just over 1,000 mg. If you encounter a powder that is substantially less potent than that, it may contain fillers. Choose accordingly.

I have told my students for a long time, "If they didn't listen to Linus Pauling, don't be too surprised that they don't line up to hear what you have to say." But Pauling's two unshared Nobel prizes (he is the only person in history with that distinction) are no protection from critics who slam ascorbic acid C without first considering some basic biochemistry.

Atomically Correct

Vitamin C is ascorbic acid, $C_6H_8O_6$, and that's pretty much all there is to it. If you really want to impress your friends, ascorbic acid can also be called (5R)-5-[(1S)-1,2-Dihydroxyethyl]-3,4-dihydroxy-2(5H)-furanone. As I liked to tell my university students, now there is something for you to answer when your parents ask what you learned in school today.

Even if this molecule comes from GMOs, which I disapprove of, it is still molecularly OK. You cannot genetically modify carbon, hydrogen, or oxygen atoms.

There are two ways the atoms can arrange themselves to make $C_6H_8O_6$. One is ascorbic acid. The other is erythorbic acid, also known as isoascorbic acid or D-araboascorbic acid. It is a commercial antioxidant, but cannot be utilized by the body as an essential nutrient.

Acidity

That word *acid* gets us going, but in fact ascorbic acid is a weak acid. If you can eat three oranges, if you can drink a carbonated cola, or if you can add vinegar to your fish fry or to your salad, there is little to worry about. In fact, your normal stomach acid is over 50 times stronger than vitamin C. The stomach is designed to handle strong acid, and nutrients are not destroyed by this strong stomach acid. If they were, all mammals would be dead. Have you ever noticed when you throw up you can feel the burn in your throat? That's stomach acid. A little gross, but we need it to live. People who have a lot of problems with hiatal hernias or reflux can actually regurgitate enough acid over a period of months to damage and scar the throat.

Vitamin C could not do that on a bet. It's impossible. You couldn't start your car if you put vinegar in your automobile's battery. It requires sulfuric acid, which is a very strong acid. The hydrochloric acid in the stomach is only slightly weaker than car-battery acid. Vitamin C is almost as weak as lemonade. That's a huge difference.

Probiotics

If you eat yogurt or take probiotic capsules, they end up in your stomach. There they are subjected to this strong stomach acid, and they survive it easily. Acidophilus bacteria, such as are found in yogurt, are literally so named because they are "acid-loving." Many studies show that eating yogurt and taking other probiotic supplements is a good idea and that it works. If a strong acid does not kill them, then neither will a weak acid.

Furthermore, your body secretes a highly alkaline substance right where your small intestine starts, just past the stomach. This neutralizes stomach acid and automatically keeps the rest of your gut from being acidic. If the body can neutralize a strong acid, ascorbic acid is virtually irrelevant.

Buffering

Ascorbic acid can be buffered, and if you have a sensitive stomach, it should be. There are a variety of nonacidic forms. I do not sell vitamins or any other health products, and do not make brand recommendations.

Don't be bluffed or blustered about ascorbic acid. It is cheap and it works. Aside from intravenous sodium ascorbate, the vast majority of research showing that vitamin C is effective in prevention and treatment of disease has used plain ascorbic acid. Yes, the cheap stuff.

Remember what Ward Cleaver, TV father on *Leave it to Beaver*, said to his young son, "A lot of people go through life trying to prove that the things that are good for them are wrong."

About "Objections" to Vitamin C Therapy

Excerpted from the *Orthomolecular Medicine News Service,* October 12, 2010.

In massive doses, vitamin C (ascorbic acid) stops a cold within hours, stops influenza in a day or two, and stops viral pneumonia (pain, fever, cough) in two or three days.[1] It is a highly effective antihistamine, antiviral, and antitoxin. It reduces inflammation and lowers fever. Administered intravenously, ascorbate kills cancer cells without harming healthy tissue. Many people therefore wonder, in the face of statements like these, why the medical professions have not embraced vitamin C therapy with open and grateful arms.

Probably the main roadblock to widespread examination and utilization of this all-too-simple technology is the equally widespread belief that there *must* be unknown dangers to tens of thousands of milligrams (mg) of ascorbic acid. Yet, since the time megascorbate therapy was introduced in the late 1940s by Fred R. Klenner, MD,[2] there has been an especially safe and extremely effective track record to follow.

Still, for some, questions remain:

Q: Is 2,000 mg per day of vitamin C a megadose?

A: No. Decades ago, Linus Pauling, PhD, and biochemist Irwin Stone showed that most animals make at least that much (or more) per human equivalent body weight per day.[3,4]

Q: Then why has the government set the "Safe Upper Limit" for vitamin C at 2,000 mg per day?

A: Perhaps the reason is ignorance. According to nationwide data compiled by the American Association of Poison Control Centers, vitamin C (and the use of any other dietary supplement) does not kill anyone.[5]

Q: Does vitamin C damage DNA?

A: No. If vitamin C harmed DNA, why do most animals make (not eat, but *make*) between 2,000 and 10,000 mg of vitamin C per human equivalent body weight per day? Evolution would never so favor anything that harms vital genetic material. White blood cells and male reproductive fluids contain unusually high quantities of ascorbate. Living, reproducing systems love vitamin C.

Q: Does vitamin C cause low blood sugar, B_{12} deficiency, birth defects, or infertility?

A: Vitamin C does not cause birth defects, nor infertility, nor miscarriage. According to an article in the *Journal of the American Medical Association:* "Harmful effects have been mistakenly attributed to vitamin C, including hypoglycemia, rebound scurvy, infertility, mutagenesis, and destruction of vitamin B_{12}. Health professionals should recognize that vitamin C does not produce these effects."[6]

Q: Does vitamin C . . . ?

A: Subjects in a randomized, double-blind, placebo-controlled 14-day trial of 3,000 mg per day of vitamin C reported greater frequency of sexual intercourse. The vitamin C group (but not the placebo group) also experienced a quantifiable decrease in depression. This is probably due to the fact that vitamin C "modulates catecholaminergic activity, decreases stress reactivity, approach anxiety and prolactin release, improves vascular function, and increases oxytocin release. These processes are relevant to sexual behavior and mood."[7]

Q: Does vitamin C cause kidney stones?

A: No. The myth of the vitamin C–caused kidney stone is rivaled in popularity only by that of the loch ness monster. A factoid-crazy medical media often overlooks the fact that William J. McCormick, MD, demonstrated that vitamin C actually *prevents* the formation of kidney stones. He did so in 1946, when he published a paper on the subject.[8] His work was confirmed by University of Alabama professor of medicine Emanuel Cheraskin, MD, DMD. Dr. Cheraskin showed that vitamin C inhibits the formation of oxalate stones.[9]

Other research reports that, "Even though a certain part of oxalate in the urine derives from metabolized ascorbic acid, the intake of high doses of vitamin C does not increase the risk of calcium oxalate kidney stones. . . In the large-scale Harvard Prospective Health Professional Follow-Up Study, those groups in the highest quintile of vitamin C intake (greater than 1,500 mg per day) had a lower risk of kidney stones than the groups in the lowest quintiles."[10]

Robert F. Cathcart, MD, said, "I started using vitamin C in massive doses in patients in 1969. By the time I read that ascorbate should cause kidney stones, I had clinical evidence that it did not cause kidney stones, so I continued prescribing massive doses to patients. Up to 2006, I estimate that I have put 25,000 patients on massive doses of vitamin C and none have developed kidney stones. Two patients who had dropped their doses to 500 mg a day developed calcium oxalate kidney stones. I raised their doses back up to the more massive doses and added magnesium and B_6 to their program and no more kidney stones. I think they developed the kidney stones because they were not taking enough vitamin C."

"The ascorbic acid kidney stone story is a myth."

—FREDERICK R. KLENNER, MD

Q: Why did Linus Pauling die from cancer if he took all that vitamin C?

A: Dr. Pauling, megadose vitamin C advocate, died in 1994 from prostate cancer. Mayo Clinic cancer researcher Charles G. Moertel, MD, critic of Pauling and vitamin C, also died in 1994, and also from cancer (lymphoma). Dr. Moertel was 66 years old. Dr. Pauling was 93 years old. One needs to make up one's own mind as to whether this does or does not indicate benefit from vitamin C.

A review of the subject indicates that "vitamin C deficiency is common in patients with advanced cancer . . . Patients with low plasma concentrations of vitamin C have a shorter survival."[11]

Q: Does vitamin C narrow arteries or cause atherosclerosis?

A: Abram Hoffer, MD, PhD, has said, "I have used vitamin C in megadoses with my patients since 1952 and have not seen any cases of heart disease develop even after decades of use. Dr. Robert Cathcart with experience on over 25,000 patients since 1969 has seen no cases of heart disease developing in patients who did not have any when first seen. He added that the thickening of the vessel walls, if true, indicates that the thinning that occurs with age is reversed. . . The fact is that vitamin C *decreases* plaque formation according to many clinical studies. Some critics ignore the knowledge that thickened arterial walls in the absence of plaque formation indicate that the walls are becoming stronger and therefore less apt to rupture. . . Gokce, Keaney, Frei et al gave patients supplemental vitamin C daily for 30 days and measured blood flow through the arteries. Blood flow *increased nearly fifty percent* after the single dose and this was sustained after the monthly treatment."[12]

> *"Indeed, if supplemental vitamin C is harmful, clear indications would have emerged by now, since thousands of people have been consuming large doses for decades."*
>
> —STEPHEN LAWSON, "THE TRIALS AND TRIBULATIONS OF VITAMIN C"

Q: What about blood pressure?

A: A randomized, double-blind, placebo-controlled study showed that hypertensive patients taking supplemental vitamin C had lower blood pressure.[13]

So why the flurry of anti–vitamin C reporting in the mass media? Negative news gets attention. Positive vitamin studies do not. Is this a conspiracy? Of course not. It is nevertheless an enormous public health problem with enormous consequences.

Approximately 150 million Americans take supplemental vitamin C every day. This is as much a political issue as a scientific issue. What would happen if everybody took vitamins? Perhaps doctors, hospital administrators, and pharmaceutical salespeople would all be lining up for their unemployment checks. A skeptic might conclude that there is at least some evidence that the politicians are on the wrong side of this. After all, the US Recommended Dietary Allowance for vitamin C for humans is only 10 percent of the United States Department of Agriculture vitamin C standards for guinea pigs.[14] But conspiracy against nutritional medicine? Certainly not. Couldn't be.

REFERENCES FOR "ABOUT 'OBJECTIONS' TO VITAMIN C THERAPY"

1. Cathcart RF. Vitamin C, titration to bowel tolerance, anascorbemia, and acute induced scurvy. *Medical Hypothesis* 1981;7:1359–1376.

2. Saul AW. Hidden in plain sight: The pioneering work of Frederick Robert Klenner, MD. *J Orthomolecular Med* 2007;22(1):31–38.

3. Pauling L. *How to Live Longer and Feel Better.* Corvallis, OR: Oregon State University Press, 2006.

4. Stone I. *The Healing Factor: Vitamin C Against Disease.* New York: Grosset & Dunlapp, 1972.

5. Mowry JB, Spyker DA, Brooks DE et al. 2014 Annual Report of the American Association of Poison Control Centers' National Poison Data System (NPDS): 32nd Annual Report. *Clinical Toxicology* 2015; (53)10: 962–1147. Available at: http://dx.doi.org/10.3109/15563650.2015.1102927.

6. Levine M, Rumsey SC, Daruwala R, et al. Criteria and recommendations for vitamin C intake." *JAMA* 1999; 281(15):1415–1423.

7. Brody S. High-dose ascorbic acid increases intercourse frequency and improves mood: A randomized controlled clinical trial. *Biol Psychiatry* 2002; 52(4):371–374.

8. McCormick WJ. Lithogenesis and hypovitaminosis. *Med World (New York)* 1946;159:410–413.

9. Cheraskin E, Ringsdorf, Jr. M, and Sisley E. *The Vitamin C Connection: Getting Well and Staying Well with Vitamin C.* New York: Harper and Row, 1983. Also paperback, 1984: New York, Bantam Books. Ringsdorf WM Jr, Cheraskin E. Nutritional aspects of urolithiasis. *South Med J* 1981; 74(1):41–3, 46.

10. Gerster H. No contribution of ascorbic acid to renal calcium oxalate stones. *Ann Nutr Metab* 1997;41(5): 269–82.

11. Mayland CR, Bennett MI, Allan K. Vitamin C deficiency in cancer patients. *Palliat Med* 2005;19(1):17–20.

12. Gokce N, Keaney JF, Frei B, et al. Long-term ascorbic acid administration reverses endothelial vasomotor dysfunction in patients with coronary artery disease. *Circulation* 1999; 99(25):3234–3240.

13. Duffy SJ, Gokce N, Holbrook M, et al. Treatment of hypertension with ascorbic acid. *Lancet* 1999;354(9195):2048–2049.

14. Saul AW. RDA for vitamin C is 10% of USDA standard for guinea pigs. *Orthomolecular Medicine News Service,* February 4, 2010. Available at: http://orthomolecular.org/resources/omns/v06n08.shtml.

VITAMIN C DOES NOT CAUSE KIDNEY STONES

by Steve Hickey, PhD, and Hilary Roberts, PhD

From the *Orthomolecular Medicine News Service*, July 5, 2012.

It is strange how some medical authors seem desperate to show that vitamin C causes harm. One recurrent scare story is that vitamin C might cause kidney stones. However, although such warnings pop up regularly, these reports do not demonstrate an increase in the number or size of stones; instead, they rely on vague indicators of improbable risk.

The authors of such uncritical papers have probably not read the literature, for this is an old story. Decades ago, the idea that vitamin C causes kidney stones formed part of the medical attack on Linus Pauling. While it was initially a reasonable hypothesis, unexpected kidney stones are not found in people taking large amounts of vitamin C.[1,2]

There is no evidence that vitamin C causes kidney stones. Indeed, in some cases, high doses may be curative.[3] A recent, large-scale, prospective study followed 85,557 women for 14 years and found no evidence that vitamin C causes kidney stones.[4] There was no difference in the occurrence of stones between people taking less than 250 milligrams per day and those taking 1.5 grams or more. This study was a follow up of an earlier study on 45,251 men. This earlier study indicated that doses of vitamin C above 1.5 grams reduce the risk of kidney stones.[5] The authors of these large studies stated that restriction of higher doses of vitamin C because of the possibility of kidney stones is unwarranted.

People with recurrent stone formation may have an unusual biochemistry, leading to increased production of oxalate from vitamin C.[6] Oxalate and urate can accumulate in kidney stones. In practice, there is an increased excretion of both oxalate and urate with gram-level doses of vitamin C (ascorbate). Various authors over the years have used this increase to predict that vitamin C will cause kidney stones; however, these predictions have never been confirmed.

Around three quarters of all kidney stones are composed of calcium oxalate; unlike some other stone types, these can form in acidic urine. Although vitamin C does increase the production of oxalate in the body, there is no evidence that it increases stone formation. It could even have the reverse effect, for several reasons. Firstly, vitamin C tends to bind calcium, which could decrease its availability for formation of calcium oxalate. Secondly, vitamin C has a diuretic action: it increases urine flow, providing an environment that is less suitable for formation of kidney stones. Finally, stone formation appears to occur around a nucleus of infection. High concentrations of vitamin C are bactericidal and might prevent stone formation by removing the bacteria around which stones form.

Vitamin C could also prevent other types of kidney stones. Less common forms of stone include uric acid stones (8 percent), which form in gout, and cystine stones (1 percent), which can occasionally be formed in children with a hereditary condition; these stones are not side effects of vitamin C. Other stones include those made from calcium phosphate (5 percent), which dissolve in a vitamin C solution. Acid urine, produced by ascorbate, will also dissolve the struvite stones (magnesium ammonium phosphate) that often occur in infected urine.

Recently, Linda Massey and colleagues from Washington State University have claimed that vitamin C increases the risk of kidney stones.[7] Their paper illustrates how the claims of risk have little basis in fact. Massey claims that vitamin C supplementation can increase the amount of oxalate. Vitamin C can increase oxalate absorption and, if degraded in the body, ascorbate can be converted into oxalate. However, while oxalate is a constituent of some types of kidney stone, an increase in its concentration does not mean that more or larger kidney stones will be formed. The formation of kidney stones is influenced by many factors and, as we have seen, vitamin C might be predicted to inhibit several aspects of stone generation. Massey suggests that this increase in oxalate may increase the risk of stones. This is a weak suggestion, which is contradicted by substantial evidence, quoted above.

This evidence suggests that a high vitamin C intake has no effect on the number of kidney stones, or may even be protective.

Massey links oxalate to risk by use of a measure called the Tiselius Risk Index or TRI.[8] However, this measure is applied incorrectly. Indeed, in the presence of high doses of vitamin C, this index should be modified to accommodate the formation of calcium ascorbate in urine. The TRI measure was developed for subjects who had not been supplemented with vitamin C and, on the basis of simple chemistry, requires modification for use with ascorbate supplementation. Since vitamin C might affect many stages of stone formation and growth, application of the TRI measure to supplemented individuals is suspect. The TRI is applied in this case as a predictive measure, for which it has not been validated. Furthermore, the TRI is derived from the concentration of calcium oxalate, making the argument for increased risk rather circular. Even more importantly, Massey uses the TRI to predict an increased theoretical risk, which substantial evidence indicates is absent.

In Massey's study, 29 stoneformers and 19 non-stoneformers were supplemented with one gram of vitamin C, twice each day. After five days on a low-oxalate diet, the subjects were challenged before breakfast with 136 mg oxalate, including 18 mg oxalic acid. They remained on the low-oxalate diet for the remainder of the day. Of the 48 people, 12 stoneformers and 7 non-stoneformers had an increased total oxalate excretion of greater than 10 percent after supplementation.

However, the number or size of kidney stones did not increase.

Also, we can note that seven of the subjects who showed an increased level of oxalate were not stoneformers. The important question of why some people form kidney stones, and others do not, was neatly sidestepped.

Massey's argument boils down to the vague idea that there could possibly be an increase in kidney stone formation in some rare people. This might be the case if vitamin C increased oxalate without affecting any other part of the process; this is known to be false. If this is the sort of evidence presented as acceptable, we can be comfortable with the claim that the areas of the moon not yet visited by man may be made of green cheese.

REFERENCES FOR "VITAMIN C DOES NOT CAUSE KIDNEY STONES"

1. Hickey S, Roberts H. *Ascorbate: The Science of Vitamin C.* Raleigh, NC: Lulu Press, 2004.

2. Hickey S, Roberts H. *Ridiculous Dietary Allowance.* Raleigh, NC: Lulu Press, 2004.

3. McCormick WJ. Lithogenesis and hypovitaminosis, *Medical Record* 1946; 159: 410–413.

4. Curhan GC, Willett WC, Speizer FE, et al. Megadose Vitamin C consumption does not cause kidney stones. Intake of vitamins B6 and C and the risk of kidney stones in women. *J Am Soc Nephrol* 1999; 10(4): 840–845.

5. Curhan GC, Willett WC, Rimm EB, et al. A prospective study of the intake of vitamins C and B6, and the risk of kidney stones in men. *J Urol* 1996; 155(6): 1847–1851.

6. Chalmers AH, Cowley DM, Brown JM. A possible etiological role for ascorbate in calculi formation. *Clin Chem* 1986; 32(2): 333–336.

7. Massey LK, Liebman M, Kynast-Gales SA. Ascorbate increases human oxaluria and kidney stone risk. *J Nutr* 2005; 135(7): 1673–1677.

8. Tiselius HG. Stone incidence and formation. *Clinical Urology* 2000; 26(5): 452–462.

VITAMIN C REDUCES VACCINATION SIDE EFFECTS

Few physicians know and fewer will tell you: high-dose vitamin C is absolutely essential before, during (yes, right at the doctor's office), and after vaccination. Keeping our children safe is our number-one priority. As states and countries continue to increase their vice grip of control mandating more and more vaccines for our children, we must find a way to make them safer. Not only does high-dose vitamin C help prevent vaccine side effects, vitamin C actually makes shots work better.

DON'T VACCINATE WITHOUT VITAMIN C

by Helen Saul Case

From the *Orthomolecular Medicine News Service,* October 22, 2015.

My husband and I chose to have our children vaccinated. We think some immunizations are worthwhile. We are not in favor of others, but the law is not set up in such a way where doctors and parents can make decisions together about which particular vaccines children receive. Only with our continued insistence did our children's pediatricians separate the administration of the shots. Otherwise our kids would have been exposed to as many as seven diseases at a clip. And unless your child has a sound medical reason not to get a particular shot, such as a known allergy to certain vaccine ingredients or he or she has a compromised immune system, it is unlikely a doctor will allow a medical exemption. So in many cases a reaction must occur first, and only *then* might a child be excused from further dosages of a particular vaccine. That's like putting up a traffic light at a dangerous intersection only after people are seriously hurt. Right now, it's a ready, fire, aim approach. It feels like a game of trial and error—of wait and see. That's simply not good enough, and that's why I give my kids vitamin C, and lots of it.

Vitamin C and Vaccine Reactions

At fifteen months old, hours after she received two shots for four diseases, DPT (diphtheria, pertussis, and tetanus) and Hib (Haemophilus influenzae type b), my baby daughter was screaming, falling over and uncoordinated, and spiked a fever that registered as high as 103.5 degrees on our temporal thermometer. Knowing that in large doses, vitamin C is an antipyretic (fever reducer) in addition to being an antibiotic, antiviral, and antitoxin,[1] I acted fast and got the fever under control with very large doses of ascorbic acid and calcium ascorbate (or buffered vitamin C) to bowel tolerance, and a tepid bath. At bowel tolerance of vitamin C, she was no longer screaming and uncoordinated. Within the first hour her fever was down by a degree; in the second hour, another degree. For the remainder of the evening her fever hovered around 100.5.

> *"When it happens to your child, the risks are 100 percent."*
>
> —BARBARA LOE FISHER,
> NATIONAL VACCINE INFORMATION CENTER

Her severe reaction was not recorded in her medical record by her doctor. It simply stated, "Called service last pm withh fever"—misspelling and all. None of her other symptoms were recorded. During the call, they recommended that I give her children's Tylenol (acetaminophen), especially if her fever went above 101 degrees. Seeing as her fever was below 101, I put her to bed and continued to monitor her temperature each hour. Her fever fluctuated inversely with her intake of vitamin C, so I continued to give her regular doses (250–500 milligrams [mg]) every two hours or so), keeping the Tylenol handy just in case. By the next morning, her temperature registered normal and she was a normal, happy little girl again. While a mild fever indicates the body's natural *immune response* is in good working order combating vaccines, a high fever that spikes during a *vaccine reaction* is very serious and must be brought down right away. Acetaminophen can do this, but so can high-dose vitamin C. We watched it work.

It would be years later before we were told which vaccine was to blame for our daughter's severe vaccine reaction at fifteen months of age. Her third, and hopefully last, pediatrician determined, based on my detailed written record of her severe reaction (the only record we had), that it was due to the pertussis component of the DPT shot.

Vitamin C Makes Shots Safer and More Effective

I believe every doctor should be telling parents to give kids vitamin C when they get vaccinations. In addition to vitamin C's antitoxin properties (for example, its ability for "neutralizing the toxic nature of mercury in all of its chemical forms"), Thomas Levy, MD, says, "There is another compelling reason to make vitamin C an integral part of any vaccination protocol: Vitamin C has been documented to augment the antibody response of the immune system. As the goal of any vaccination is to stimulate a maximal antibody response to the antigens of the vaccine while causing minimal to no toxic damage to the most sensitive of vaccine recipients, there would appear to be no medically sound reason not to make vitamin C a part of all vaccination protocols."[2]

Over forty years ago, Archie Kalokerinos, MD, found that giving infants doses of vitamin C stopped them dying from complications of inoculations.[3] Over forty years ago, Frederick R. Klenner, MD, recommended children under ten take daily "at least one gram (1,000 mg) of ascorbic acid for each year of life."[4] In preparation for immunizations, Dr. Levy recommends "[i]nfants under ten pounds can take 500 mg daily in some fruit juice, while babies between ten and twenty pounds could take anywhere from 500 mg to 1,000 mg total per day, in divided doses. Older children can take 1,000 mg daily per year of life (5,000 mg for a five year-old child, for example, in divided doses)."[5] A sick child, or one suffering vaccine side effects, would require much more.

"Ideally, the vitamin C would be given prior to vaccination and continue afterwards," says Levy. "For optimal antibody stimulation and toxin protection, it would be best to dose for three to five days before the shot(s) and to continue for at least two to three days following the shot. . . . Even taking a one-time dose of vitamin C in the dosage range suggested above directly before the injections can still have a significant toxin-neutralizing and antibody-stimulating effect. It's just that an even better likelihood of having a positive outcome results from extending the pre- and post-dosing periods of time."[6]

As for the kind of vitamin C to give little ones, our children have done well with a mixture of about 80 percent ascorbic acid crystals buffered with 20 percent calcium ascorbate powder added to their favorite juice. As infants, we gave it to them using a dropper.

> *"When I was in active pediatric practice, I wish I had known what I know now about vitamin C's ability to greatly modify vaccination side effects. The 103-degree fever worried me much less than the screaming and unsteadiness, which are markers of cerebral irritation."*
>
> —RALPH CAMPBELL, MD

Giving Vitamin C Before, During, and After Vaccinations

My kids take vitamin C every day, and always have. Now, in preparation for shots, they receive numerous, regular doses of vitamin C before, during (yes right at the doctor's office), and for weeks after administered immunizations. This is what experience and our daughter's vaccine reaction has taught us. While we had given her vitamin C all along, we weren't nearly as diligent about frequent, timely dosing at vaccination time. We thought we were doing enough. As many folks come to find out, what they think is "a lot" of vitamin C isn't always enough vitamin C. You take enough to get the job done.

To avoid vaccine reactions and side effects, days before, the day of, and for days after vaccination, we give our children enough vitamin C to get them just to the point of saturation. After immunizations, their immune system needs all the help it can get. They will get C as often as every hour until they get gassy, a telltale sign that they are getting adequate amounts. The goal is to get them to the point just before "bowel tolerance," or loose bowels. For example, when our daughter was four, we started her with a relatively large loading dose in the morning, 2,000 mg or so, then gave her 1,000 to 2,000 mg every couple of hours throughout the day. We wait until there is a rumbling tummy or softened or loose stool. Once that point is reached, we throttle back the dose. We continue to give C, but give less. The next day, we do it again.

Amazingly, the day of and for several days after our four-year-old daughter's last vaccination, the first shot she had received since her severe reaction years before, she comfortably held 15 to 20 grams, that's 15,000 to 20,000 milligrams, of vitamin C each day. She had no reaction whatsoever to the vaccination. No swelling. No fever. No redness. Nothing. She was happy. We were happy. That may sound like a lot of C for a child who only weighed about 33 pounds, but it got the job done. Perhaps your child won't need that much.

You might be surprised how much vitamin C a three-month-old can hold after a couple of vaccinations. I was. We don't allow the kids to get diarrhea and dehydrate, but we do want them to have the vitamin C their bodies require when tackling sickness or immunization side effects. Since gassiness comes before loose bowels, it's a helpful indicator. If bowel tolerance is reached and stools become frequent, liquid, or, as was the case for my breastfed three-month-old, frequent and greenish in color (since they are always liquid-like), we reduced the frequency and dose, but continued to give it regularly, ramping the frequency and dose up and down as the situation requires. This takes a little practice, but we know we're not hurting our children with extra C. It is a very, very safe vitamin.

Vitamin C Works

Vitamin C is incredibly safe and effective. We are very comfortable giving both of our kids high doses of C. Older, bigger children may hold more C, and younger ones not as much. Saturation becomes a helpful indicator of how much your child can hold.

I don't believe it is fair to let children get vaccines without vitamin C. I also do not believe it is it fair to let them acquire natural immunity through exposure to disease without vitamin C. Always give C. As to the quantity of C to give, when in doubt, give more.

Dr. Levy is convinced of vitamin C's safety. He says, "Except in individuals with established, significant renal insufficiency, vitamin C is arguably the safest of all nutrients that can be given."[7] And it works. Over forty years ago, Robert F. Cathcart, MD, discovered that bowel tolerance of vitamin C resolved illness more quickly.[8] Neither of our children has yet to need an antibiotic. We use vitamin C instead.

For any parent worried about vaccine reactions and side effects, knowing about vitamin C should provide some real comfort. It sure does for us.

REFERENCES FOR "DON'T VACCINATE WITHOUT VITAMIN C"

1. *Orthomolecular Medicine News Service.* Antibiotics put 142,000 into emergency rooms each year. U.S. Centers for Disease Control waits 60 years to study the problem. Oct 13, 2008. Available at: http://www.orthomolecular.org/resources/omns/v04n14.shtml (accessed May 2016). See also: Saul AW. "Notes on orthomolecular (megavitamin) use of vitamin C." Available at: http://www.doctoryourself.com/ortho_c.html.

2. Levy TE. Vitamin C prevents vaccination side effects; increases effectiveness. *Orthomolecular Medicine News Service,* Feb 14, 2012. Available at: http://orthomolecular.org/resources/omns/v08n07.shtml.

3. Kalokerinos A. *Every Second Child.* New Canaan, CT: Keats Publishing, 1981.

4. Klenner FR. Observations on the dose and administration of ascorbic acid when employed beyond the range of a vitamin in human pathology. *Journal of Applied Nutrition* 1971; 23(3 & 4):61–87.

5. Levy TE. Vitamin C prevents vaccination side effects; increases effectiveness. *Orthomolecular Medicine News Service,* Feb 14, 2012. Available at: http://orthomolecular.org/resources/omns/v08n07.shtml.

6. Ibid.

7. Ibid.

8. Cathcart RF. Vitamin C, titration to bowel tolerance, anascorbemia, and acute induced scurvy. *Medical Hypotheses* 1981; 7:1359–1376.

VACCINATIONS, VITAMIN C, AND "CHOICE"

by Helen Saul Case

From the *Orthomolecular Medicine News Service,* February 13, 2016.

Some folks are pretty appalled that my husband and I had our children vaccinated. People write and tell me that vaccinations are dangerous. They warn me about the side effects of this vaccine and that one. They share alternative, natural ways to improve immunity. What we've got here is a failure to communicate. I am sorry that I did not explain myself better the first time. (See "Don't Vaccinate Without Vitamin C.")

Let's fix that.

Vaccinations Can Be Dangerous

You don't have to tell me this. I already know. I watched my child suffer a severe vaccine reaction before my very eyes. Seeing my 15-month-old baby, screaming, trying to walk to me but not being able to because she was stumbling and falling over and uncoordinated, is a vision I will *never* be able to get out of my mind. It was horrific.

I also watched high-dose, saturation-level vitamin C return her to normal. I will never forget this either.

But why didn't I just stop the shots right then and there?

"Choosing" to Vaccinate

In the article I wrote, "My husband and I chose to have our children vaccinated." We did. We *could* have chosen not to.

We could have said no to *all* shots by *choosing* a religious exemption stating that shots are against our sincerely held religious beliefs. We chose not to make this our religion.

Philosophical, personal, or conscientiously held belief exemptions to vaccinations are not lawful in New York State, where our family lives. We could have *chosen* to move to a different state where philosophical exemptions are allowed. But we chose not to move.

We could have *chosen* to just flat-out refuse immunizations and go face to face against state government and school districts and child protective services. Ultimately, we chose to comply only with state-mandated vaccinations, but just the ones required for school, and no more.

So yes, we *chose* to have our children vaccinated. Truly, though, we didn't feel we had much choice. Nobody really does. "Choice" can be taken away in an instant.

Shots for Every Child

Pay attention: this is important. As states push stronger and more stringent immunization laws onto their citizens, mandatory vaccination is quickly becoming the rule rather than the exception. You can argue about the dangers of vaccinations, but I will just agree with you. That doesn't change the fact that children are still getting shots every day. Vaccine reactions and side effects are a real danger. Doctors agree. This is the cold, hard reality.

I do not agree with all of the shots recommended for children. I do not agree with the timing of shots for children. I do not agree that toddlers and babies and infants should be given shots so early in their life, so many at a clip, and three, and four, and five doses of the same ones over and over again. I do not agree that pregnant mothers of developing babies should be given shots. And I do not condone the fact that no medical or governmental authority instructs parents how to protect against vaccination damage by giving massive doses of vitamin C.

> *"A young child may receive 49 doses of 14 vaccines before age 6, and 69 doses of 16 vaccines before age 18. It is also worrying when you examine the various ingredients that are present in these vaccines. What does make sense is the use of bowel tolerance amounts of oral vitamin C to counter the toxic effects of vaccines."*
>
> —KEN WALKER, MD

My opinion notwithstanding, every year more than ten million vaccines are given to children less than a year of age.[1] Only somewhere between 1 and 10 percent of vaccine reactions are ever reported.[2] That one comes as no surprise to us. Our daughter's pediatrician did not report her vaccine reaction. We did.

In most states, when it comes to vaccinations, you must become an extremist or you must comply. Parents in my state are not allowed to postpone shots for their children past state mandates without medical exemptions. We can only delay them and spread them out within these limitations. Saying yes to some shots and no to others is not permitted; the law does not allow families a "buffet" approach. As states look to tighten the screws on medical exemptions, eliminate philosophical and conscientious exemptions, and even try to (unconstitutionally) limit religious exemptions, it is becoming more likely than not: a needle is going into your child.

And we had all better be ready.

> *"I feel strongly that vaccinations have to be considered separately as applied to the individual and tracked for effectiveness. There will never be a good vaccine for every infectious disease. I would hope that many will heed the fact that high-dose C does wonders in reducing vaccine side effects."*
>
> —RALPH CAMPBELL, MD

High-Dose Vitamin C for Everybody

High-dose vitamin C safely prevents and treats vaccine side effects.[3] This has been evident in our experience. We watched high-dose, saturation-level vitamin C bring our daughter back to health after a vaccine reaction. We watched high-dose, saturation-level vitamin C prevent vaccination side effects. We give both of our children saturation levels of C before, during (yes, right at the doctor's office), and after immunizations. We don't give the amount of vitamin C we *think* might work; we give enough to get the job done.

This is no small task. It takes determination like you have never had before to get your children to take very high amounts of vitamin C again and again, day after day. It also takes love, patience, understanding, praise, yummy "chasers" after taking vitamin C powder in juice, and when all else fails: straight up bribery.

Keeping kids as healthy as possible takes a great deal of effort. And it is worth it. Even our doctor marvels that our children only visit the office for wellness appointments and vaccinations.

I see it this way: when you are a parent and are breastfeeding or giving a bottle, you don't just give up if your child doesn't eat. You see to it that your baby gets the nutrition he or she needs. You do it *until*. That's how we feel about vitamin C. It is that important.

No Shots Until My Twenties

In my article I say "We (my husband and I) believe some immunizations to be worthwhile." And I do. Two, in fact.

In in my twenties, I received a single tetanus shot after I stepped on a nail that went up through my foot while I was walking through an old barn. Horse dung naturally carries tetanus bacteria, which can survive dormant encased in spores for decades.[4] While the chance was probably quite slim that I would actually end up with tetanus, I thought it a "good idea" to get a tetanus shot under such circumstances. So did my doctor. I got the shot and took lots of vitamin C, too.

I also received a single dose of an MMR (measles, mumps, rubella) vaccine years before I became pregnant. My doctor made a case for this one being a good idea if I wanted to have a family. Getting measles while pregnant can result in serious problems for a developing baby. We discussed if any other shots would also be worth the inherent risk. The answer was no. Again, I took vitamin C to bowel tolerance. I was spared any ill effects from the MMR inoculation.

So yes, this would mean I believe some shots are worthwhile. I, myself, have had two. But there's more to it than that. I did not have a single shot as a child. My parents chose to use vitamins and nutrition as the answers to (and more often for the prevention of) our health problems. Not surprisingly, we were really healthy kids. I was raised all the way into college with no shots, and no antibiotics either. They used vitamins instead because they are safe and they work. But this was a very tough road for my parents and for me to travel. That road is even more difficult to navigate now with so much more pressure to vaccinate and more vaccinations to be pressured for.

We All Want Healthy Kids

We must meet parents where they are. While we work to mandate vaccine safety, demand informed consent, and advocate for real choice when it comes to whether or not to vaccinate, let's minimize any chance of vaccine damage *now*. Children are powerless. We aren't. Whether we have a choice to vaccinate or not, let's choose to give them vitamin C and lots of it.

REFERENCES FOR "VACCINATIONS, VITAMIN C, AND 'CHOICE'"

1. Vaccine Adverse Event Reporting System. https://vaers.hhs.gov/data/index.

2. National Vaccine Information Center. Frequently asked questions. Topic: vaccine reactions. Available at: http://www.nvic.org/faqs/vaccine-reactions.aspx.

3. Levy TE. Vitamin C prevents vaccination side effects; increases effectiveness. *Orthomolecular Medicine News Service*, Feb 14, 2012.

4. U.S. National Library of Medicine. National Institutes of Health. Medline Plus. Tetanus. Available at: https://www.nlm.nih.gov/medlineplus/ency/article/000615.htm. See also: Centers for Disease Control and Prevention. Epidemiology and prevention of vaccine-preventable diseases. Available at: http://www.cdc.gov/vaccines/pubs/pinkbook/tetanus.html.

CHAPTER 7

Vitamin A

"Potentially large numbers of Americans may consume levels of vitamin A below the Recommended Dietary Allowance (RDA)."
—JACK CHALLEM, *THE NUTRITION REPORTER*

The benefits of getting adequate vitamin A in your diet are immense. A great way to do that is by drinking fresh, raw vegetable juice. Getting vitamins from veggies is ideal. You may also choose to take a supplement for extra protection.

VITAMIN A AND BETA-CAROTENE

by Bradford S. Weeks, MD

Excerpted from *J Orthomolecular Med* 2003;18(3 & 4):131–145.

Vitamins, as we know them today, serve four primary biological functions—membrane stabilization, potentiation of hormonal activity, hydrogen/electron donors/acceptors and co-enzyme functions. Vitamin A is the generic term for that class of compounds with the biologic activity of retinal and it occurs in nature in three primary forms: retinol, retinal and retinoic acid—the alcohol, aldehyde and acid forms respectively. Possessing a large number of double bonds, vitamin A distinguishes itself as being the only known human molecule that can absorb photonic energy (light) and create a new physical bond *de novo* along its backbone of conjugated polyene systems. That, itself, merits our incredulity, being as close as we come to photosynthesis.

Forms of Vitamin A

Vitamin A was discovered by E.V. McCollum at the University of Wisconsin (1913–1915)–he also discovered vitamin D and was named Mr. Vitamin by *Time* magazine in 1951—after noting that this new substance prevented xerophthalmia (dry eyes) and night blindness in laboratory rats. Accordingly, the most common physiological association with vitamin A has been visual function which utilizes the retinal form exclusively. However, subsequent research demonstrated that vitamin A deficient animals died prematurely. We now know that the vital effects of systemic vitamin A require primarily the long chain fatty acid retinyl ester (predominately retinyl palmitate) form. Both vitamin A and beta-carotene are available for consumption in natural forms (foods and food extracts) as well as in synthetic and analogue forms.

Sources

Vitamin A can occur naturally in animal tissue as the bio-available, preformed isoprenoid compounds (retinoids). Animal foods highest in vitamin A include: beef liver, 10,503 international units (IU) per 100 grams (g); butter, 754 IU per 100 g; egg, 552 IU per 100 g; and fish flesh, such as mackerel, which contains 130 IU per 100 g. Of course, unless these animal products are organic, they can accumulate pesticides, heavy metals, and other toxins and therefore are typically unsafe to consume on a regular basis. Another consideration in sourcing vitamin A is quite simply that most anything that goes rancid has some vitamin A.

Things that inhibit absorption of vitamin A include: high-protein diets, antacids (especially those containing aluminum), and most rampantly, in the elderly population, laxatives, which inhibit absorption of all fat-soluble vitamins, including A, D, and E.

Another source of vitamin A is the class of isoprenoid plant pigments, the carotenoids. There are over 500 carotenoids, but beta-carotene is of primary importance to humans. Good food sources are orange or yellow vegetables and fruits. One cantaloupe offers four times as much beta-carotene as one carrot. Broccoli is another good source of vitamin A, but the chlorophyll (green) camouflages the yellow carotene color. If it weren't for chlorophyll, broccoli would be yellow or orange.

We accept dietary vitamin A in two distinct forms: "ready-made" retinoids from tissues or milk of animals, or "disassembly-required" beta-carotene or pro-vitamin A from vegetables. Both the free retinal and the intact beta-carotene diffuse passively across our mucosal membranes in a process facilitated by dietary fat and inhibited by starvation (actual starvation involving inadequate fats and proteins; iatrogenic starvation involving laxatives such as mineral oil, cholesterol-lowering statin drugs, and antacids, which inhibit digestion and absorption). Biliary, pancreatic, or hepatic diseases can also inhibit absorption and compromise utilization of fat-soluble vitamins A, D, E, and K via similar mechanisms. Primary among the rate-limiting minerals for the utilization of vitamin A include zinc, selenium, and manganese. Nonetheless, the most common source from which most of us get our Recommended Dietary Allowance (RDA) of 5,000 IU of vitamin A is our own liver, which has the capacity to store up to two years' worth of vitamin A at a time.

Consideration of Vitamin A's Risk/Benefit Ratio

One cannot read about vitamin A without being warned against taking too much of this substance, and yet "too much" remains poorly defined and is currently a source of much debate within nutritional circles. The rationale for caution is easily understood. Fat-soluble vitamins, A, D, E and K, are not excreted as copiously and frequently as are the water-soluble vitamins, the Bs, folate, biotin, and C, so they tend to accumulate and may reach toxic levels over time. The logic for limiting vitamin A dosage to 10,000 IU a day is quite clear. However, clinical practice yields a more ambiguous picture. Reports of megadosing of vitamin A palmitate for specific orthomolecular indications have informed us of vitamin A's remarkable abilities when given in high doses. Typical of these prescriptions is 200,000 IU given daily over ten years by Frederick R. Klenner, MD (as reported in the *Medical Tribune*), which at the time of printing, had restored healthy skin to what had been a case of ichthyosis (dry, scaly, thick skin). Dr. Klenner himself took at least 75,000 IU of vitamin A daily for 15 years with no toxicity.

These are extreme cases, which are worth considering in that they remind us of Roger J. Williams's tenet of biochemical individuality. Those doses may not be appropriate for everyone, and the practice of taking far more than the RDA for vitamin A should not be done without the consultation of a knowledgeable health care practitioner. Sometimes, however, a conservative low dose consistent with the RDA is not enough to achieve a targeted therapeutic effect.

Vitamin A and vitamin D can act antagonistically in general (competition for fat absorption) and in particular (as regards bone metabolism).[1] Any study which discussed vitamin A and fracture risk without addressing the variables of seasonal light and its degree of activation of endogenous vitamin D_3 (cholecalciferol) as compared with vitamin D_2 (the yeast ergosterol, which is often used to fortify dairy products) should be deemed preliminary at best.

Studies[2,3] that attempted to link vitamin A and beta-carotene to an increased incidence of fracture and cardiac risk were seriously flawed, and their uncritical acceptance in the referenced prestigious journals is cause for not a little concern.

Vitamin A Toxicity

In considering the risks of overdosing on vitamin A, let's remember the wise words of Hippocrates: "Poison is a matter of dosage." Doctors should seek to practice "medicine by Braille" meaning, give a dose and then stay in "close touch" with the patient in order to gather ample data with which to modify protocols responsibly. We can agree that Mae West's famous quotation, "Too much of a good thing is wonderful," applies delightfully to many things in life but not to vitamin A, which history teaches us can be lethal above a certain dose.

We recall the story of hungry arctic explorers who made the potentially deadly mistake of eating polar bear liver, which contains 1 *million* units of vitamin A per *gram.* Animal sources of vitamin A (retinal) are six times more potent than vegetable sources (beta-carotene). Explorer V. Stefansson learned from natives not to eat the liver of arctic animals. In his book *My Life with the Eskimos* (1906), Stefansson records the best way to cook arctic meat: "[A]ccording to Eskimo custom, you put the meat into cold water, bring it to a boil, take it off the heat and allow it to cool. You then scrape the fat off the top of the water, drink the remaining juice and eat the meat." In this way, without knowing the name of the fat-soluble vitamin so concentrated in livers, Stefansson kept the vitamin A dosage well within a tolerable range for consumption.

Levels above 100,000 IU of vitamin A are considered toxic, but clinical protocols for skin problems (acne, psoriasis [dry, patchy skin], hyper-keratosis, ichthyosis), visual problems (xerophthalmia [dry eyes], night blindness), and immune deficiencies (viral infections, bronchitis, mucosal resilience) require much higher doses for a discrete period of time in order to bolster vitamin A–dependent metabolisms.

The signs of excess vitamin A include hair loss, erythema (painful skin bumps), desquamation (skin peeling), myalgias (muscle pain), and headaches, as well as mucous membrane reactions, including cheilitis (lip inflammation), stomatitis (mouth sores), and conjunctivitis (pink eye). The warning signs of vitamin A saturation in the liver include developing a yellow/orange tint to the skin and even the whites of eyes. If this happens, discontinue the vitamin A supplements and the yellow coloring in the whites of your eyes, palms of your hands, and soles of your feet will go away in a few months—except for infants. In their case, excessive vitamin A can be lethal. However, carotene is not. Generally, carotene will turn the skin yellow when the intake is above 20 mg per day (about 34,000 IU), and when consumption is discontinued, no damage results.

Vitamin A Benefits

In answer to the question, "Who would benefit from supplementation with vitamin A?" we can simply respond from the orthomolecular perspective: "Everyone who is deficient in vitamin A would experience enhanced health and vitality when given a dosage that replenishes their deficiency." Who are these people? You and I, perhaps? The clinical signs of vitamin A deficiency are all around us, and they include a generalized loss of appetite and muscular stamina, retarded growth, a drying and kerotinization of skin and mucous membranes, as well as dry and rough-feeling hair. X-rays may show periosteal overgrowth, which can manifest as sciatica since vertebral foraminae can narrow in this condition. The ocular signs, however, are as tragic as they are pathognomonic: xerophthalmia (dryness of conjunctiva), crusting, and the eventual Bitot's spots ("cheesy" deposits on the conjunctiva near the cornea) all presage easily preventable infant and childhood blindness. If those visual signs are not sufficient, one could have the laboratory quantify liver stores of the vitamin. Dr. T. Keith Murray did just this when he examined the livers of deceased Canadians for vitamin A storage and learned that 30 percent of the specimens had less vitamin A in their livers than would be expected at birth. Additionally, of 500 deceased Canadians, 33 percent had less than 40 mcg (about 130 IU) of vitamin A in the liver, and 20 percent had no measurable vitamin A stores at all. This scenario worsens with age as other factors conspire to inhibit absorption of vitamin A—laxatives and cholesterol-binding drugs as well as hypochlorhydria, resulting in frank protein deficiency and malabsorption.

Vitamin A Requirements Through Life

One way to appreciate the benefits of vitamin A is to start at the beginning of a life and create a timeline for vitamin A requirements from conception on.

Conception. Adequate vitamin A is required for fertility and conception. Vitamin A gradients in uterine mucosal tissue also determine where in the uterus the fertilized egg will implant—a highly significant factor, as any obstetrician or midwife will agree.

Embryogenesis. Once fertilization is accomplished, embryogensis and cell differentiation will not proceed normally in the absence of adequate vitamin A and carotenoids.[4] Subsequent neural growth and development in utero and on through infancy rely to a great degree upon vitamin A and beta-carotenes, just as children rely upon these vitamins to support skeletal growth.

Infancy. In order to survive infancy and grow into childhood, vitamin A is required in a very dramatic manner.

In 1982, Alfred Sommer, a 40-year-old Johns Hopkins ophthalmologist doing research in infant blindness from vitamin A deficient xerophthalmia (dry eyes), noted that most of the 4,000 Indonesian children in his study had died of infant diarrhea or bronchitis. Wondering which was causal, he crunched numbers and discovered that a child with night blindness when the study began was three times more likely to die by the end of the study than a child with normal vision. If the child had Bitot's spots, the risk of death was six times higher. With both symptoms, death was nine times more likely. His subsequent publication[5] was met with indifference, but his clinical trials (Indonesia 1984 and Nepal from 1989 to 1991 demonstrating 34 percent and 30 percent less death in vitamin A–supplemented groups) got some attention. Researchers have also observed[6] that vitamin A deficiency leads to a strong reduction of certain enterocyte enzymatic activities, which in turn precipitates a lethal dysbiosis (microbial imbalance) with increased bacterial translocation and consequent diarrhea.

Vitamin A deficiency has been implicated in sudden infant death syndrome (SIDS). Researchers[7] found an association between low or no vitamin A supplementation and an increased risk of sudden infant death syndrome during infants' first year of life. This effect persisted when an adjustment was made for potential confounders, including socioeconomic factors.

Adolescence. Once safely into adolescence, people require vitamin A for its antiviral and antiacne effect as well as to minimize the unsightly hyperkeratosis (those bumps on the back of your arms), which you thought was "just something you have to live with." Not so. You can live without it if you avoid saturated fats and sugar and take adequate amounts of vitamin A and flaxseed oil. Vitamin A comes to the rescue with its more generally appreciated benefit—the enhancement of night vision now that the kids are borrowing the car and staying out too late at night. If your visual acuity is diminished in the dark beyond what is expected, try vitamin A as well as selenium and zinc.

Young Adulthood. The college students in my practice all have vitamin A palmitate in their first aid kits. We know that stress is an immune suppressant, and given the velocity of life at this age with the inevitable "all-nighters," my college students know to take a megadose of vitamin A palmitate at the first sign of sore throat, cough, or that ominous feeling of "I am going to be sick tomorrow." They report, however, that after taking the megadose of vitamin A before going to sleep, they invariably awaken the next morning feeling great. Their chief complaint becomes, "I never get any sick days . . ." The exception to this treatment protocol, of course, is pregnant or potentially pregnant women who understand that megadoses of vitamin A can be dangerous for the fetus. Women enjoy another benefit of vitamin A, however, that the men cannot: rapid, painless resolution of that terrifying Pap smear result: cervical dysplasia. Like most virus-related illnesses, cervical dysplasia is effectively treated with vitamin A along with other complementary nutrients such as selenium, vitamin E, and beta-carotene.

Middle Age. Years ago, Abram Hoffer, MD, PhD, pioneer orthomolecular scientist and physician, noted that niacin cured his bleeding gums (gingivitis). This simple observation ultimately resulted in collaborative research demonstrating the role of niacin as the gold standard for treatment of high cholesterol. Vitamin A is a heart-healthy nutrient that can also treat gingivitis. Furthermore, patients with related and compounding diseases such as diabetes and glaucoma also tend to be deficient in vitamin A. Retinoids minimize experimental vessel wall narrowing due to atherosclerosis, postballoon injury stenosis, and bypass graft failure. Retinoids also promote a differentiated phenotype in smooth muscle cells. Given the similarities in the pathogenesis of neoplasia and vascular disease, we ought not be surprised to learn that many in vitro studies report beneficial effects of retinoids on cell migration, proliferation, apoptosis, matrix remodeling, fibrinolysis, coagulation, and inflammation, all of which should make the cardiologists sit up and take notice.[8]

Old Age. Another illness that plagues us as we age is bronchitis. This, too, is humbled before the immune-enhancing and antiviral power of vitamin A. How does vitamin A protect the mucous membranes and thereby reinforce our barrier immunological defense system? Conceptually speaking, you can understand vitamin A as the protector and nurturer of mucous membranes. That includes the entire gastrointestinal tract, as well as syptoms ranging from sniffles to diarrhea. In addition, vitamin A protects the urogenital tract, most specifically the female cervix and vagina, which can be successfully treated with vitamin A if ulcers or dysplasia occur. If your vitamin A level is low, you are not immunologically "buffed." Any mucous vulnerability, including nasal allergies, sore throat, gastritis, ulcers (including Crohn's disease and ulcerative colitis), and cervical dysplasia, signals a deficiency of vitamin A, and all benefit from a simple nutrient. Third-world doctors have long called vitamin A "the anti-infection vitamin." These doctors are not concerned with vitamin A toxicity; rather they see patients dying of vitamin A deficiency as it manifests in a great variety of infectious diseases which ravage poor countries, including fatal diarrhea, many respiratory ailments, tuberculosis, ear and eye infections, and malaria. One common side effect of malaria is vitamin A deficiency.[9]

Antiviral Effects

Antiviral effects are especially important as the flu season approaches, but there is more. Professor Richard Semba, MD, of the prestigious Johns Hopkins University Hospital, presented his research demonstrating that pregnant women infected with HIV (AIDS virus) who also were vitamin A deficient were much more likely to transmit the virus to their newborn infants than were HIV-infected mothers who had adequate amounts of this important vitamin. Specifically, with low vitamin A, the transmission rate between mother and infant was 32 percent, whereas with adequate levels the rate was only 7 percent. Additionally, 93 percent of the infants born to the vitamin A deficient women died in the first year of life compared to only 14 percent of those born to women with adequate levels of vitamin A. The cost of the vitamin A in Dr. Semba's study was only two cents a day.

If you are pregnant and infected with HIV, you are in a dangerous situation, but more vulnerable still is your unborn child. Doctors and scientists have long sought a way to interrupt the viral replication of sexually transmitted diseases so that a baby can be born while escaping infection from its mother. Vitamin A is our best bet so far, according to recent research.

In another study,[10] HIV type 1–infected women from Tanzania (1,078 in number) were randomized in a placebo-controlled trial to examine the effects of supplementation with vitamin A (preformed vitamin A and beta-carotene) and/or multivitamins (vitamins B, C, and E). The investigators found that maternal receipt of vitamin A significantly reduced the risk that the child would have cough and pneumonia. The study concluded that providing multivitamin supplements (including those with vitamins B, C, and E) to HIV-infected, lactating women may be a low-cost intervention to improve their children's health.

Cancer and Vitamin A

Fundamentals (diet and lifestyle) aside, vitamin A does have proven benefit in the treatment of cancer. Intriguing is the role of vitamin A in preventing the metastatic disease process as described by Weinzweig and colleagues.[11] They found that vitamin A stimulates collagenous encapsulation around several murine breast and lung tumor systems. Tumor encapsulation such as this can allow for easier surgical excision at the least and optimally afford lifesaving benefit. To quote from their findings:

"Vitamin A could promote the encapsulation of a murine melanoma. Sixty days after tumor inoculation, a 60% survival rate was observed in the control group as opposed to the vitamin A-supplemented animals, which demonstrated a 100% survival rate in both groups (n=5 in each group). Decreased mean tumor size and gross tumor in most vitamin A-supplemented animals were statistically significant when compared with the control animals. The control animals had a mean tumor size of 26.1 mm, whereas the post-vitamin A group had a mean tumor size of 5.7 mm. One hundred percent of the control group exhibited tumor; one animal had distant metastases. The pre-vitamin A group did not exhibit any tumor growth, and the post-vitamin A group exhibited tumor growth in 40% of animals. Neither vitamin A-supplemented group showed any evidence of distant metastases. The animals supplemented with vitamin A demonstrated decreased tumor growth and metastasis."

The authors concluded that vitamin A offers a potential prophylactic (preventive) and therapeutic role in the treatment of malignant melanoma (skin cancer). Another study concluded that treatment with retinoic acid significantly alleviates autoimmune renal disorder and prolongs survival in lupus-prone mice, thus suggesting a novel approach to the treatment of patients with lupus nephritis.[12]

Vitamin A and the Flu

Want to avoid the flu this season? If so, at the next sign of a cold coming on, consider a cheap, easy, and highly effective remedy for you and those you love. My recommendation is to take vitamin A. That's right: vitamin A. I prescribe high doses for a short period of time: 100,000 IU of vitamin A palmitate (retinyl palmitate, a stable esterified form of retinol) at onset of symptoms and another 100,000 IU at bedtime. Typically, that aborts the flu, and my patients awaken feeling great the next morning. For those who need more immune support, continue that protocol of 100,000 IU twice a day for no more than a week (to be on the safe side). Remember that toxic levels of vitamin A are determined not only by amount, but by duration of exposure. Therefore, 100,000 IU for a day or two is not only safe, it's highly effective. Don't continue taking that dosage for more than a week as it can, in some cases, saturate the liver storage capacity. Do not use this protocol in pregnancy or for women of childbearing age who might be pregnant since too much vitamin A can be teratogenic to the fetus. Also, to reiterate, this protocol works best if started at the *onset* of the flu and not as well after the symptoms are already wreaking havoc with you. I teach patients to use high-dose vitamin A at the onset of an acute immune challenge, but they all know to use vitamin C chronically. Once the flu is underway, vitamin C is your best friend, as Dr. Linus Pauling wrote in *Vitamin C and the Common Cold*. So remember: Vitamin "A" for "acute" and vitamin "C" for "chronic."

Editor's note: To read the unabridged version of this important article go to: http://orthomolecular.org/library/jom/2003/pdf/2003-v18n0304-p131.pdf.

REFERENCES FOR "VITAMIN A AND BETA-CAROTENE"

1. Johanson S, Melhus H. Vitamin A antagonizes calcium response to vitamin D in man. *J Bone Mineral Res* 2001; 16 (10): 1899–1905.

2. Feskanich D, Singh V, Willett WC, Coulditz GA. Vitamin A intake and hip fractures among postmenopausal women. *JAMA* 2002; 287: 47–54.

3. Michaelsson K, Lithell H, Vessby B, Melhus H. Serum retinal levels and risk of fracture. *N Engl J Med* 2003; 248; 287–294.

4. Lampert JM, Holzschuh J, Hessel S, et al. Provitamin A conversion to retinal via the beta, beta-carotene15,15'-oxygenase (bcox) is essential for pattern formation and differentiation during zebrafish embryogenesis. *Development* 2003; 130 (10): 2173–2186.

5. Sommer A, Tarwotjo I, Hussaini G, et al. Increased mortality in children with mild vitamin A deficiency. *Lancet* 1983; 2(8350): 585–588.

6. Kozakova H, Hanson LA, Stepankova R, et al. Vitamin A deficiency leads to severe functional disturbance of the intestinal epithelium enzymes associated with diarrhoea and increased bacterial translocation in gnotobiotic rats. *Microbes Infect* 2003; 5: 405–411.

7. Alm B, Wennergren G, Norvenius SG, et al. Nordic Epidemiological SIDS Study. Vitamin A and sudden infant death syndrome in Scandinavia 1992–1995. *Acta Paediatr* 2003; 92(2): 162–164.

8. Streb JW, Miano JM. Retinoids: Pleiotropic agents of therapy for vascular diseases? *Curr Drug Targets Cardiovasc Haematol Disord* 2003; 3(1): 31–57.

9. Mizuno Y, Kawazu SI, Kano S, et al. In-vitro uptake of vitamin A by Plasmodium falciparum. *Ann Trop Med Parasitol* 2003; 97(3): 237–243.

10. Fawzi WW, Msamanga GI, Wei R, et al. Effect of providing vitamin supplements to human immunodeficiency virus-infected, lactating mothers on the child's morbidity and CD4+ cell counts. *Clin Infect Dis* 2003; 36(8): 1053–1062.

11. Weinzweig J, Tattini C, Lynch S, et al. Investigation of the growth and metastasis of malignant melanoma in a murine model: The role of supplemental vitamin A. *Plast Reconstr Surg* 2003; 112(1): 152–158. Discussion: 159–161.

12. Kinoshita K, Yoo BS, Nozaki Y, et al. Retinoic acid reduces autoimmune renal injury and increases survival in NZB/W F(1) Mice. *J Immunol* 2003; 170(11): 5793–5798.

LYCOPENE: ITS ROLE IN HEALTH AND DISEASE

by James A. Jackson, PhD, Hugh D. Riordan, MD, Chris Revard, and Jerry Tiemeyer

From *J Orthomolecular Med* 2000; 15(2): 103–104.

To date, about 600 different carotenoids have been discovered. Carotenoids are fat-soluble nutrients that help give orange, red, and yellow color to various plants and, in some cases, are associated with chlorophyll.[1] Since these compounds were first isolated from carrots, they are called carotenoids. There are about 20 different carotenoids present in human plasma. The five most abundant in human plasma are lutein, lycopene, beta-cryp-toxanthin, alpha-carotene, and beta-carotene.[2] The best known member of the carotenoids is beta-carotene. It is an antioxidant that helps stimulate the immune system and protects against some types of cancer. In addition to acting as an antioxidant on its own, beta-carotene has the ability to produce two molecules of vitamin A. Other carotenoids lack this ability. Alpha-carotene, for example, is only half as efficient in producing vitamin A as beta-carotene, while lycopene lacks the ability to form any vitamin A.[3]

Lycopene has a strong antioxidant effect and has been shown to be effective in neutralizing singlet oxygen, a very potent free radical. Additional studies have shown that lycopene has a higher tissue concentration than the other carotenoids.[4] The highest level has been found in the testes, followed by the adrenal, liver, serum, ovary, fat, and kidneys.[5] Another study confirmed the high tissue level of lycopene in the lung, colon, breast, and skin as compared to alpha-carotene, beta-carotene, cryptoxanthin, and lutein.[6] The high tissue levels may help explain the recent findings that lycopene is protective against certain cancers, especially prostate cancer.

Lycopene Protects Against Cancer

A six-year study of 800 men compared the incidence of prostate cancer to their intake of five different carotenoids. Of the five, lycopene was the only one shown to have a significant preventive effect. Another important finding dealing with diet and prostate cancer is that men from Mediterranean countries eating a diet high in tomatoes or tomato sauce have lower rates of prostate cancer than men in other countries. Two or more servings of tomato products a week resulted in a 35 percent reduction in prostate cancer risk. The serum lycopene level in people from Italy is about six times higher than those from Ireland and about three times higher than those from England. Tomato sauce was more effective than tomato juice or tomato fruits in providing protection against prostate cancer.[7] Lycopene has also been shown to be effective in preventing cervical intraepithelial neoplasia and as an inhibitor to cancer cells of the breast, endometrium, and lung.[8] Foods high in lycopene are tomato catsup, tomato paste, and the raw tomato fruit, guava, watermelon, grapefruit, and papaya. Lycopene supplements are available from several commercial companies as an extract from tomatoes. Lycopene is best absorbed when taken with oil.

At the Riordan Clinic, a procedure was developed for measuring vitamin A, vitamin E, beta-carotene, and lycopene on a single sample using high-performance liquid chromatography (HPLC). This is a very accurate and fast way of determining plasma levels of these fat-soluble substances in a patient. Center physicians prescribe nutrients based upon actual plasma, serum, tissue (red blood cell, whole blood, hair), or urine levels of these nutrients. Reference values (for healthy individuals) established for the patient population (194 adult males and females) on the four nutrients described above are:

- vitamin A 30 to 110 micrograms (mcg) per deciliter (dL)
- beta-carotene 5 to 65 mcg per dL
- lycopene 10 to 50 mcg dL
- vitamin E 0.6 to 2.7 milligrams per dL.

To access the complete article, go to: http://www.orthomolecular.org/library/jom/2000/articles/2000-v15n02-p103.shtml.

REFERENCES FOR "LYCOPENE"

1. *The Merck Index*, Martha Windholz, Editor. Rathway, NJ, Merck & Co., Inc, 1983; 258–259.

2. Talwar D, Ha T KK, Cooney J, et al. A routine method for the simultaneous measurement of retinol, alpha-tocopherol and five carotenoids in human plasma by reverse phase HPLC. *Clinica Chimica Acta* 1998; 270:85–100.

3. Scheer JF. Lycopene: One of the most important carotenoids. In *Tomato Power*. Hauppauge, NY, Advanced Research Press, Inc., 1999, 19–23.

4. Conn PF, Schalch W, Truscott TG. The singlet oxygen and carotenoid interaction. *J Photochem Photobiol* 1991; 11:41–47.

5. Kaplan LA, Lau JM, Stein EA. Carotenoid composition, concentrations, and relationships in various human organs. *Clin Physiol Biochem* 1990; 8:1–10.

6. Nierenberg DW, Nann S. A method for determining concentrations of retinol, tocopherol, and five carotenoids in human plasma and tissue samples. *Am J Clin Nutr* 1992; 56: 417–426.

7. Rao AV, Agarwal S. Bioavailability and in vivo antioxidant properties of lycopene from tomato products and their possible role in the prevention of cancer. *Nutr Canc* 1998; 199–203.

8. Levy J, et al. Lycopene is a more potent inhibitor of human cancer cell proliferation than either a-carotene or b-carotene. *Nutr Canc* 1995; 24(3): 257–266.

Which Kills Smokers: "Camels" or Carrots? Are Smokers Getting Lung Cancer from Beta-Carotene?

by Andrew W. Saul, PhD

From the *Orthomolecular Medicine News Service,* November 18, 2008.

If one is to believe the media,[1] carotene is a killer. Carotene? As in carrots? Nope: just the carotene in vitamin tablets. A study published in *Cancer* is critical, very critical, of beta-carotene in dietary supplements. The study authors wrote, "High-dose beta-carotene supplementation appears to increase the risk of lung cancer among current smokers."[2] The "high doses" they say are harmful are only 20–30 milligrams (mg) per day. To come up with this sensational conclusion, they chose only four studies for their analysis. All four were selected from the Medline database; none were from non-Medline-indexed nutritional medicine journals such as the *Journal of Orthomolecular Medicine.*[3]

Why did the authors choose to target only those "high doses" obtained from supplements? As the headlines do not differentiate between natural and "synthetic" beta-carotene, they are in effect saying that it does not matter whether it is in a tablet or in carrot cake: carotene looks bad for smokers.

Smokers Need More Antioxidants

Actually, smoking is bad for carotene. It destroys carotene's beneficial antioxidant properties. So it is much more likely that smokers need higher doses of antioxidants than nonsmokers. Smoking burns tobacco. Burning is fast oxidation. Smoking also oxidizes essential substances in the body, including carotenes. These long molecules have many carbon-carbon double bonds that are vulnerable to free-radical attack. A smoker's antioxidants are consumed in trying to protect him or her from the toxins in tobacco. As smokers persist in smoking, they need more antioxidants, not less. R. F. Cathcart, MD, found this to be true with the antioxidant vitamin C. When the vitamin is oxidized into dehydroascorbate, he said, patients need more of it, not fewer. Vitamin C, Dr. Cathcart said, is a non-rate-limited free-radical scavenger.[4] Similarly, Drs. Wilfrid and Evan Shute treated patients with very high doses of antioxidant vitamin E.[5] Giving smokers a greatly increased amount of supplemental antioxidants (carotene, vitamins E and C, plus the mineral selenium) would likely change things for the better. Studies purporting to try this with smokers, without success, usually employed low doses of these nutrients.[6,7] A small dose is an ineffective dose.

High Doses Get Results

Researchers using higher doses get better results. Carotene in high doses has been specifically shown to strengthen the immune system by helping the body to build more helper T cells.[8] The amount used in one well-controlled study was 180 milligrams of beta-carotene per day. This is the equivalent of nearly three dozen carrots per day. And nobody died. How about that.

Perhaps it is because beta-carotene is such a vital antioxidant. Says one review paper, "Numerous animal and laboratory studies have substantiated beta-carotene's ability to inhibit tumor cell growth and the progression of carcinogenesis."[9] Another large study showed that men consuming the beta-carotene equivalent of just one carrot each day, over 25 years, had a 28 percent lower risk of death from all causes compared with men eating less.[10] *USA Today* comments that you should "keep eating beta carotene-rich foods. Nobody disputes that the beta carotene in food is healthful and safe."[11]

Beta-Carotene Is Safe. Very Safe.

Safe in food, but perhaps not safe in supplements? You cannot have it both ways: either beta-carotene in doses of only 20 to 30 mg per day is harmful to smokers, as the study claims, or it is not. Whether it is derived from pills or your plate should not matter, unless synthetic beta-carotene is not as good for you as natural, food-source beta-carotene. Research still has that to determine.[9] In the meantime, people uncritically accepting what the study purports to say may, unfortunately, stop consuming supplemental beta-carotene. For smokers, ceasing would be a genuine risk. About one-quarter of North America's adult population consists of smokers. Their diet, like everybody else's, is generally devoid of carrots. We are not eating vegetables in general, smoker or not. According to the American Heart Association, nine out of ten Americans do not meet the (rather low) government recommendations of fruit or vegetables. And one-quarter of Americans do not eat even one single serving of a fruit or vegetable in a given day, according to the National Cancer Institute.

Smokers Need More Carotene

Everywhere you look you see cancer-fighting recommendations for all of us to eat more green and yellow vegetables. For smokers, the stakes are higher. For them, six carrots, or their supplemental equivalent of 20 to 30 mg of carotene a day, is too little too late. Indeed, cigarette smoking is "significantly related to lower beta-carotene concentrations (even) after supplementation."[12] Smokers should not send the proverbial boy to do a man's job. They need more carotene, not less. And they need it any way they can get it.

Smokers can start by eating their vegetables. Beta-carotene is abundant in orange fruits and vegetables, such as pumpkin, squash, and apricots, as well as dark green leafy vegetables like spinach. One medium carrot has only about 30 calories. It has zero cholesterol. It has zero fat. It is an excellent source of potassium and fiber. A single medium sweet potato contains about 10 milligrams of beta carotene. Do you really think that two or three sweet potatoes a day is harmful? Do you really think that six carrots a day are bad for you? Does spinach kill smokers? Then why are supplements with exactly that amount of beta-carotene a problem? The answer is, they aren't. Smoking is what is harmful to smokers. Carrots are good for you. Cigarettes aren't.

Smokers Need More Vitamin C Too

One might say that this analysis actually shows that smoking probably destroys at least 20 to 30 mg of beta-carotene a day. To conclude that smokers need less seems a bit odd, doesn't it? What other antioxidant nutrients do smokers need less of? Certainly they cannot do with less vitamin C. Nearly 55 years ago, William J. McCormick, MD, wrote that smoking just one single cigarette neutralizes in the body approximately 25 mg of ascorbic acid. That is 500 mg of vitamin C deficit per pack. The doctor wrote, "The ability of the heavy smoker to maintain normal vitamin C status from dietary sources is obviously questionable."[13] This was quite a statement in 1954, at a time when physicians were literally endorsing their favorite cigarette in magazines and on television commercials.

No Deaths from Beta-Carotene

Some nutritional supplement preparations may, notes the media, contain "high" doses of beta-carotene. Once again, the analysis defines "high" as only 20 to 30 mg, and only from supplements. At 6 to 7 mg of beta-carotene per typical carrot, the study is saying that the amount of beta-carotene equivalent to four carrots per day is potentially dangerous to smokers. That is a bit counterintuitive. Where are all these carrot-eating corpses? Where are the bodies? If you search decades of the medical literature, and also search the American Association of Poison Control Centers' collected data,[14] you will find there have been no deaths whatsoever from beta-carotene. None. Zip. Nada. Zero. Evidently it must be singularly difficult to kill yourself with carrots. Or with carotene supplements.

Excess carotene causes the skin to turn slightly orange, once succinctly described as resembling an artificial suntan. The medical name for this condition is "hypercarotenosis" or just "carotenosis." "Hypercarotenemia" refers to elevated blood levels of carotene, and is also called just "carotenemia." Both are harmless.

Cigarettes Kill Smokers, Not Carrots

In performing their limited four-study review, the authors said that they looked at many "national brands" of carotene-containing vitamin supplements. The "national brands" they should have been looking at are Marlboro, Winston, and Camel. The authors are finding fault with the wrong plant. It's not carrots that hurt smokers; it's tobacco.

Given all this, it is no surprise that the study found that ex-smokers were not at all negatively affected by beta-carotene. Why? Because they stopped smoking, that's why. The preeminent danger is smoking itself. Stop today, and go have plenty of carotene.

REFERENCES FOR "WHICH KILLS SMOKERS"

1. Harding A. Vision vitamins may be harmful for smokers. *Reuters* Thu Jul 10, 2008. Available at: http://www.reuters.com/article/healthNews/idUSCOL06955420080710.

2. Tanvetyanon T, Bepler G. Beta-carotene in multivitamins and the possible risk of lung cancer among smokers versus former smokers: A meta-analysis and evaluation of national brands. *Cancer* 2008; 113(1):150–157.

3. The Journal of Orthomolecular Medicine archives are posted for free access at http://orthomolecular.org/library/jom.

4. Cathcart RF. Vitamin C, the nontoxic, non-rate-limited antioxidant free radical scavenger. *Med Hypothesis* 1985 18:61–77.

5. Shute WE. *Complete Updated Vitamin E Book.* New Canaan, CT: Keats, 1975. And: Shute WE. *Health Preserver.* Emmaus, PA: Rodale Press, 1977. Also: Shute WE. *The Vitamin E Book.* New Canaan, CT: Keats, 1978.

6. Heinonen OP, et al. The effect of vitamin E and beta carotene on the incidence of lung cancer and other cancers in male smokers. *N Engl J Med* 1994;330:1029–1035.

7. Vivekananthan DP, Penn MS, Sapp SK, et al. Use of antioxidant vitamins for the prevention of cardiovascular disease: Meta-analysis of randomised trials. *Lancet* 2003; 361(9374):2017–2023. Also: Bjelakovic G, Nikolova D, Simonetti RG, et al. Antioxidant supplements for prevention of gastrointestinal cancers: A systematic review and meta-analysis. *Lancet* 2004; 364: 1219–1228.

8. Alexander M, et al: Oral beta-carotene can increase the number of OKT4 cells in human blood. *Immunol Lett* 1985; 9:221–224.

9. Patrick L. Beta-carotene: The controversy continues. *Altern Med Rev* 2000; 5(6): 530–545.

10. Pandey DK, Shekelle R, Selwyn BJ, et al. Dietary vitamin C and beta-carotene and risk of death in middle-aged men. The Western Electric Study. *Am J Epidemiol* 1995; 142(12):1269–1278.

11. Carper J. Revisiting beta-carotene. USA Weekend: April 5–7, 1996. *Rome News Tribune,* Apr 7, 1996: 10–11.

12. McLarty JW, Holiday DB, Girard WM, et al. Beta-Carotene, vitamin A, and lung cancer chemoprevention: Results of an intermediate endpoint study. *Am J Clin Nutr* 1995;62(6 Suppl):1431S-1438S.

13. Saul AW. Taking the cure: The pioneering work of William J. McCormick, M.D. *J Orthomolecular Med* 2003;18(2): 93–96.

14. American Association of Poison Control Centers. http://www.aapcc.org/annual-reports/.

VITAMIN A: CANCER CURE OR CANCER CAUSE? MEDIA TELLS A ONE-SIDED STORY

by Andrew W. Saul, PhD

From the *Orthomolecular Medicine News Service,* August 20, 2008.

Vitamin A "pushes," "promotes," and even "incites" cancer growth, say the headlines! Is this yet another instance of vitamin bashing, or are you supplement-takers killing yourselves? Let's take a look.

Let's Take a Better Look at the Test Tube

A few researchers are claiming that vitamin A, in a test-tube experiment, will "push" stem cells to change into cells that can build blood vessels. This, they say, may increase cancer. So when "structures similar to blood vessels developed within the tumor masses grown in culture," they concluded that vitamin A promotes carcinogenesis.[1] That is a bit of a leap. An in vitro (test-tube) project is far from clinical proof. Even the study authors admit "vitamin A is known to be necessary for embryonic development precisely because it helps to 'differentiate' stem cells, pushing them to become required tissue."

There is an anticancer drug that specifically acts by blocking the breakdown of retinoic acid, derived from vitamin A. This approach has been found to be "surprisingly effective in treating animal models of human prostate cancer. . . Daily injections of the agent VN/14–1 resulted in up to a 50 percent decrease in tumor volume in mice implanted with human prostate cancer cells. . . No further tumor growth was seen during the five-week study."[2] It seems that when cancerous tumors have more vitamin A available, they shrink. And there is a good reason tumors shrink. "Keeping more retinoic acid available within cancer cells. . . redirects these cells back into their normal growth patterns, which includes programmed cell death. . . This potent agent causes cancer cells to differentiate, forcing them to turn back to a non-cancerous state." So vitamin A seems to induce positive, healthy cell changes. Indeed, this is why vitamin A derivatives are already in wide use to fight skin cancer. Vitamin A fights cancer. It does not "push," "promote," or "incite" it.

Sensational warnings and outright misstatements that natural vitamin A may "incite" cancer actually serve to incite newspaper readers and television viewers. Upon closer examination, a "vitamin promotes cancer" study often has the appearance of being conducted to prove an intended point. As the authors fuel fears about vitamin A, they also give away their goal, in their own words stating that "these findings open a new door to drug development." New marketing avenues for the development of patentable vitamin A–like drugs are a commercial opportunity that the pharmaceutical industry has not overlooked.

Vitamins Work Together

A vitamin A derivative "could protect against lung cancer development" in former smokers, says another report.[3] Significantly, the vitamin A derivative is used "combined with alpha-tocopherol (vitamin E), in order to reduce toxicity known to be associated with 13-cis-RA (the vitamin A derivative) therapy." This illustrates why orthomolecular (nutritional) physicians do not use high doses of vitamin A by itself, but rather give it in context with other important, synergistic nutrients. A baseball team entirely made up of pitchers might get a lot of strikeouts while in the field, but not hit many home runs when at bat. All nutrients are needed in a living body. Vitamin A is an essential part of the team.

Here is an example: "A study published in the *Journal of Nutritional Biochemistry* found that administering both vitamin A and vitamin C to cultured human breast cancer cells was more than three times as effective as the administration of either compound alone (since) the combination of the two vitamins inhibited proliferation by 75.7 percent compared to untreated cells. . . The ability of retinoic acid (vitamin A) to inhibit tumor cell proliferation is well known, although its mechanism has not been defined. The authors suggest that the synergistic effect observed in this study is due to ascorbic acid's ability to slow the degradation of retinoic acid, thereby increasing vitamin A's cell proliferation inhibitory effects."[4] Vitamin C helps vitamin A do its work even better, a clear team advantage.

Vitamin A Prevents Cancer

Doctors' experience and clinical evidence both show that vitamin A helps prevent cancer. This has been known for a long time. "The association of vitamin A and cancer was initially reported in 1926 when rats, fed a vitamin A–deficient diet, developed gastric carcinomas. . . The first investigation showing a relationship between vitamin A and human cancer was performed in 1941 by Abelsetal who found low plasma vitamin A levels in patients with gastrointestinal cancer."[5] Moon and colleagues reported that daily supplemental doses of 25,000 international units (IU) of vitamin A prevented squamous cell carcinoma. And de Klerk and colleagues reported "findings of significantly lower rates of mesothelioma among subjects assigned to retinol. . . Studies that use animal models have shown that retinoids (including vitamin A) can act in the promotion-progression phase of carcinogenesis and block the development of invasive carcinoma at several epithelial sites, including the head and neck and lung."[5] The Linus Pauling Institute adds, "Studies in cell culture and animal models have documented the capacity for natural and synthetic retinoids to reduce carcinogenesis significantly in skin, breast, liver, colon, prostate, and other sites."[6]

Vitamin A Is Safe and Essential

National data from the American Association of Poison Control Centers repeatedly fails to show even one death from vitamin A per year.[7] Vitamin A is very safe. However, pregnancy is a special case in which prolonged intake of too much preformed oil-form vitamin A might be harmful to the fetus, even at relatively low levels (under 20,000 IU per day). Interestingly enough, you can get over 100,000 IU of vitamin A from eating only seven ounces of beef liver. Have you ever yet seen a pregnancy overdose warning on a supermarket package of liver?

A lack of vitamin A, especially during pregnancy and in infancy, poses far greater risks. Deficiency of vitamin A in developing babies is known to cause birth defects, poor tooth enamel, a weakened immune system, and literally hundreds of thousands of cases of blindness per year worldwide. This is why developing countries safely give megadoses of vitamin A to newborns to prevent infant deaths and disease.[8]

There will always be people bent on believing that vitamins must be harmful, somehow. For them, it only remains to set up some test tubes to try to prove it. Such has been done with other vitamins, perhaps most notably a famous if silly experiment that claimed that vitamin C promoted cancer. The study, reported in *New Scientist,* 22 September 2001, was a prime example of sketchy science carelessly reported. The article would have readers uncritically extend the questionable findings of a highly artificial, electrical-current-vibrated quartz crystal test-tube study, and conclude that 2,000 milligrams of vitamin C can (somehow) do some sort of mischief to human DNA in real life. If two thousand milligrams of vitamin C were harmful, the entire animal kingdom would be dead. Our nearest primate relatives all eat well in excess of 2,000 milligrams (mg) of vitamin C each day. And, pound for pound, most animals actually manufacture from 2,000 to 10,000 mg of vitamin C daily, right inside their bodies. If such generous quantities of vitamin C were harmful, evolution would have had millions of years to select against it. Same with vitamin A. If it "promoted" cancer, every animal eating it would get cancer. They don't, of course. And, if we consume enough vitamin A, perhaps neither do we.

Vitamin A Lowers Cancer Risk

The National Institutes of Health says, "Dietary intake studies suggest an association between diets rich in beta-carotene and vitamin A and a lower risk of many types of cancer. A higher intake of green and yellow vegetables or other food sources of beta carotene and/or vitamin A may decrease the risk of lung cancer."[9] A study of over 82,000 people showed that high intakes of vitamin A reduce the risk of stomach cancer by one-half.[10] Dr. Jennifer Brett comments that "Vitamin A helps to fight cancer by inhibiting the production of DNA in cancerous cells. It slows down tumor growth in established cancers and may keep leukemia cells from dividing."[11] A derivative of the vitamin has been shown to kill CEM-C7 human T lymphoblastoid leukemia cells and P1798-C7 murine T lymphoma cells.[12]

Vitamin A is very far from being a cancer "promoter." Rather, it is very near to the cancer solution.

REFERENCES FOR "VITAMIN A: CANCER CURE OR CANCER CAUSE?"

1. Georgetown University Medical Center. Vitamin A pushes breast cancer to form blood vessel cells. *ScienceDaily* Jul 17, 2008.

2. American Association for Cancer Research. Drug slows prostate tumor growth by keeping vitamin A active. *ScienceDaily* Nov 8, 2007.

3. Chemical cousin of vitamin A restores gene function in former smokers. *ScienceDaily* Feb 6, 2003.

4. Dye D. Vitamin A and C synergistically fight breast cancer cell growth. Life Extension. May 3, 2006. Available at: http://www.lifeextension.com/whatshot/2006/5/lower-dose-of-garlic-extract-more-effective/page-01#vaac . See also: Kim KN, Pie JE, Park JH, et al. Retinoic acid and ascorbic acid act synergistically in inhibiting human breast cancer cell proliferation. *J Nutr Biochem* 2006; Jul;17(7):454–462.

5. http://www.bccancer.bc.ca/PPI/UnconventionalTherapies/VitaminARetinol.htm (no longer available).

6. Linus Pauling Institute. Micronutrient Information Center. Vitamin A. Available at: http://lpi.oregonstate.edu/infocenter/vitamins/vitaminA/.

7. American Association of Poison Control Centers (AAPCC). Annual reports. Available at: http://www.aapcc.org/annual-reports/.

8. Basu S, Sengupta B, Paladhi PK. Single megadose vitamin A supplementation of Indian mothers and morbidity in breastfed young infants. *Postgrad Med J* 2003 ;79(933):397–402. And: Rahmathullah L, Tielsch JM, Thulasiraj RD, et al. Impact of supplementing newborn infants with vitamin A on early infant mortality: Community based randomized trial in southern India. *BMJ* 2003;327(7409):254.

9. National Institutes of Health. Office of Dietary Supplements. Vitamin A: fact sheet for health professionals. Available at: http://ods.od.nih.gov/factsheets/vitamina.asp.

10. Larsson SC, Bergkvist L, Näslund I, et al. Vitamin A, retinol, and carotenoids and the risk of gastric cancer: A prospective cohort study. *Am J Clin Nutr* 2007;85(2):497–503.

11. Vitamin A overview. HowStuffWorks.com. Available at: http://recipes.howstuffworks.com/vitamin-a.htm.

12. Chan LN, Zhang S, Shao J, et al. N-(4-hydroxyphenyl)retinamide induces apoptosis in T lymphoma and T lymphoblastoid leukemia cells. *Leuk Lymphoma* 1997;25(3–4):271–280.

CHAPTER 8

Vitamin E

"Toxic levels of vitamin E in the body simply do not occur."
—MARET TRABER, MD

The first time I watched vitamin E work in a dramatic way, I was 16. A friend and I were at the lake in July. We wanted to go for a long swim and ended up being in the water for about three hours in midday rays, swimming around the lake. I had on SPF 50 sunblock everywhere, but did not reapply. She had on none.

I was pretty pink that evening. You can imagine how she looked.

Of course, too much sun exposure is not a good idea, and you should wear sunblock if you plan on being in the sun for a long time. If you end up getting burned anyway, vitamin E helps you heal. (I just discovered this again when I missed some spots with sunscreen during a long sunny day at the beach.) I always pack extra vitamin E to take on summer trips.

While I was growing up, my parents taught me that vitamin E would help keep sunburned skin from blistering. I told my friend she may want to spread vitamin E all over her red skin. She did. So did I. By morning, she looked much better. I did too. However, she forgot to put vitamin E on her lips. They swelled and blistered and looked positively awful for days. She imagined how awful the *rest* of her skin might have looked had she not applied it. She was so impressed by how well the E worked, she became a believer in vitamins that very day. I find this is the case with vitamin therapy more often than not: first there is a need, then a decision to try the vitamin, and finally the realization that this stuff really does work.

Vitamin E and Sunburn

Poke a hole in several natural vitamin E capsules and really slather the contents on your burned skin. Rub it in well. Do this after (not before) you shower and before bed. Wear old clothing to protect your sheets. Apply more vitamin E again the next evening. You should see (and feel) marked improvement by the first morning. Repeat as needed for the next day or two.

Vitamin E is not only an effective topical treatment for sunburn; it is also great for treating dry, sore, or cracked skin. But this is only the beginning. What vitamin E can do to protect your heart is nothing short of extraordinary. For most healthy people, 200 to 400 international units (IU) a day is sufficient. Therapeutic doses may be twice that or higher. Presented here are two papers that discuss the clear benefits and safety of supplemental vitamin E.

VITAMIN E: A CURE IN SEARCH OF RECOGNITION

by Andrew W. Saul, PhD

From *J Orthomolecular Med* 2003; 18(3 & 4):205–212.

"Some doctors claim that vitamin E helps many heart cases, but the official view is that the substance has not been proved of value in treating heart disease."

This statement could have been taken verbatim from any of a number of recent news media reports. But in fact, this particular quote is from a 1953 article in *Maclean's Magazine* entitled "The Fight over Vitamin E."[1]

Half a century later, it would seem that little has changed. "[W]e do not support the continued use of vitamin E treatment and discourage the inclusion of vitamin E in future primary and secondary prevention trials in patients at high risk of coronary artery disease."[2]

This statement is from a 2003 analysis that looked at studies employing daily treatment dosages between 50 and 800 international units (IU). Yet since the 1940s, clinicians have been reporting that vitamin E dosages between 450 and 1,600 IU or more are required to effectively treat cardiovascular disease. I would enjoy seeing a meta-analysis of the work of Drs. Wilfrid and Evan Shute, who treated coronary thrombosis (arterial clot blocking blood flow to the heart) with 450 to 1,600 IU; angina (chest pain due to reduced blood flow to the heart) with 450 to 1,600 IU; and thrombophlebitis (blood clots in a vein) with 600 to 1,600 IU of vitamin E daily.[3] The *Lancet* meta-analysis did not include them. There is nothing capricious about either study selection or dosage choice. Researchers and analysts know full well that high dosage will obtain different results than low dosage. Statistical analysis of meaningless studies will rarely enable a meaningful conclusion.

Double Standard

Countless comedians have made fun of the incompetent physician who, when called late at night during a life-threatening disease crisis, says, "Take two aspirin and call me in the morning." Now it's no longer funny. One of the largest pharmaceutical conglomerates in the world ran prime-time national television commercials that declared, "Bayer aspirin may actually help stop you from dying if you take it during a heart attack." The company also promotes such use of its product on the Internet.[4] This statement comes forth after a century of widespread aspirin consumption. Cardiovascular disease remains the number-one killer of men and women, and there are over a million heart attacks annually in the US alone.

If you produced a TV ad that said that megadoses of wheat germ oil, or the vitamin E in it, could save your life by preventing a heart attack, not only would people disbelieve you, you'd also be subject to arrest for breaking federal law. Foods and vitamins may not be advertised as treatments for specific diseases. "All statements of nutritional support for dietary supplements must be accompanied by a two-part disclaimer on the product label: that the statement has not been evaluated by FDA and that the product is not intended to 'diagnose, treat, cure or prevent any disease.'"[5]

Yet even traditional nutrition textbooks acknowledge the extensive scientific proof of successful treatment of intermittent claudication with vitamin E. "This therapy helps reduce the arterial blockage," says *Nutrition and Diet Therapy*, seventh edition, a standard dietetics work.[6] Unless there be something absolutely unique about arterial real estate between the knee and the ankle, would not vitamin E also help "reduce the blockage" in other arteries? This is rationale the Shutes used when, 65 years ago, they employed vitamin E to successfully treat circulatory diseases in thousands of patients, using daily dosages as high as 3,200 IU. For that achievement, they were praised by their patients and ostracized from the ranks of orthodox physicians.

By 1971, it was increasingly clear that the Shutes had gotten it right. Intermittent claudication, now regarded as a reliable sign of peripheral arterial disease, was shown by double-blind study to be diminished 66 percent with the use of vitamin E. The dosage administered was 1,600 mg per day.[7]

A Torrid History

The USSR was formed in 1922, the same year the comic strip *Little Orphan Annie* debuted. Trumpeter Al Hirt and future heart transplant pioneer Christiaan Barnard were born. Alexander Graham Bell died. And vitamin E was discovered by H. M. Evans and K. S. Bishop.[8]

In 1936, Evans' team had isolated alpha-tocopherol from wheat germ oil; vitamin E was beginning to be widely appreciated, and the consequences of deficiency better known. *Health Culture Magazine* in January 1936 said, "The fertility food factor (is) now called vitamin E. Excepting for the abundance of that vitamin in whole grains, there could not have been any perpetuation of the human race. Its absence from the diet makes for irreparable sterility occasioned by a complete degeneration of the germinal cells of the male generative glands. [T]he expectant mother requires vitamin E to insure the carriage of her charge to a complete and natural term. If her diet is deficient in vitamin E . . . the woman is very apt to abort. . . It is more difficult to insure a liberal vitamin E supply in the daily average diet than to insure an adequate supply of any other known vitamin."[9]

And that very same year, 1936, the Shutes were already at work employing tocopherol from wheat germ oil to relieve angina symptoms.[10]

Since the word "tocopherol" is taken from the Greek words for "to carry offspring" or "to bring forth childbirth," it is easy enough to see how Evan Shute and other obstetricians were drawn into the work. As early as 1931, Vogt-Moller of Denmark successfully treated habitual abortion in human females with wheat germ oil vitamin E. By 1939 he had treated several hundred women with a success rate of about 80 percent. In 1937, both Young in England and the Shutes in Canada reported success in combating threatened abortion and pregnancy toxemias as well. A. L. Bacharach's 1940 statistical analysis of published clinical results "show quite definitely that vitamin E is of value in recurrent abortions."[11] And also in 1940, the Shutes were curing atherosclerosis with vitamin E. By 1946, they were also curing thrombosis (blood clots), phlebitis (vein inflammation), and claudication (pain due to reduced blood flow).

Yet when the MDRs (Minimum Daily Requirements) first came out in 1941, there was no mention of vitamin E. It was not until 1959 that vitamin E was recognized by the US Food and Drug Administration as necessary for human existence, and not until 1968 that any government recommendation for vitamin E would be issued. That year, the Food and Nutrition Board of the US National Research Council offered its first Recommended Daily Allowance: 30 IU. It has been as low as 15 IU in 1974. In 2000, it was set at 22 IU (15 mg) for all persons, including pregnant women. This is somewhat odd in view of a 70-year established research history showing how vital vitamin E is during gestation. It is another curious fact that today, when the public has been urged to increase its consumption of unsaturated fats, the official dietary recommendation for vitamin E is substantially lower than it was 35 years ago. "The requirement for vitamin E is related to the amount of polyunsaturated fatty acids (PUFAs) consumed in the diet. The higher the amount of PUFAs, the more vitamin E is required."[12]

One reason the Recommended Dietary Allowance (RDA) was lowered is that "dieticians were having difficulty devising diets of natural foods which had the recommended amount (30 IU) of vitamin E."[13] There are about 39 IU of vitamin E in an

8-ounce cup of olive oil. A full pound of peanuts yields 34 IU. Professor Max K. Horwitt, PhD, who spent 15 years serving on the Food and Nutrition Board's RDA committees, said in an interview that "The average intake by adults, without supplements, seems to be about 8 milligrams of alpha-tocopherol per day, or 8 tocopherol equivalents. This is equivalent to 12 International Units (IU)."[14] So it might be said that, in the end, the accommodation was not to raise the bridge but rather to lower the river.

Vitamin E is the body's chief fat-soluble antioxidant. It is a powerful one indeed, when you consider that 22 IU is presumed adequate to protect each one of the tens of trillions of body cells in a human being. Even though there has been a veritable explosion in antioxidant research since 1968, the RDA for vitamin E has been decreased.

Postal Fraud

"Any claim in the labeling of drugs or of foods offered for special dietary use, by reason of Vitamin E, that there is need for dietary supplementation with Vitamin E, will be considered false." (United States Post Office Department Docket No. 1/187, March 15, 1961)

On October 26, 1959, the US government charged an organization known as the Cardiac Society with postal fraud for selling 30 IU vitamin E capsules through the mail. Specifically, the charge was "the operation of a scheme or device for obtaining money through the mails by means of false and fraudulent pretenses, representations or promises . . . that Respondent's product 'E-FEROL 30 I.U.' (containing vitamin E) is therapeutically effective and beneficial in the treatment of heart and cardiovascular diseases for any person so afflicted; that Respondents said product will prevent heart disease;" that "It (vitamin E) is the key both to the prevention and treatment of all those conditions in which a lack of blood supply due to thickened or blocked blood vessels or a lack of oxygen is a part or the whole story of the disease"; that "Vitamin E seems to be a natural anti-thrombin in the human blood stream. . . It is the only substance preventing the clotting of blood which is not dangerous"; that the book "Your Heart and Vitamin E" tells you "What Vitamin E Is and Does, How It Treats Heart Disease, Its Success In Circulatory Diseases, Your Foods' Deficiency in Vitamin E"; That "It (the book) explains medical facts in every-day language concerning the help that is available for sufferers from diseases of the heart and blood vessels such as Coronary Heart Disease, Angina Pectoris, Phlebitis, Buerger's Disease, Diabetes, Strokes, etc."[15]

A four-day hearing in Washington, D.C., generated sufficient testimony to fill "four volumes totaling 856 pages. Seventy-six exhibits were received in evidence. . . for the consideration of the Hearing Examiner. His Initial Decision covers forty-two pages."

It is an oddity of history that, at the height of the Cuban Missile Crisis, the United States of America found both the reason and the resources to prosecute such a case as this.

"The record here shows that the consensus of medical opinion is that Respondent's claims are false and that this is the universality of medical opinion on the subject. Numerous tests and experiments have been conducted to attempt to substantiate the claims made by Respondent that Vitamin E is efficacious for treatment of a number of conditions but these have failed to substantiate the claims. It appears perfectly clear from the testimony of the expert witnesses that Respondent's claims and representations are devoid of scientific support... The Hearing Examiner correctly found that the Respondent intends to deceive by its false representation and that actual fraud under established law is proven. . . A fraud order shall issue forthwith forbidding the delivery of mail and the payment of money orders incident to such scheme, to the Respondent, its agents and representatives, all in accordance with 39 U.S.C. 259 and 732."[15]

After this, all mail addressed to the Cardiac Society was returned to the sender, with "Fraudulent" stamped on the envelope.

Dosage and Utility

Vitamin E has many clinically important and seemingly unrelated properties. In their books[16–21] the Shutes discuss a number of them.

1. Vitamin E strengthens and regulates heartbeat, like digitalis and similar drugs, at a dose adjusted between 800 and 3,000 IU daily.
2. Vitamin E reduces inflammation and scarring when frequently applied topically to burns or to sites of lacerations or surgical incisions. Internally, vitamin E helps to very gradually break down thrombi at a maintained oral dose of between 800 IU and 3,000 IU.
3. Vitamin E has an oxygen-sparing effect on the heart, enabling the heart to do more work on less oxygen. The benefit for recovering heart attack patients is considerable. A dose of 1,200 to 2,000 IU daily relieves angina very well. My father, duly diagnosed with angina, gradually worked up to 1,600 IU over a period of a few weeks. He never had an angina symptom again. In this, he had the identical success that thousands of Shute patients had.
4. Vitamin E moderately prolongs prothrombin clotting time, decreases platelet adhesion, and has a limited "blood thinning" effect. This is the reason behind the Shutes' using vitamin E (1,000–2,000 IU/day) for thrombophlebitis and related conditions. The pharmaceutical industry and the medical profession are well aware of vitamin E's anticoagulant property and that "very high doses of this vitamin may act synergistically with anticoagulant drugs."[21] However, this also means that vitamin E can, entirely or in part, substitute for such drugs but do so more safely. Perhaps this is best summed up by surgeon Edward William Alton Ochsner, MD (1896–1981), who said, "Vitamin E is a potent inhibitor of thrombin that does not produce a hemorrhagic tendency and therefore is a safe prophylactic against venous thrombosis."[23]

5. Vitamin E is a modest vasodilator, promotes collateral circulation, and consequently offers great benefits to diabetes patients.[24] The Shutes used a dose of about 800 IU or more, tailored to the patient. For this, among other reasons, Evan Shute, author of over 100 scientific papers, was literally judged to be a fraud by the United States Post Office Department. The 1961 court decision said, "Vascular degenerations in a diabetic are not effectively treated in the use of vitamin E in any dosage . . . Vitamin E has been thoroughly studied and that there is no doubt whatsoever as to its lack of utility."[15]

This statement was premature to say the least. The "thorough study" of vitamin E was not quite completed by 1961. Thirty-eight years later, a crossover study of 36 patients who had type 1 diabetes, and retinal blood flows that were significantly lower than nondiabetics, showed that those taking 1,800 IU of vitamin E daily obtained normal retinal blood flow. The patients with the worst initial readings improved the most. "[V]itamin E may potentially provide additional risk reduction for the development of retinopathy or nephropathy in addition to those achievable through intensive insulin therapy alone. Vitamin E is a low-cost, readily available compound associated with few known side effects; thus, its use could have a dramatic socioeconomic impact if found to be efficacious in delaying the onset of diabetic retinopathy and/or nephropathy."[25] Vitamin E also works synergistically with insulin to lower high blood pressure in diabetics.[26]

Quantity and Quality

The most common reason for irreproducibility of successful vitamin E cures is either a failure to use enough of it, or a failure to use the natural form (D-alpha, plus mixed natural tocopherols), or both. For example, in an oft-quoted negative study,[27] researchers who gave 300 milligrams of synthetic vitamin E to patients who had recently had a heart attack saw no beneficial effect. Such failure is to be expected. You can set up any experiment to fail. The Shutes would have used only the natural form, and four times as much.

Natural vitamin E is always the dextro- (right-handed) form. On the other hand, "[S]ynthetic vitamin E is a mixture of eight isomers in equal proportions containing only 12.5% of d-alpha tocopherol. One mg of dl-alpha tocopherol has the lowest Vitamin E equivalence of any of the common vitamin E preparations."[28]

There may be other differences. "Vitamin E derived from natural sources is obtained by molecular distillation and, in most cases, subsequent methylation and esterification of edible vegetable oil products. Synthetic vitamin E is produced from fossil plant material (coal tar) by condensation of trimethylhydroquinone with isophytol."[12]

While personal philosophy is the only possible basis for a decision to conduct a study using only the synthetic form of a vitamin, the use of low dosage is generally explained away by alleging doubts about safety.

Safety

The most elementary of forensic arguments is, where are the bodies? Poison control statistics report no deaths from vitamin E.[29] There is a reason for this. Vitamin E is a safe and remarkably non-toxic substance. Even the 2000 report by the Institute of Medicine of the National Academy of Sciences, which actually recommends against taking supplemental vitamin E, specifically acknowledges that 1,000 mg (about 1,500 IU) is a "tolerable upper intake level . . . that is likely to pose no risk of adverse health effects for almost all individuals in the general population."[30] The Shutes observed no evidence of harm with doses as high as 8,000 IU per day. In fact, "toxicity symptoms have not been reported even at intakes of 800 IU per kilogram of body weight daily for 5 months" according to the Food and Nutrition Board.[31] This demonstrated safe level would work out to be around 60,000 IU daily for an average adult, some 2,700 times the RDA!

In addition to an awareness of anticoagulation medications, "Dr. Shute advises starting with small doses for patients who have rheumatic heart disease. He starts with 90 IU and very slowly works up the dose. The reason for this is that if too much is given at the beginning the increased strength of the heartbeat may create some difficulty. The same applies to heart failure. The initial dose should be small and gradually increased. If this is done the final dose can safely reach 800 to 1200 IU."[31]

Safety in the Elderly

A Columbia University study reported that progression of Alzheimer's disease was significantly slowed in patients taking high daily doses (2,000 IU) of vitamin E for two years.[32] The vitamin worked better than the drug selegiline did. The patients in the Alzheimer's study tolerated their vitamin E doses well. Perhaps the real story is that 2,000 IU per day for two years is safe for the elderly.

Safety in Children

Children using antiepileptic medication have reduced plasma levels of vitamin E, a sign of vitamin E deficiency. So doctors at the University of Toronto gave epileptic children 400 IU of vitamin E per day for several months, along with their medication. This combined treatment reduced the frequency of seizures in most of the children by over 60 percent. Half of them "had a 90 to 100 percent reduction in seizures."[33] This extraordinary result is also proof of the safety of 400 IU of vitamin E per day in children (equivalent to at least 800 to 1,200 IU per day for an adult). "There were no adverse side effects," said the researchers. It also provides a clear example of pharmaceutical use creating a vitamin deficiency, and an unassailable justification for supplementation.

Safety in Infants

Overexposure to oxygen has been a major cause of retrolental fibroplasia (retinopathy of prematurity) and subsequent blindness in premature infants. Incubator oxygen retina damage is now prevented by giving preemies 100 mg E per kilogram body weight. That dose is equivalent to an adult dose of about 7,000 IU for an average-weight adult. "There have been no detrimental side effects" from such treatment, said the *New England Journal of Medicine,* Dec. 3, 1981.[34] Nevertheless, the 1989 (sixth) edition of the textbook *Nutrition and Diet Therapy*[6] advised that "healthy persons stand the chance of developing signs of toxicity with the megadoses that are recommended in these studies" (p. 225). That incorrect statement was dropped in the book's next edition. Instead, the seventh edition (1993) said under "Toxicity Effects" that "[v]itamin E is the only one of the fat-soluble vitamins for which no toxic effect in humans is known. Its use as a supplement has not shown harmful effects" (p. 186).

Immune Function

Worst Pills, Best Pills is a monthly newsletter published by Public Citizen, Ralph Nader's "Health Research Group" (http://www.citizen.org/hrg/). The October, 2002 issue (vol. 8, no. 10) contained this statement by editor Sidney M. Wolfe, MD: "You should not take dietary supplements. These products have not been tested or shown to be effective for any use, and their safety is unknown. The only exception to this advice is an inexpensive vitamin or mineral preparation" (p. 80). On page 77, the doctor presents a *JAMA* study[35] alleging that a mere 200 mg of vitamin E is somehow detrimental to patients over the age of 60 with respiratory tract infections.

But there are other studies that Public Citizen might do well to present to its readership. Emanuel Cheraskin, MD, writes, "The effect of daily vitamin E supplementation (800 IU alpha-tocopherol for 30 days) on immune responses of 32 healthy subjects (60+ years old) was examined in a placebo-controlled, double-blind trial in a metabolic research unit. The data suggest that vitamin E supplementation improves immune responsiveness in healthy elderly."[36] In a second study, "using a double blind protocol, immune response was studied in a group receiving vitamin E (800 mg per day) versus placebo. The increased immunocompetence was matched by blood vitamin E levels which jumped from 1.1 to 3.1 mg%. No such change in blood vitamin E occurred in the control group (1.1 to 1.0 mg%)."[37]

Perhaps an even more important study looked at patients with colon cancer "who received a daily dose of 750 mg of vitamin E during a period of 2 weeks. Short-term supplementation with high doses of dietary vitamin E leads to increased CD4:CD8 ratios and to enhanced capacity by their T cells to produce the T helper 1 cytokines interleukin 2 and IFN-gamma. In 10 of 12 patients, an increase of 10% or more (average, 22%) in the number of T cells producing interleukin 2 was seen after 2 weeks of vitamin E supplementation." The authors concluded that "dietary vitamin E may be used to improve the immune functions in patients with advanced cancer." That the improvement was achieved in only two weeks merits special attention.[38]

Note that the doses in these positive studies were nearly four times the dose used in the negative *JAMA* study cited by Dr. Wolfe.

Hypertension

Research has indicated that Vitamin E normalizes high blood pressure.[39–41] In some hypertensive persons, commencement of very large vitamin E doses may cause a slight temporary increase in blood pressure, although maintained supplementation can then be expected to lower it. The solution is to increase the vitamin gradually, along with the proper monitoring that hypertensive patients should have anyway. High blood pressure has been called the "silent killer," and nearly one-third of adults have it. It is all too frequently unrecognized and untreated.

Nearly half of all deaths are due to cardiovascular diseases, and often the first symptom is death. Advocating daily supplementation with several hundred IUs of vitamin E would be good public health policy. Yet vitamin E, for decades lampooned as a "cure in search of a disease," remains virtually the "silent healer" for as much as the public has been advised of its benefits.

Back in 1985, Linus Pauling wrote, "The failure of the medical establishment during the last forty years to recognize the value of Vitamin E in controlling heart disease is responsible for a tremendous amount of unnecessary suffering and for many early deaths. The interesting story of the efforts to suppress the Shute discoveries about Vitamin E illustrates the shocking bias of organized medicine against nutritional measures for achieving improved health." (10, vii)

Dr. Pauling would most likely have appreciated this comment from a *Harvard Health Letter*: "A consistent body of research indicates that vitamin E may protect people against heart disease. . . The data generally indicate that taking doses ranging from 100 to 800 IU (International Units) per day may lower the risk of heart disease by 30%–40%."[42] Over half a century ago, the Shute brothers and their colleagues showed that, with even higher doses than those, and with an insistence on the use of natural vitamin E, the results are better still.

A bibliography of selected books and papers by Wilfrid and Evan Shute is posted at http://www.doctoryourself.com/biblio_shute.html.

REFERENCES FOR "VITAMIN E: A CURE IN SEARCH OF RECOGNITION"

1. Hutton, E. The fight over vitamin E. *Maclean's Magazine,* Jun 15, 1953.

2. Vivekananthan DP, Penn MS, Sapp SK, et al. Use of antioxidant vitamins for the prevention of cardiovascular disease: Meta-analysis of randomised trials. *Lancet* 2003; 361: 2017–2023.

3. Saul, AW. Natural alpha tocopherol (vitamin E) in the treatment of cardiovascular and renal diseases. Available at: http://www.doctoryourself.com/shute_protocol.html.

4. http://www.bayeraspirin.com/news/heart_attack.htm.

5. Dietary Supplements: An Advertising Guide for Industry, Part 3. Federal Trade Commission. Available at: http://www.ftc.gov/bcp/conline/pubs/buspubs/dietsupp.htm#Application.

6. Williams SR. *Nutrition and Diet Therapy,* Seventh Edition. St. Louis: Mosby, 1993 (p 186). Sixth edition, 1989 (p 225).

7. Williams HTG, Fenna D, MacBeth RA. Alpha Tocopherol in the treatment of intermittent claudication. *Surg Gynecol and Obstet* 1971; 132(4): 662–666.

8. Evans HM, Bishop KS. On the existence of a hitherto unrecognized dietary factor essential for reproduction. *Science* 1922; 56(1458): 650–651.

9. Pacini AJ. Why we need vitamin E. *Health Culture Magazine,* January, 1936.

10. Shute E, Shute JCM (ed). *The vitamin E story.* Burlington, Ontario: Welch Publishing, 1985.

11. *British Medical Journal,* i, 890, 1940 (cited in Bicknell & Prescott. *The vitamins in medicine.* Milwaukee: Lee Foundation, 1953, p 632).

12. Roche Vitamins: Vitamin E in human nutrition. http://www.roche-vitamins.com/home/what/what-hnh/what-hnh-vitamins/what-hnh-vitamin-e (accessed 2003). See also: Valk EE, Hornstra G. Relationship between vitamin E requirement and polyunsaturated fatty acid intake in man: A review. *Int J Vitam Nutr Res* 2000;70(2):31–42. Available at: http://www.ncbi.nlm.nih.gov/pubmed/10804454.

13. Horwitt MK. Vitamin E: A reexamination. *Am J Clin Nutr* 1976;29(5):569–578.

14. HealthWorld Online Interviews with Nutritional Experts: "Vitamin E and the RDA" http://www.healthy.net.

15. United States Post Office Department Docket No. 1/187. March 15, 1961. http://www.usps.gov/judicial/1961deci/1–187.htm.

16. Shute EV, et al. *The heart and vitamin E.* London, Canada: Shute Foundation for Medical Research, 1963.

17. Shute WE. *(Dr. Wilfred Shute's) Complete updated vitamin E book.* New Canaan, CT: Keats, 1975.

18. Shute WE, Taub HJ. *Vitamin E for ailing and healthy hearts.* New York: Pyramid House, 1975.

19. Shute WE. *Health Preserver.* Emmaus, PA: Rodale Press, 1977.

20. Shute WE. *The Vitamin E Book.* New Canaan, CT: Keats Publishing, 1978.

21. Shute WE. *Your Child and Vitamin E.* New Canaan, CT: Keats Publishing, 1979.

22. Butterworth, Jr. CE. *Vitamin Safety: A current appraisal.* Backgrounder, Vol 5, No 1. Vitamin Nutrition Information Service, 1994.

23. Letter. *New England Journal of Medicine* 271(4); July 23, 1964.

24. Shute, Vogelsang, Skelton and Shute. *Surg Gyn Obst* 1948; 86:1.

25. Bursell SE, Clermont AC, Aiello LP, et al. High-dose vitamin E supplementation normalizes retinal blood flow and creatinine clearance in patients with type 1 diabetes. *Diabetes Care* 1999; 22(8):1245–1251.

26. Koo JR, Ni Z, Oviesi F, et al. Antioxidant therapy potentiates antihypertensive action of insulin in diabetic rats. *Clin Exp Hypertens* 2002;24(5):333–344.

27. Gruppo Italiano per lo Studio della Sopravvivenza nell'Infarto miocardico. Dietary supplementation with n-3 polyunsaturated fatty acids and vitamin E after myocardial infarction: Results of the GISSI-Prevenzione trial. *Lancet* 1999;354(9177):447–455.

28. Hoffer A. Personal communication, June 2003.

29. Rosenbloom M. Vitamin toxicity. http://www.eMedicine.com. October 23, 2001.

30. Vita-Mania: RDA for C, E Raised; Limits Set. The Associated Press, Washington, April 11, 2000.

31. Rosenberg H, Feldzamen AN. *The book of vitamin therapy.* New York: Berkley Publishing Corp, 1974.

32. Sano M, Ernesto C, Thomas RG, et al. A controlled trial of selegiline, alpha-tocopherol, or both as treatment for Alzheimer's disease. The Alzheimer's Disease Cooperative Study. *N Engl J Med* 1997;336(17):1216–1222.

33. Ogunmekan AO, Hwang PA. A randomized, double-blind, placebo-controlled, clinical trial of D-alpha-tocopheryl acetate (vitamin E), as add-on therapy, for epilepsy in children. *Epilepsia* 1989; 30(1):84–89.

34. Hittner HM, Godio LB, Rudolph AJ, et al. Retrolental fibroplasia: Efficacy of vitamin E in a double-blind clinical study of preterm infants. *N Engl J Med* 1981; 305(23):1365–1371.

35. Graat JM, Schouten EG, Kok FJ. Effect of daily vitamin E and multivitamin-mineral supplementation on acute respiratory tract infections in elderly persons: A randomized controlled trial. *JAMA* 2002;288(6): 715–721.

36. Cheraskin E. Antioxidants in health and disease: The big picture. *J of Orthomolecular Medicine* 1995;10(2): 89–96, citing Meydani SN, Barklund MP, Liu S, et al. Effect of vitamin E supplementation on immune responsiveness of healthy elderly subjects. *FASEB Journal* 1989; 3: A1057.

37. Meydani SN, Barkiund MP, Liu S, et al. Vitamin E supplementation enhances cell-mediated immunity in healthy elderly subjects. *Am J Clin Nutr* 1990; 52(3), 557–563.

38. Malmberg KJ, Lenkei R, Petersson M, et al. A short-term dietary supplementation of high doses of vitamin E increases T helper 1 cytokine production in patients with advanced colorectal cancer. *Clin Cancer Res* 2002; 8(6):1772–1778.

39. Vasdev S, Gill V, Parai S, et al. Dietary vitamin E supplementation lowers blood pressure in spontaneously hypertensive rats. *Mol Cell Biochem* 2002; 238(1–2):111–117.

40. Vaziri ND, Ni Z, Oveisi F, et al. Enhanced nitric oxide inactivation and protein nitration by reactive oxygen species in renal insufficiency. *Hypertension* 2002; 39(1):135–141.

41. Galley HF, Thornton J, Howdle PD, et al. Combination oral antioxidant supplementation reduces blood pressure. *Clin Sci (Lond)* 1997;92(4):361–365.

42. President and Fellows of Harvard College. Antioxidants: what they are and what they do. *Harvard Health Letter* 1999; 24(5).

Vitamin E Attacked Again. Of Course. Because It Works.

by Andrew W. Saul, PhD

From the *Orthomolecular Medicine News Service,* October 14, 2011.

The very first Orthomolecular Medicine News Service release was on the clinical benefits of vitamin E.[1] In fact, the battle over vitamin E has been going full-tilt for over 60 years.[2]

One accusation against vitamin E is that somehow it increases risk of prostate cancer.[3] That is nonsense. If you take close look at the numbers, you will see that "[c]ompared with placebo, the absolute increase in risk of prostate cancer per 1000 person-years was 1.6 for vitamin E, 0.8 for selenium, and 0.4 for the combination." That works out to be a claimed 0.63 percent increase risk with vitamin E alone, 0.24 percent increase in risk with vitamin E and selenium, and 0.15 percent increase in risk for selenium alone.

Note the decimal points: these are very small figures. But more importantly, note that the combination of selenium with vitamin E resulted in a much smaller number of deaths. If vitamin E were really the problem, vitamin E with selenium would have been a worse problem. Selenium recharges vitamin E, recycling it and effectively rendering it more potent. Something is wrong here, and it isn't the vitamin E. Indeed, a higher dose of vitamin E might work as well as E with selenium, and be more protective.

And, in fact, this study did show that supplementation was beneficial. Vitamin E and selenium reduced risk of all-cause mortality by about 0.2 percent, and also reduced the risk of serious cardiovascular events by 0.3 percent. Vitamin E reduced risk of serious cardiovascular events by 0.7 percent. But what you were told, and just about all you were told, was "Vitamin E causes cancer!"

Specifically in regards to prostate cancer, new research published in the *International Journal of Cancer* has shown that gamma-tocotrienol, a cofactor found in natural vitamin E preparations, actually kills prostate cancer stem cells.[4] As you would expect, these are the very cells from which prostate cancer develops. They are or quickly become chemotherapy-resistant. And yet natural vitamin E complex contains the very thing to kill them. Mice given gamma-tocotrienol orally had an astonishing 75 percent decrease in tumor formation. Gamma-tocotrienol also is effective against existing prostate tumors.[5,6]

Additionally:

- Vitamin E reduces mortality by 24 percent in persons 71 or older. Even persons who smoke live longer if they take vitamin E.[7]

- Taking 300 IU vitamin E per day reduces lung cancer risk by 61 percent.[8]
- Vitamin E is an effective treatment for atherosclerosis. Drs. Wilfrid and Evan Shute knew this half a century ago.[1] In 1995, JAMA published research that confirmed it, saying, "Subjects with supplementary vitamin E intake of 100 IU per day or greater demonstrated less coronary artery lesion progression than did subjects with supplementary vitamin E intake less than 100 IU per day." [9]
- 400 to 800 IU of vitamin E daily reduces risk of heart attack by 77 percent.[10]
- Increasing vitamin E with supplements prevents COPD.[11] Chronic obstructive pulmonary disease includes emphysema and chronic bronchitis.
- 800 IU vitamin E per day is a successful treatment for fatty liver disease.[12]
- Alzheimer's patients who take 2,000 IU of vitamin E per day live longer.[13]
- 400 IU of vitamin E per day reduces epileptic seizures in children by more than 60 percent.[14]
- Vitamin E supplements help prevent amyotrophic lateral sclerosis (ALS).[15] This important finding is the result of a ten-year-plus Harvard study of over a million persons.
- Vitamin E is more effective than a prescription drug in treating chronic liver disease (nonalcoholic steatohepatitis).[16] Said the authors of this study, "The good news is that this study showed that cheap and readily available vitamin E can help many of those with this condition."

What Kind of Vitamin E?

Which work best: natural or synthetic vitamins? The general debate might not end anytime soon. However, with vitamin E, we already know. The best E is the most natural form, generally called "mixed natural tocopherols and tocotrienols." This is very different from the synthetic form, DL-alpha-tocopherol. In choosing a vitamin E supplement, you should carefully read the label—the entire label. It is remarkable how many natural-looking brown bottles with natural-sounding brand names contain a synthetic vitamin. And no, we do not make brand recommendations.

Unfortunately, that's not the case with some authors of the negative vitamin E paper.[3] You will not see this in the abstract at the *JAMA* website, of course, but if you read the entire paper, and get to the very last page (p. 1556), you'll find the "Conflict of Interest" section. Here you will discover that a number of the study authors have received money from pharmaceutical companies, including Merck, Pfizer, Sanofi-Aventis, AstraZeneca, Abbott, GlaxoSmithKline, Janssen, Amgen, Firmagon, and Novartis. In terms of cash, these are some of the largest corporations on the planet.

Well how about that: a "vitamins are dangerous" article, in one of the most popular medical journals, with lots of media hype . . . and the pharmaceutical industry's fingerprints all over it.

So How Much Vitamin E?

More than the RDA, and that's for certain. A common dosage range for vitamin E is between 200 and 800 IU per day. Some orthomolecular physicians advocate substantially more than that. The studies cited above will give you a ballpark idea. However, this is an individual matter for you and your practitioner to work out. Your own reading and research, before you go to your doctor, will help you determine optimal intake. If your doctor quotes a negative vitamin study, then haul out the positive ones. You may start with this article.

REFERENCES FOR "VITAMIN E ATTACKED AGAIN"

1. Saul, AW. Vitamin E: Safe, effective and heart-healthy. Available at: http://orthomolecular.org/resources/omns/v01n01.shtml.

2. Saul AW. Vitamin E: A cure in search of recognition. *J Orthomolecular Med* 2003;18(3 & 4):205–212.

3. Klein EA, Thompson Jr, IM, Tangen CM, et al. Vitamin E and the risk of prostate cancer. *JAMA* 2011;306(14):1549–1556. Also, as an example of many media spins: http://www.webmd.com/prostate-cancer/news/20111011/vitamin-e-supplements-may-raise-prostate-cancer-risk.

4. Luk SU, Yap WN, Chiu YT, et al. Gamma-tocotrienol as an effective agent in targeting prostate cancer stem cell-like population. *Int J Cancer* 2011;128(9):2182–2191.

5. Nesaretnam K, Teoh HK, Selvaduray KR, et al. Modulation of cell growth and apoptosis response in human prostate cancer cells supplemented with tocotrienols. *Eur J Lipid Sci Technol* 2008; 110(1): 23–31.

6. Conte C, Floridi A, Aisa C, et al. Gamma-tocotrienol metabolism and antiproliferative effect in prostate cancer cells. *Ann N Y Acad Sci* 2004;1031: 391–394.

7. Hemilä H, Kaprio J. Vitamin E may affect the life expectancy of men, depending on dietary vitamin C intake and smoking. *Age Ageing* 2011; 40(2): 215–220.

8. Mahabir S, Schendel K, Dong YQ, et al. Dietary alpha-, beta-, gamma- and delta-tocopherols in lung cancer risk. *Int J Cancer* 2008;123(5):1173–1180.

9. Hodis HN, Mack WJ, LaBree L, et al. Serial coronary angiographic evidence that antioxidant vitamin intake reduces progression of coronary artery atherosclerosis. *JAMA* 1995; 273:1849–1854.

10. Stephens NG et al. Randomized controlled trial of vitamin E in patients with coronary artery disease: Cambridge Heart Antioxidant Study (CHAOS). *Lancet* 1996; 347:781–786.

11. Agler AH et al. Randomized vitamin E supplementation and risk of chronic lung disease (CLD) in the Women's Health Study. American Thoracic Society 2010 International Conference, May 18, 2010.

12. Sanyal AJ, Chalasani N, Kowdley KV, et al. Pioglitazone, vitamin E, or placebo for nonalcoholic steatohepatitis. *N Engl J Med* 2010;362(18):1675–1685.

13. Pavlik VN, Doody RS, Rountree SD, et al. Vitamin E use is associated with improved survival in an Alzheimer's disease cohort. *Dement Geriatr Cogn Disord* 2009;28(6):536–540. See also: Grundman M. Vitamin E and Alzheimer disease: The basis for additional clinical trials. *Am J Clin Nutr* 2000;71(2):630S-636S.

14. Ogunmekan AO, Hwang PA. A randomized, double-blind, placebo-controlled, clinical trial of D-alpha-tocopheryl acetate [vitamin E], as add-on therapy, for epilepsy in children. *Epilepsia* 1989; 30(1):84–89.

15. Wang H, O'Reilly EJ, Weisskopf MG, et al. Vitamin E intake and risk of amyotrophic lateral sclerosis: A pooled analysis of data from 5 prospective cohort studies. *Am J Epidemiol* 2011;173(6): 595–602.

16. Sanyal AJ, Chalasani N, Kowdley KV, et al. Pioglitazone, vitamin E, or placebo for nonalcoholic steatohepatitis. *N Engl J Med* 2010;362(18):1675–1685.

CHAPTER 9

Vitamin D

"Go outside and play."
—EVERYBODY'S PARENTS

Research indicates that we need far more vitamin D than the Recommended Dietary Allowance (RDA). The optimal dose of vitamin D for most adults falls somewhere between 1,000 international units (IU) and 5,000 IU per day when we aren't getting adequate exposure to sunshine. However, correction of vitamin D deficiency may require as much as 10,000 IU per day.

WHY YOU NEED MORE VITAMIN D. A LOT MORE.

by William B. Grant, PhD

From the *Orthomolecular Medicine News Service,* September 16, 2011.

Vitamin D has emerged as the nutrient of the decade. Numerous studies have found benefits for nearly 100 types of health conditions, including bone diseases, many types of cancer, cardiovascular disease (CVD), diabetes mellitus, bacterial and viral infectious diseases, autoimmune diseases such as multiple sclerosis,[1] and neurological conditions such as cognitive dysfunction.[2] It has also been shown to improve athletic and physical performance.[3]

Sunshine, Skin, Sunburn, and Sunscreen

The primary source of vitamin D for most people is solar ultraviolet-B (UVB) light. Skin pigmentation has adapted to the location where a population lives for a thousand years or more as those with skin that is too dark or light for the geographical region do not survive as well as those with the appropriate skin pigmentation.[4] Dark skin protects against the harmful effects of UV, but also blocks the UVB from penetrating deeply enough into the skin to produce vitamin D from 7-dehydrocholesterol. Those with lighter skin can produce vitamin D more rapidly, but are more prone to melanoma and other skin cancer. Sunscreens block UVB and thus limit vitamin D production. While sunscreens are useful in reducing risk of sunburning, they do not block the long-wave UV (UVA) as well as they do UVB. UVA is linked to risk of melanoma. Wearing sunscreen when there is no danger of burning can actually increase the risk of melanoma.[5]

Understanding Vitamin D Research

Since the body's own vitamin D production is the primary source of vitamin D, ecological and observational studies have been very useful in teasing out the effects of vitamin D on health. There are two types of ecological studies, based on geographical and temporal (over time) variations. In geographical studies, populations are defined geographically and both health outcome and risk-modifying factors are averaged for each geographical unit. Statistical analyses are then used to determine the relative importance of each factor. The first paper linking UVB and vitamin D to reduced risk of colon cancer was published in 1980.[6] This link has now been extended to about 15 types of cancer in the United States with respect to average noontime solar UVB doses in July.[7] Solar UVB doses in July are highest in the Southwest and lowest in the Northeast.[8] Mortality rates are generally lowest in the Southwest and highest in the Northeast.[9] Similar results have been found in Australia, China, France, Japan, Russia, and Spain, and the entire world.[10]

In temporal studies, seasonal variations in health outcomes are sought. A good example of a seasonal effect linked to solar UVB doses and vitamin D is influenza, which peaks in winter.[11]

Observational studies are generally of three types: case-control, cohort, and cross-sectional. In case-control studies, those diagnosed with a disease have serum 25-hydroxyvitamin D [25(OH)D] level or oral vitamin D intake determined at that time and are compared statistically with others with similar characteristics but without that disease. In cohort studies, people are enrolled in the study and the vitamin D index determined at that time. The cohort is followed for a number of years, and those who develop a specific disease are compared statistically with matched controls who did not. The main problem with cohort studies is that the single value of the vitamin D index may not relate to the time in the individual's life when vitamin D had the most impact on the disease outcome. Cross-sectional studies are essentially snapshots of a population and look at various factors in relation to the prevalence of health conditions. As biochemistry can be affected by health status, such studies provide less reliable information on the role of UVB and vitamin D on health outcome.

The role of vitamin D in CVD and diabetes mellitus type 2 have largely been studied using cohort studies. Significantly reduced risk of CVD and diabetes mellitus incidence have been reported in a number of studies in the past three years.[12]

Health policy officials like to see randomized controlled trials (RCTs) reporting health benefits with limited adverse effects. RCTs are certainly appropriate for pharmaceutical drugs which, by definition, are artificial substances that the human body has no experience with. RCTs with vitamin D are problematic for a number of reasons. For one, many RCTs used only 400 international units (IU) per day of vitamin D_3, which is much lower than the 10,000 IU per day that can be produced with whole-body exposure to the midday sun in summer, or 1,500 IU per day from casual sunlight exposure in summer.[13] For another, there are both oral and UVB sources of vitamin D, so the amount taken in the study will compete with the other sources. There is considerable individual variation in serum 25(OH)D for a given oral vitamin D intake.[14] Unfortunately, serum 25(OH)D levels are generally not measured in oral vitamin D RCTs.

Nonetheless, there have been several vitamin D RCTs that found significant health benefits beyond preventing falls and fractures.[15] These include ones for cancer,[16,17] influenza and colds,[18] type A influenza,[19] and pneumonia.[20]

Important Benefits of Vitamin D

The evidence of beneficial roles of UVB and vitamin D for a large number of health conditions have been posted at the Vitamin D Council's website: http://www.vitamindcouncil.org/health-conditions/.

In addition to an overview of the literature, the website also includes a feature allowing the user to pull up a large number of titles on each condition from www.pubmed.gov.

Sufficient information is currently available from observational studies with support from ecological studies and RCTs to determine relationships between serum 25(OH)D levels and incidence rates for breast and colorectal cancer,[21] CVD,[22] and influenza.[23] Risk decreases rapidly for small increases in 25(OH)D for those with initial values below 10 nanograms (ng) per milliliter (ml) (25 nanomoles [nmol] per liter [L]), then decreases at a slower rate to levels above 40 ng/ml (100 nmol/L). These relations have been used to estimate the change in mortality rates and life expectancy if population mean serum 25(OH)D levels were raised from current levels of 20 to 25 ng/ml (50 to 63 nmol/L) to 45 ng/ml (113 nmol/L). For the US, it was estimated that 400,000 deaths per year could be delayed,[24] which is about 15 percent of all deaths per year. For the entire world, it was estimated that the reduction in all-cause mortality rates would correspond to an increased life expectancy of two years.[22]

The mechanisms whereby vitamin D reduces the risk of disease are largely understood. For cancer, they include effects on cellular differentiation and proliferation, angiogenesis, and metastasis.[25] For infectious diseases, they include induction of cathelicidin and defensins[26] and shifting cytokine production from proinflammatory T-helper 1 (Th1) cytokines to Th2 cytokines.[27] For CVD, they may include reducing blood pressure and keeping calcium in the bones and teeth and out of the vascular tissues.[28] For diabetes mellitus type 2, they may include improving insulin sensitivity.[29]

Current Government-Sponsored Recommendations Are Too Low

In spite of the large and expanding body of scientific evidence that vitamin D has many health benefits, the US Institute of Medicine issued a report in November 2010 claiming that the evidence was strong only for effects on bones.[30,31] The reason given was lack of convincing randomized controlled trials on other health conditions. The one on cancer showing a 77 percent reduced risk of all-cancer incidence between the ends of the first and fourth years involved 1,100 IU per day of vitamin D plus 1,450 mg per day of calcium.[16] However, the Institute of Medicine (IOM) Committee relied on the findings from the start of the study, which were not statistically significant. In addition, the IOM Committee pointed to observational studies reporting a U-shaped serum 25(OH)D–disease incidence relation as a reason to be concerned about higher doses of vitamin D. However, these studies used a single serum 25(OH)D value from the time of enrollment followed by follow-up times as long as 17 years. Two studies reported that the sign of the correlation between disease outcome and serum 25(OH)D level changes from negative to positive after seven to 15 years.[32,33] Thus, the U-shaped relations are not reliable and should not be used as the basis for policy decisions, especially since the Committee refused to consider the largely beneficial findings from observational studies.

How Much Vitamin D Do We REALLY Need?

The IOM committee set the recommended vitamin D intake at 600 IU/day for those under the age of 70 years and 800 IU/day for those over 70, and stated that 20 ng/ml (50 nmol/L) was an adequate level. The vitamin D research community has responded to the Institute of Medicine report on vitamin D with over 60 letters and articles in peer-reviewed journals pointing out the absurdity and illogic of the IOM recommendations.[34]

The scientific consensus is that oral intake should be 1,000–5,000 IU per day of vitamin D with a goal of 30 to 40 ng/ml (75–100 nmol/L).[35] The Endocrine Society published a paper recommending 1,500–2,000 IU per day and 30 ng/ml.[36]

REFERENCES FOR "WHY YOU NEED MORE VITAMIN D"

1. Holick MF. Vitamin D deficiency. *N Engl J Med* 2007;357(3):266–281.

2. Llewellyn DJ, Lang IA, Langa KM, et al. Vitamin D and cognitive impairment in the elderly U.S. population. *J Gerontol A Biol Sci Med Sci* 2011;66(1):59–65.

3. Cannell JJ, Hollis BW, Sorenson MB, et al. Athletic performance and vitamin D. *Med Sci Sports Exerc* 2009;41(5):1102–1110.

4. Jablonski NG, Chaplin G. Colloquium paper: Human skin pigmentation as an adaptation to UV radiation. *Proc Natl Acad Sci* U S A. 2010;107 Suppl 2:8962–8968.

5. Gorham ED, Mohr SB, Garland CF, et al. Do sunscreens increase risk of melanoma in populations residing at higher latitudes? *Ann Epidemiol* 2007;17(12):956–963.

6. Garland CF, Garland FC. Do sunlight and vitamin D reduce the likelihood of colon cancer? *Int J Epidemiol* 1980;9(3):227–231.

7. Grant WB, Garland CF. The association of solar ultraviolet B (UVB) with reducing risk of cancer: Multifactorial ecologic analysis of geographic variation in age-adjusted cancer mortality rates. *Anticancer Res* 2006;26(4A):2687–2699.

8. Leffell DJ, Brash DE. Sunlight and skin cancer. *Sci Am* 1996; 275(1): 52–53, 56–59.

9. Devesa SS, Grauman DJ, Blot WJ, et al. Atlas of Cancer Mortality in the United States, 1950–1994. *NIH Publication* No. 99–4564, 1999. http://ratecalc.cancer.gov/ratecalc//.

10. Grant WB, Mohr SB. Ecological studies of ultraviolet B, vitamin D and cancer since 2000. *Ann Epidemiol* 2009;19(7):446–454.

11. Cannell JJ, Vieth R, Umhau JC, et al. Epidemic influenza and vitamin D. *Epidemiol Infect* 2006;134(6):1129–1140.

12. Parker J, Hashmi O, Dutton D, et al. Levels of vitamin D and cardiometabolic disorders: Systematic review and meta-analysis. *Maturitas* 2010;65(3):225–236.

13. Hyppönen E, Power C. Hypovitaminosis D in British adults at age 45 y: Nationwide cohort study of dietary and lifestyle predictors. *Am J Clin Nutr* 2007;85(3):860–868.

14. Garland CF, French CB, Baggerly LL, et al. Vitamin D supplement doses and serum 25-hydroxyvitamin D in the range associated with cancer prevention. *Anticancer Res* 2011:31:617–622.

15. Bischoff-Ferrari HA, Willett WC, Wong JB, et al. Prevention of nonvertebral fractures with oral vitamin D and dose dependency: A meta-analysis of randomized controlled trials. *Arch Intern Med* 2009;169(6):551–561.

16. Lappe JM, Travers-Gustafson D, Davies KM, et al. Vitamin D and calcium supplementation reduces cancer risk: Results of a randomized trial. *Am J Clin Nutr* 2007;85(6):1586–1591.

17. Bolland MJ, Grey A, Gamble GD, et al. Calcium and vitamin D supplements and health outcomes: A reanalysis of the Women's Health Initiative (WHI) limited-access data set. *Am J Clin Nutr* 2011; 94(4):1144–1149. [Epub ahead of print].

18. Aloia JF, Li-Ng M. Re: epidemic influenza and vitamin D. *Epidemiol Infect* 2007;135(7):1095–1096; author reply 1097–1098.

19. Urashima M, Segawa T, Okazaki M, et al. Randomized trial of vitamin D supplementation to prevent seasonal influenza A in schoolchildren. *Am J Clin Nutr* 2010;91(5):1255–1260.

20. Manaseki-Holland S, Qader G, Isaq Masher M, et al. Effects of vitamin D supplementation to children diagnosed with pneumonia in Kabul: A randomised controlled trial. *Trop Med Int Health* 2010;15(10):1148–1155.

21. Grant WB. Relation between prediagnostic serum 25-hydroxyvitamin D level and incidence of breast, colorectal, and other cancers. *J Photochem Photobiol B* 2010;101:130–136.

22. Grant WB. An estimate of the global reduction in mortality rates through doubling vitamin D levels. *Eur J Clin Nutr* 2011;65:1016–1026.

23. Sabetta JR, DePetrillo P, Cipriani RJ, et al. Serum 25-hydroxyvitamin D and the incidence of acute viral respiratory tract infections in healthy adults. *PLoS One* 2010;5(6):e11088.

24. Grant WB. In defense of the sun: An estimate of changes in mortality rates in the United States if mean serum 25-hydroxyvitamin D levels were raised to 45 ng/mL by solar ultraviolet-B irradiance. *Dermato-Endocrinology* 2009;1(4):207–214.

25. Krishnan AV, Feldman D. Mechanisms of the anti-cancer and anti-inflammatory actions of vitamin D. *Annu Rev Pharmacol Toxicol* 2011;51:311–336.

26. Liu PT, Stenger S, Tang DH, et al. Cutting edge: Vitamin D-mediated human antimicrobial activity against Mycobacterium tuberculosis is dependent on the induction of cathelicidin. *J Immunol* 2007;179(4):2060–2063.

27. Cantorna MT, Mahon BD. Mounting evidence for vitamin D as an environmental factor affecting autoimmune disease prevalence. *Exp Biol Med (Maywood)* 2004;229(11):1136–1142.

28. Zagura M, Serg M, Kampus P, et al. Aortic stiffness and vitamin D are independent markers of aortic calcification in patients with peripheral arterial disease and in healthy subjects. *Eur J Vasc Endovasc Surg* 2011 Aug 24 [Epub ahead of print].

29. Alvarez JA, Ashraf AP, Hunter GR, et al. Serum 25-hydroxyvitamin D and parathyroid hormone are independent determinants of whole-body insulin sensitivity in women and may contribute to lower insulin sensitivity in African Americans. *Am J Clin Nutr* 2010;92(6):1344–1349.

30. Institute of Medicine (US) Committee to Review Dietary Reference Intakes for Vitamin D and Calcium; Ross AC, Taylor CL, Yaktine AL, Del Valle HB, editors. *Dietary Reference Intakes for Calcium and Vitamin D.* Washington (DC): National Academies Press (US); 2011.

31. Ross AC, Manson JE, Abrams SA, et al. The 2011 report on dietary reference intakes for calcium and vitamin D from the Institute of Medicine: What clinicians need to know. *J Clin Endocrinol Metab* 2011;96(1):53–58.

32. Lim U, Freedman DM, Hollis BW, et al. A prospective investigation of serum 25-hydroxyvitamin D and risk of lymphoid cancers. *Int J Cancer* 2009;124(4):979–986.

33. Robien K, Cutler GJ, Lazovich D. Vitamin D intake and breast cancer risk in postmenopausal women: The Iowa Women's Health Study. *Cancer Causes Control* 2007;18(7):775–782.

34. Heaney RP, Ahmed AH, Gordon R. The IOM Report on Vitamin D misleads. *J Clin Endocrinol Metab* eLetter. (4 March 2011). Available at: http://press.endocrine.org/e-letters/10.1210/jc.2010–2704.

35. Souberbielle JC, Body JJ, Lappe JM, et al. Vitamin D and musculoskeletal health, cardiovascular disease, autoimmunity and cancer: Recommendations for clinical practice. *Autoimmun Rev* 2010;9:709–715.

36. Holick MF, Binkley NC, Bischoff-Ferrari HA, et al. Evaluation, treatment, and prevention of vitamin D deficiency: An Endocrine Society clinical practice guideline. *J Clin Endocrinol Metab* 2011;96(7):1911–1930.

Latest Research on Vitamin D Shows Remarkable Range of Health Benefits

by Jack Challem

From *The Nutrition Reporter* 22(9), 2011.

Research on the health benefits of vitamin D is growing at a breathtaking pace. These are summaries of some of the latest studies.

Vitamin D and Type 2 Diabetes Risk

Claudia Gagnon, MD, of the University of Melbourne, Australia, and her colleagues studied 5,200 men and women whose glucose tolerance was assessed in 1999–2000.[1] Five years later, their glucose tolerance and insulin sensitivity were reassessed, and 199 of the subjects were diagnosed with type 2 diabetes.

People with low blood levels of vitamin D and low calcium intake were more likely to develop type 2 diabetes. Each increase of 10 ng/ml (25 nmol/L) in blood vitamin D levels was associated with a 24 percent lower risk of diabetes. Calcium intake did not influence the risk of diabetes.

Vitamin D and Insulin Function

Anastassios G. Pittas, MD, of the Tufts University Medical Center, Boston, enrolled 92 prediabetic men and women in a 16-week study.[2] The subjects had an average age of 57 years, were obese, and had an average glycated hemoglobin (HbA1c) of 5.9 percent. They were given one of the following: vitamin D (2,000 IU/day) and calcium (400 mg/day), vitamin D or placebos, calcium or placebos, or placebos.

People taking vitamin D, but not calcium or placebo, had improvements in pancreatic function and significant increases in insulin secretion. In addition, their HbA1c was slightly less compared with that of those not receiving vitamin D. Pittas noted that the improvement in insulin secretion with vitamin D might have benefits in people with type 1 diabetes, but that studies were needed to confirm this benefit.

Vitamin D and Metabolic Syndrome

Metabolic syndrome, also known as syndrome X, is a cluster of symptoms that increases the risk of type 2 diabetes and heart disease. These symptoms include elevated blood sugar or insulin, abdominal obesity, hypertension, and elevated total or low-density lipoprotein cholesterol.

Researchers at Georgia State University, Atlanta, studied 5,867 adolescents, ages 12 to 19 years old, and found that those with the lowest blood levels of vitamin D were 71 percent more likely to have signs of metabolic syndrome, including greater waist circumference, higher systolic blood pressure, and poorer glucose tolerance.[3]

Vitamin D During Pregnancy

Pregnant women can feel safe taking up to 4,000 IU of vitamin D during pregnancy, according to a study conducted at the Medical University of South Carolina, Charleston. Bruce Hollis, PhD, and his colleagues gave 350 women supplements containing 400 IU, 2,000 IU, or 4,000 IU of vitamin D daily, starting at 12 to 16 weeks of gestation and continuing until delivery. Women receiving 4,000 IU of vitamin D were more likely to achieve normal levels of vitamin D, as were their newborn babies.[4]

Vitamin D and Allergies

A deficiency of vitamin D is associated with greater risk of IgE (immunoglobulin E) mediated allergies to pollens and some foods. In a study conducted at Rush University Medical Center, Chicago, doctors measured vitamin D levels and IgE allergic sensitization in 3,100 US children and 3,400 adults.[5] Seventeen allergens were tested, and 11 were more common in children and adolescents with vitamin D deficiencies. Peanut, ragweed, and oak allergies were most strongly associated with vitamin D deficiencies.

Vitamin D and Skin Cancer

Some studies have suggested that high blood levels of vitamin D protect against both melanoma and nonmelanoma skin cancer. Jean Y. Tang, MD, of the Stanford University School of Medicine, Redwood City, California, and her colleagues tracked 36,282 postmenopausal women who were asked to take 400 IU of vitamin D and 1,000 mg of calcium or placebos daily for an average of seven years.[6]

Although the overall incidence of skin cancer did not differ among women getting vitamin D and calcium, benefits were found in a specific subgroup of women. Women with a history of nonmelanoma skin cancer had a 57 percent lower risk of developing melanoma if they took vitamin D and calcium supplements.

How Much Vitamin D for You?

Late last year, a committee of researchers at the US Institute of Medicine (IOM) decided that the vast majority of Americans didn't need to take more than 600 IU of vitamin D daily and that everyone was fine as long as their blood level of vitamin D was above 20 ng/ml.

The question most vitamin D experts asked was: What on earth was going through their heads? After all, a blood level of 20 ng/ml is a sign of vitamin D deficiency.

Finally, the Endocrine Society, whose members are hormone specialists, weighed in with more rationale guidelines: infants less than one year old get 400 to 1,000 IU of vitamin D daily, older children and teenagers get 600 to 1,000 IU daily, and adults get 1,500 to 2,000 IU daily.

The Endocrine Society went a step further. It advised doctors that up to 10,000 IU daily might be needed to correct vitamin D deficiency in adults.

The ideal approach is to ask your doctor to measure your blood level of vitamin D. If it's less than 30 ng/ml, you're deficient. An optimal range is most likely between 40 and 60 ng/ml, though many people have higher amounts without any ill effects. If you are deficient, you may need between 2,000 and 10,000 IU daily to bring your level up to normal.[7]

REFERENCES FOR "LATEST RESEARCH ON VITAMIN D"

1. Gagnon C, Lu ZX, Magliano DJ, et al. Serum 25hydroxyvitamin D, calcium intake, and risk of type 2 diabetes after 5 years. *Diabetes Care* 2011;34(5):1133–1138.

2. Mitri A, Dawson-Hughes B, Hu FB, et al. Effects of vitamin D and calcium supplementation on pancreatic beta cell function, insulin sensitivity, and glycemia in adults at high risk of diabetes: The calcium and vitamin D for diabetes mellitus (CaDDM) randomized controlled trial. *Am J Clin Nutr* 2011; 94(2):486–494. doi 10.3945/ajcn.111.011684.

3. Ganji V, Zhang X, Shaikh N, et al. Serum 25hydroxyvitamin D concentrations are associated with prevalence of metabolic syndrome and various cardiometabolic risk factors in US children and adolescents based on assay-adjusted serum 25-hydroxyvitamin D data from NHANES 2001–2006. *Am J Clin Nutr* 2011;94(1):225–233.

4. Hollis BW, Johnson D, Hulsey TC, et al. Vitamin D supplementation during pregnancy: Double blind, randomized clinical trial of safety and effectiveness. *J Bone Miner Res* 2011; 26(10): 2341–2357 [Epub ahead of print].

5. Sharief S, Jariwala S, Kumar J, et al. Vitamin D levels and food and environmental allergies in the United States: Results from the national health and nutrition examination survey 2005–2006. *J Allergy Clin Immunol* 2011;127(5):1195–1202.

6. Tang JY, Fu T, LeBlanc E, et al. Calcium plus vitamin D supplementation and the risk of nonmelanoma and melanoma skin cancer: Post hoc analyses of the women's health initiative randomized controlled trial. *J Clin Oncol* 2011;29(22):3078–3084.

7. Holick MF, Binkley NC, Bischoff-Ferrari HA, et al. Evaluation, treatment, and prevention of vitamin D deficiency: An endocrine society clinical practice guideline. *J Clin Endocrinol Metab* 2011;96(7):1911–1930.

TOP VITAMIN D RESEARCH OF 2014

by William B. Grant, PhD

From the *Orthomolecular Medicine News Service,* February 3, 2015.

Higher vitamin D blood levels may reduce the risk of many types of disease, including autoimmune diseases, cancers, cardiovascular disease, dementia, diabetes mellitus, and falls and fractures.

Research into the health effects associated with vitamin D continued to be strong in 2014. The number of publications with vitamin D in the title or abstract listed at pubmed.gov increased from 3,119 in 2011 to 3,919 in 2014. Seven vitamin D researchers (listed after this report) worked together to pick the 20 papers from 2014 that made the most contribution to understanding the health effects of vitamin D.

Papers are not in priority order, but instead grouped by type of study. For the purpose of this article "vitamin D" in the blood is a measurement of 25-hydroxyvitamin D or 25(OH)D.

RANDOMIZED CONTROL TRIALS IN 2014

No one refutes the fact that vitamin D is beneficial to the skeletal system. There are many studies (randomized controlled trials [RCTs] and also epidemiological) that support this hypothesis. What is at odds is whether or not vitamin D is beneficial to the nonskeletal system. There are many observational (epidemiological, or association) studies that show vitamin D is beneficial, and many RCTs that show it isn't. Does that mean that vitamin D does not aid in disease prevention? Or does it mean that the RCT model does not work for nutrients?

Vitamin D_3 and COPD

A vitamin D trial in the United Kingdom in which patients with chronic obstructive pulmonary disease (COPD) were given 120,000 international units (IU) vitamin D_3 every two months for a year found that vitamin D_3 supplementation was protective against moderate or severe exacerbation in those with baseline 25(OH)D concentrations less than 50 nanomoles per liter (nmol/L) (20 nanograms per milliliter [ng/mL]) but not for those with concentrations greater than 50 nmol/L.[1] Vitamin D_3 supplementation had no effect on upper respiratory infections. This is consistent with previous RCTs that used high doses at infrequent intervals, every two months in this case; however, other trials that used an adequate dose given daily have shown reduction in upper respiratory tract infections.

Vitamin D Promotes Vascular Regeneration

This study[2] demonstrated that vitamin D improved cardiovascular disease. The German team investigated this effect several ways. They showed that supplementation with 4,000 IU per day of vitamin D_3 increased the number of circulating angiogenic myeloid cells, which promote growth and vascular regeneration necessary for a healthy cardiovascular system. A similar result was found in a mouse model, which also demonstrated restoration of impaired angiogenesis (new vessel formation) function. They also examined the mechanisms by which vitamin D acted.

Vitamin D and Depression

This paper[3] reported on a statistical average of many studies of vitamin D RCTs without methodological flaws and found that vitamin D supplementation resulted in a statistically significant improvement in clinical depression. However, the same analysis of vitamin D RCTs with methodological flaws found a statistically significant worsening of depression. The major flaws identified included not increasing 25(OH)D concentrations and not measuring baseline or final 25(OH)D concentrations. Vitamin D supplementation of greater than 800 IU per day was somewhat favorable in the management of depression.

Vitamin D and Decreased Antibiotic Use

A post hoc (conducted after the study was completed) analysis of a vitamin D RCT involving 644 Australian residents aged 60 to 84 years found a significant reduction in prescribed antibiotics if they were over the age of 70 years and taking 60,000 IU of vitamin D_3 monthly compared with the placebo groups.[4] The effect was not significant for those less than 70 years of age. This study suggests that taking an average of 2,000 IU per day of vitamin D_3 reduces the risk of infections, most likely respiratory infections, in older adults.

OBERVATIONAL STUDIES OF VITAMIN D

Observational studies provide some of the strongest evidence to date for beneficial health outcomes related to vitamin D. Observational studies measure vitamin D status and health outcomes for every participant. Blood samples are taken at the time of enrollment and people are followed for several years. Vitamin D is said to be effective if positive health outcomes result.

Vitamin D and Specific Death Reduction

This paper was a review of observational and RCT studies that showed a correlation between vitamin D and specific mortality outcomes.[5] One conclusion was that supplementation with vitamin D_3 significantly reduces overall mortality among older adults. They used data from 73 cohort studies (849,412 participants) and 22 RCTs (30,716 participants). In the RCTs, all-cause mortality rate was reduced by 11 percent for vitamin D_3 supplementation but increased by 4 percent for vitamin D_2 supplementation. In addition, their meta-analysis of cancer-specific incidence and mortality rates comparing those who started in the lowest third of vitamin D blood concentrations against those in the highest third suggests that vitamin D may have a much stronger impact on survival after developing cancer than on reducing the risk of developing cancer to start with.

Vitamin D and All-Cause Mortality

An analysis of 32 observational studies found that as 25(OH)D concentrations increased from 13 nmol/L (5 ng/ml) to 90 nmol/L (36 ng/ml), there was a linear reduction in all-cause mortality.[6] At concentrations greater than 90 nmol/L (36 ng/ml), no further improvement was observed. This finding is important in that it did not find any evidence for a U-shaped relationship showing higher risk for both low and high 25(OH) D concentrations, as has been reported in some studies. Furthermore, the risk for all-cause mortality for those with 25(OH)D concentration less than 25 nmol/L (10 ng/mL) was 1.9 compared to that for those with concentrations greater than 100 nmol/L (40 ng/mL).

Low Vitamin D and *Clostridium Difficile*–Associated Diarrhea

A study in New York found that 25(OH)D concentration and age were the only independent predictors of response to the highly fatal *Clostridium difficile*–associated diarrhea (CDAD).[7] Subjects with 25(OH)D concentration less than 53 nmol/L (21 ng/mL) were 4.75 times more likely to fail to resolve CDAD after 30 days than subjects with 25(OH)D concentrations greater than 75 nmol/L (30 ng/mL). This is an important finding since CDAD rates are increasing due to antibiotic-resistant strains of CD.

Avoidance of Sun Exposure Is a Risk Factor for All-Cause Mortality

An observational study in Sweden involving 29,518 women followed for up to 20 years with 2,545 reported deaths found that the mortality rate for those who avoided sun exposure was approximately twice as high as those who were most exposed to the sun.[8] This difference explained 3 percent of all deaths and is important since UVB doses in Sweden are generally low and virtually absent for six months of the year. Production of vitamin D may explain most of the differences between sun exposure amounts, although other beneficial effects of solar UV exist, such as release of nitric oxide, resulting in reduction of blood pressure, as well as vitamin D–independent effects on the immune system.

Vitamin D and Kidney Stones

GrassrootsHealth (501c3) initiated a voluntary reporting project called D*action. There are over 7,000 in the cohort, of which 2,012 have reported their data for a median of 19 months. In this cohort, there has been no evidence of an association of 25(OH)D and kidney stones.[9] What was a risk factor for kidney stones in this study was high body mass index. This study counters the Women's Health Initiative study that reported an elevated risk of kidney stones for women taking 400 IU per day of vitamin D_3 and 1,500 mg per day of calcium.

Vitamin D and Liver Cancer

An observational study involving 520,000 participants in the European Prospective Investigation into Cancer and Nutrition (EPIC) cohort, of which 138 developed hepatocellular carcinoma (HCC), or liver cancer, found that higher levels of 25(OH)D reduced incidence of HCC.[10] Each 10 nmol/L (4 ng/mL) increase in 25(OH)D concentration was associated with a 20 percent average decrease in risk of HCC. The large number of participants in the study with a very small number of cases indicates the difficulty of demonstrating the beneficial effect of vitamin D for the rare cancers. The authors noted that the result did "not change after adjustment for biomarkers of preexisting liver damage, nor chronic infection with hepatitis B or C viruses."

Vitamin D and Colorectal Cancer

A study in Ireland and Scotland involving 1,598 patients with stage I to III colorectal cancer found that 25(OH)D concentrations (measured approximately 15 weeks after diagnosis of colorectal cancer) were associated with survival rates.[11] Those in the highest third of 25(OH)D concentrations, with a median concentration of 51 nmol/L (20 ng/mL), compared to the lowest third, with a median concentration of 10 nmol/L (4 ng/mL), had a 32 percent lower risk of cancer-specific mortality and a 30 percent lower risk of all-cause mortality over a ten-year follow-up period. This study provides support for the idea that people diagnosed with cancer should raise their 25(OH)D concentration to above a minimum of 50 nmol/L (20 ng/mL).

Vitamin D and Breast Cancer

Two meta-analyses found significantly increased cancer survival rates with higher concentration of 25(OH)D at time of diagnosis.[12] For breast cancer, results from five studies found that those with 25(OH)D concentration of 75 nmol/L (30 ng/mL) had half the five- to twenty-year mortality rate as those with a concentration of 30 nmol/L (12 ng/mL).

Vitamin D and Colorectal Cancer Survival

In this meta-analysis for colorectal cancer, results from four studies found that those with 25(OH)D concentration of 80 nmol/L (32 ng/mL) had 60 percent of the six- to twenty-year mortality rate as those with 45 nmol/L (18 ng/mL).[13]

Low Vitamin D, Alzheimer's Disease, and Dementia

Two papers reported that those with low 25(OH)D concentrations had increased risk of developing vascular dementia and Alzheimer's disease. The first one is from Denmark: a study involving 418 people followed for 30 years found a 25 percent increased risk of Alzheimer's disease and a 22 percent increased risk of vascular dementia for those with baseline 25(OH)D concentration less than 25 nmol/L (10 ng/ml) compared to greater than 50 nmol/L (20 ng/ml).[14] Another study in the United States involving 1,658 participants followed for 5.6 years found a 125 percent increased risk of Alzheimer's disease for those with severely deficient 25(OH)D levels (< 25 nmol/L (10 ng/mL)), and a 53 percent increased risk for those with deficient levels (□ 25 to < 50 nmol/L) compared to participants with sufficient concentrations (□ 50 nmol/L (20 ng/mL)).[15]

PREGNANCY

Lower Risk of Preterm Birth with Higher Vitamin D

There is considerable interest in the role of vitamin D during pregnancy. In a reanalysis of results from two maternal vitamin D supplementation trials conducted in South Carolina, it was found that: "(1) maternal vitamin D status closest to delivery date was more significantly associated with preterm birth, suggesting that later intervention as a rescue treatment may positively impact the risk of preterm delivery, and (2) a serum concentration of 100 nmol/L (40 ng/mL) in the 3rd trimester was associated with a 47% reduction in preterm births."[16]

Vitamin D and Fetal Development

A study in Australia compared maternal 25(OH)D concentration at 18 weeks' pregnancy with outcomes of the children years later. The authors found that "maternal vitamin D deficiency during pregnancy was associated with impaired lung development in 6-year-old offspring, neurocognitive difficulties at age 10, increased risk of eating disorders in adolescence, and lower peak bone mass at 20 years."[17]

Vitamin D and Preeclampsia

A review of vitamin D supplementation and 25(OH)D concentrations during pregnancy found vitamin D reduces the risk of preeclampsia.[18] For 25(OH)D concentration, the combined risk reduction was 48 percent with higher level circulating vitamin D. For vitamin D RCTs, the combined risk reduction was 34 percent for vitamin D supplementation vs. a placebo. This review provides further support for the importance of vitamin D supplementation and raising 25(OH)D concentrations during pregnancy.

Conclusion

Research on the health benefits of solar UVB exposure and vitamin D continues at a rapid pace. We appear to be in the middle of the golden age of vitamin D research, a period with much progress in understanding the effects of UVB exposure and vitamin D for a large range of health outcomes. We are shifting from discovery to evaluation of previous findings and testing the role of vitamin D in prevention and treatment of various diseases.

While many of the findings from ecological and observational studies are strong, it appears that health systems and policy makers are awaiting results from large ongoing RCTs before they accept UVB exposure and vitamin D as valid factors for health. Unfortunately, most of the RCTs currently underway and due to be completed before the end of the decade, including large-scale RCTs in several countries, have not been properly designed, so they may not shed light on vitamin D's preventive powers. Thus, it may be another decade before the true health benefits of vitamin D and sunlight are accepted. Meanwhile, various types of research will continue, and it will be up to individuals and their health care providers to evaluate the available evidence and act accordingly.

REFERENCES FOR "TOP VITAMIN D RESEARCH OF 2014"

1. Martineau AR, James WY, Hooper RL, et al. Vitamin D_3 supplementation in patients with chronic obstructive pulmonary disease (ViDiCO): a multicentre, double-blind, randomised controlled trial. *Lancet* 2015; 3(2):120–130.

2. Wong MS, Leisegang MS, Kruse C, et al. Vitamin D promotes vascular regeneration. *Circulation* 2014;130(12):976–986.

3. Spedding S. Vitamin D and depression: a systematic review and meta-analysis comparing studies with and without biological flaws. *Nutrients* 2014; 6(4):1501–1518.

4. Tran B, Armstrong BK, Ebeling PR, et al. Effect of vitamin D supplementation on antibiotic use: a randomized controlled trial. *Am J Clin Nutr* 2014; 99(1):156–161.

5. Chowdhury R, Kunutsor S, Vitezova A, et al. Vitamin D and risk of cause specific death: systematic review and meta-analysis of observational cohort and randomised intervention studies. *BMJ* 2014; 348:g1903.

6. Garland CF, Kim JJ, Mohr SB, et al. Meta-analysis of all-cause mortality according to serum 25-hydroxyvitamin D. *Am J Public Health* 2014; 104(8):e43–50.

7. Wang WJ, Gray S, Sison C, et al. Low vitamin D level is an independent predictor of poor outcomes in Clostridium difficile-associated diarrhea. *Therap Adv Gastroenterol* 2014; 7(1): 14–19.

8. Lindqvist PG, Epstein E, Nielsen K, et al. Avoidance of sun exposure is a risk factor for all-cause mortality. *J Intern Med* 2016 [Epub ahead of print].

9. Nguyen S, Baggerly L, French C, et al. 25-Hydroxyvitamin D in the range of 20 to 100 ng/ml and incidence of kidney stones. *Am J Public Health* 2014;104(9):1783–1787.

10. Fedirko V, Duarte-Salles T, Bamia C, et al. Prediagnostic circulating vitamin D levels and risk of hepatocellular carcinoma in European populations: a nested case-control study. *Hepatology* 2014;60(4):1222–1230.

11. Zgaga L, Theodoratou E, Farrington SM, et al. Plasma vitamin D concentration influences survival outcome after a diagnosis of colorectal cancer. *J Clin Oncol* 2014;32(23):2430–2439.

12. Mohr SB, Gorham ED, Kim J, et al. Meta-analysis of vitamin D sufficiency for improving survival of patients with breast cancer. *Anticancer Res* 2014;34(3):1163–1166.

13. Mohr SB, Gorham ED, Kim J, et al. Could vitamin D sufficiency improve the survival of colorectal cancer patients? *J Steroid Biochem Mol Biol* 2015;148:239–44 [Epub 2014 Dec 19].

14. Afzal S, Bojesen SE, Nordestgaard BG. Reduced 25-hydroxyvitamin D and risk of Alzheimer's disease and vascular dementia. *Alzheimers Dement* 2014;10(3):296–302.

15. Littlejohns TJ, Henley WE, Lang IA, et al. Vitamin D and the risk of dementia and Alzheimer disease. *Neurology* 2014 [Epub 2014 Aug 6].

16. Wagner CL, Baggerly C, McDonnell SL, et al. Post-hoc comparison of vitamin D status at three time points during pregnancy demonstrates lower risk of preterm birth with higher vitamin D closer to delivery. *J Steroid Biochem Mol Biol* 2015;148:256–260.

17. Hart PH, Lucas RM, Walsh JP. Vitamin D in fetal development: findings from a birth cohort study. *Pediatrics* 2015;135(1):e167–73.

18. Hyppönen E, Cavadino A, Williams D, et al. Vitamin D and pre-eclampsia: original data, systematic review and meta-analysis. *Ann Nutr Metab* 2013;63(4):331–340.

CHAPTER 10

B Vitamins

"The reason that one nutrient can cure so many different illnesses is because a deficiency of one nutrient can cause many different illnesses. This has led to something of a vitamin public relations problem. When pharmaceuticals are versatile, they are called 'broad spectrum' and 'wonder drugs.' When vitamins are versatile, they are called 'faddish' and 'cures in search of a disease.' Such a double standard needs to be exposed and opposed at every turn."

—ABRAM HOFFER, MD, PHD; ANDREW W. SAUL, PHD; HAROLD FOSTER, PHD, IN *NIACIN: THE REAL STORY*

Taking a quality B complex twice a day would provide most adults with a good amount of each B vitamin. Higher, therapeutic doses of individual B vitamins such as niacin may require additional supplementation. Keep in mind: the Bs work together and should be taken together. Any particular B vitamin you wish to take should also be taken along with a B complex.

Optimal daily B-vitamin supplementation for healthy adults could include the following:[1]

- Thiamine B_1: 50 to 100 milligrams (mg)
- Riboflavin B_2: 50 to 100 mg
- Niacin B_3: 300 to 600 mg
- Pantothenic acid B_5: 100 to 200 mg
- Pyridoxine B_6: 50 to 100 mg
- Folate or folic acid B_9: 400 to 800 micrograms (mcg)
- Methylcobalamin B_{12}: 1,000 to 2,000 mcg

Adding biotin (30 to 300 mcg per day) is a good idea. In addition, 500 mg per day of choline is recommended for good health.[2]

The B vitamins are very important, and they are all remarkably safe. Because they are water soluble, excess is excreted in urine. This might cause a colorful bathroom experience. For example, you may notice that when you take riboflavin (B_2), your urine is electric yellow. Don't distress. This is normal. It simply shows that the body is flushing out the surplus. Because of this efficient process, B vitamins are not stored in the body and must be obtained from your diet or supplements, preferably both. Remember, having an abundance of essential nutrients is a good thing. It is deficiency that is a problem.

THE PIONEERING WORK OF RUTH FLINN HARRELL: CHAMPION OF CHILDREN

by Andrew W. Saul, PhD

From the *J Orthomolecular Med* 2004; 19(1):21–26.

"The person who says it cannot be done should not interrupt the person doing it."

—CHINESE PROVERB

Early in 1981, the medical and educational establishments were shaken to their socks. Ruth F. Harrell and colleagues, in *Proceedings of the National Academy of Sciences,*[1] showed that high doses of vitamins improved intelligence and educational performance in learning-disabled children, including those with Down syndrome. Though to many observers this seemingly came straight out of left field, Dr. Harrell, who had been investigating vitamin effects on learning for 40 years, was not inventing the idea of megavitamin therapy in one paper. But she had at last succeeded in focusing much-needed public attention on the role of nutrition in learning disabilities, a problem that inkwell-era US RDAs and pharmaceuticals by the lunchbox-full have failed to solve.

The start of the Second World War was breaking news when Ruth Flinn Harrell conducted her first investigations into what she called "superfeeding." Her 1942 Columbia University PhD thesis, "Effect of Added Thiamine on Learning,"[2] was published by the university in 1943 and would be followed by "Further Effects of Added Thiamine on Learning and Other Processes" in 1947.[3] Her research was not about enriched or fortified foods; "added" meant "provided by supplement tablets." World War II had just ended when Dr. Harrell stated in a 1946 *Journal of Nutrition* article[4] that "a liberal thiamine intake improved a number of mental and physical skills of orphanage children." By 1956, Dr. Harrell had investigated "The Effect of Mothers' Diets on the Intelligence of Offspring,"[5] finding that "supplementation of the pregnant and lactating mothers' diet by vitamins increased the intelligence quotients of their offspring at three and four years of age."

Thiamine (Vitamin B_1)

Most everyone has heard of beriberi, and few are all that passionate about it anymore. But beriberi, which literally means "I can't, I can't," may all too well describe the learning-disabled child. Such children, recognized as truly disabled by the Americans with Disabilities Act, are not unwilling but rather unable to perform well in school. To see the physical incapacitation thiamine deficiency causes in impoverished countries is all too easy. To see the mental incapacitation in American classrooms is not difficult, either. Yet both may be caused by thiamine deficiency, and both helped by thiamine supplementation. Harrell zeroed in on this topic sixty years ago, demonstrating that supplemental thiamine improves learning. One reporter wrote, "An experiment was conducted by Dr. Ruth Flinn Harrell which involved 104 children from nine to nineteen years of age. Half of the children were given a vitamin B_1 (thiamine) pill each day, and the other half received a placebo. The test lasted 6 weeks. It was found by a series of tests that the group that was given the vitamin gained one-fourth more in learning ability than did the other group."[6]

Carbohydrates, including sugar, increase the body's need for thiamine. Children eat a lot of sugar. An unmet increase is effectively the same as a deficiency. This may be part of the mechanism of attention-deficit hyperactivity disorder (ADHD) and other children's learning and behavior disorders, as many so-called "food faddists" or "health nuts" have proclaimed for decades. Vitamin deficiency can become vitamin dependency. Chronic subclinical beriberi may result in thiamine dependency in the same way that chronic subclinical pellagra results in niacin dependency.

The Importance of Thiamine

You need thiamine "every moment of every day," says Dr. Saul. "It plays a crucial role in carbohydrate metabolism, pregnancy, lactation, and muscular activity. Less well known is that more thiamine is needed in tissues during fevers. The US thiamine RDA of a milligram or two is not even remotely close to being enough. A very strong case can be made for 25 to 65 mg per day even for nonalcoholics." Food sources of thiamine include fortified grains, wheat germ, eggs, legumes, vegetables, and seeds.

Severe thiamine deficiency is a rare condition, but when it appears it is often seen in alcoholics. Alcohol inhibits the body's ability to absorb vitamin B_1, among other nutrients. "Continued deficiency of thiamine is very grave," says Dr. Saul. "Unchecked, beriberi is fatal. But a long-standing inadequate, marginal, or minimal thiamine supply may cause severe neurological effects, most significantly nerve irritation, diminished reflex response, prickly or deadening sensations, pain, damage to or degeneration of myelin sheaths (the fatty nerve-cell insulation material), and ultimately paralysis. Dr. Klenner, aware that this could well describe multiple sclerosis, went to work trying megadoses of thiamine. On the principle that it takes a lot of water to put out a well-established fire, Klenner ignored the US RDA of 1 to 2 milligrams per day and gave multiple sclerosis sufferers 1,000 or 2,000 milligrams of thiamine a day. He administered other vitamin megadoses as well. Patients improved."

B-Complex

The B-vitamins as a group are absolutely vital to nerve function, and it would be difficult to imagine the juvenile owner of malnourished nerves performing well in school. Specifically, it is well established that thiamine deficiency causes not only loss of nerve function and ultimately paralysis but also, according to *The Nutrition Desk Reference,*[7] "memory loss, reduced attention span, irritability, confusion and depression." Riboflavin (B_2) deficiency causes "nerve tissue damage that may manifest itself as depression and hysteria." Niacin (B_3) deficiency causes "loss of memory and emotional instability." Pyridoxine (B_6) deficiency results in "impaired production of neurotransmitters (and) mental confusion." Folic acid deficiency causes irritability, apathy, forgetfulness, and hostility. Cobalamin (B_{12}) deficiency causes "degeneration of the spinal cord, fatigue, disorientation, ataxia, moodiness, and confusion."

Though these symptoms generally appear after prolonged deficiency, they are very serious and, if untreated, the ultimate result in each case would be death. Practically speaking, a shortage of any one of the B vitamins can lead to neurological damage sufficient to contribute to learning and behavioral troubles.

Harrell recognized that thiamine and the rest of the vitamins work better as a team. She used two clinically effective but oft-criticized therapeutic nutrition techniques: simultaneous supplementation with many nutrients (the "shotgun" approach), and megadoses. Working on the reasonable assumption that learning-disabled children, because of functional deficiencies, might need higher than normal levels of nutrients, she progressed from her initial emphasis on thiamine to later providing a wide variety of supplemental nutrients.

Deficiency Debate

The only escape from the inevitability of concluding that vitamin deficiency is a serious factor in learning is the political one: declare a victory. Dodging the issue is as easy as proclaiming that, thanks to food fortification (coupled with a generous portion of wishful thinking), no child has such deficiencies. Though the processed food industry and its apologists continue to assert exactly this, statistics fail to bear it out.

An analysis of National Health and Nutrition Examination Survey (NHANES III) data from 1988 to 1994 by Gladys Block, PhD, indicates that over 85 percent of American elementary school–age children fail to eat the recommended five or more daily servings of fruits and vegetables. "NHANES III, a federally sponsored survey, shows that on any given day, 45 percent of children eat no fruit, and 20 percent eat less than one serving of vegetables. The average 6 to 11 year-old eats only 3.5 servings of fruits and vegetables each day, achieving only half the recommended 7 servings per day for this age group."[8] Additionally, Dr. Block reports, 20 percent of children's caloric intake comes from junk snacks, such as soda pop, cookies, and candy.

Though it is a stretch to say that all learning and behavioral disabilities are due to inadequate vitamin intake, it is certain that some are. Behavioral deficiency tends to show up before nutritional deficiency is recognized. Arthur Winter, MD, writes that "[i]n thiamine (vitamin B_1) deficiency, symptoms such as lack of wellbeing, anxiety, hysteria, depression, and loss of appetite preceded any clinical evidence of beriberi. Other studies using the Minnesota Multiphasic Personal Index (MMPI) have also demonstrated that adverse behavioral changes precede physical findings in thiamine deficiency."[9]

Dosage Debate

Dr. Harrell anticipated that her use of megadoses would result in "controversy and brickbats."[10] She was right. A number of well-publicized studies[11–15] conducted to "replicate" Dr. Harrell's work seemingly could not do so. Would-be "replications" fail the moment they start when they refuse to use adequate dosages. Surely it is the most basic condition for any replication that one must exactly copy the original experiment, or it is not a replication at all. When DNA replicates, it forms an exact and indistinguishable copy of the original. Even the smallest of changes can result in dysfunction, mutation, and death. Yet Harrell's "replicators" failed to adhere to her protocol, and consequently but not surprisingly, failed to get her results.[16]

Probably one of the closer replications was done by Smith and colleagues,[17] and even that study totally omitted desiccated thyroid, a component of the Harrell protocol that her coauthor, Donald R. Davis, PhD, says was "emphasized to Smith (as) Harrell's subjects received thyroid continuously."[18]

F. Jack Warner, MD, a supporter the Harrell approach,[19] writes, "Even today many medical professionals scoff at the validity of Dr. Ruth Harrell's study with nutritional supplements and the important addition of thyroid medication. Dr. Harrell pleaded with her replicators to use exactly the same chemical values of supplements and medications. To date, this still has not been accomplished."[20] In spite of obvious bias, negative "replication" studies using incomplete or low doses are the ones that have been accepted, and Harrell's work shelved. This is saying that the results of inaccurate replication are more valuable than the original successful research. Imagine cloning a sheep, getting a hedgehog, and then claiming that it was the sheep's fault. Incredible. But that is what politicized medical apologetics are capable of.

The Harrell study was successful because her team gave learning-disabled kids much larger doses of vitamins than other researchers are inclined to use: over 100 times the adult (not child's) Recommended Dietary Allowance (RDA) for riboflavin; 37 times the RDA for niacin (given as niacinamide); 40 times the RDA for vitamin E; and 150 times the RDA for thiamine. Supplemental minerals were also given, as was natural desiccated thyroid. Harrell's team achieved results that were statistically significant, some with confidence levels so high that there was less than one chance in a thousand that the results were due to chance ($P < 0.001$). Simply stated, Ruth Harrell found IQ to be proportional to nutrient dosage. This may simultaneously be the most elementary and also the most controversial mathematical equation in medicine.

There is a tone to the controversy that does more than merely suggest that Harrell's research was careless or incompetent. This is unlikely in the extreme; Dr. Harrell, formerly the chairman of the psychology department at Old Dominion University, had been studying children before many of her critics were even born. What is more likely is that Harrell's critics embrace the assumption that medicine must ultimately prove to be the better approach, and if there are any megadoses to be given, they shall be megadoses of pharmaceutical products. Vitamin therapy is unattractive to pharmaceutical companies. There is no money in products that cannot be patented. Children learn at an early age that mud pies don't sell. No investment is made, no research is done where no money is to be recovered. Drug companies do not expect to find, nor do they want to find, a cure that does not involve a drug. A tragic example is modern medicine's approach to Down syndrome.

Down Syndrome

If there is orthodox resistance to using vitamins to enhance student learning, there is positively a fortified roadblock to the suggestion that vitamins can help children with Down syndrome. Nutrition, critics say, cannot undo trisomy.[21] But nutritional therapy is not a science-fiction attempt to rearrange chromosomes. Nutritional intervention may help the body to biochemically compensate for a genetic handicap. Roger Williams, discoverer of the vitamin pantothenic acid, termed this the "genetotrophic concept." Genetotrophic diseases are "diseases in which the genetic pattern of the afflicted individual requires an augmented supply of one or more nutrients such that when these nutrients are adequately supplied the disease is ameliorated." Ruth Harrell's decades of research showed that it is plausible. Conventional Down syndrome educational material holds that it is hogwash.

As of August 2003, the National Down Syndrome Society's "Position Statement on Vitamin Related Therapies" states that "[d]espite the large sums of money which concerned parents have spent for such treatments in the hope that the conditions of their child with Down syndrome would be bettered, there is no evidence that any such benefit has been produced."[21]

At the heart of the issue are the usual, and largely philosophical, front-line disagreements of definition and interpretation. First, what precisely constitutes a "deficiency" in a society that, as nutritional legend would have it, has eliminated vitamin deficiency? Adherents of conventional dietetics presuppose that anyone who claims that there are widespread vitamin deficiencies among children must proceed from a false assumption. Those who advocate vitamin therapy would answer that Down's creates a "functional deficiency" which must be met with appropriate supplementation. The very idea that doses sufficiently high to effectively do so should be 100 times the RDA is positively repellent to most investigators. When asked about whether she had received National Institutes of Health funding for her study, Dr. Harrell replied, "Heavens, no! Nobody knows anything about the area of dietary supplementation, but the National Institutes of Health knows for sure it's impossible."[10]

Some reviews of Down's nutrition studies actually state that doses as low as 500 milligrams (mg) of vitamin C are unsafe, and that other Harrell-sized dosages are harmful as well. In one such article posted at the Down Syndrome Information Network, the authors conclude that "[i]f it is necessary for additional vitamins to be given to someone with Down syndrome, all that is usually needed is a multivitamin tablet, not more than once a day, at a cost of about one penny per tablet. Meanwhile, the best nutritional advice anyone can honestly offer is to consume a varied and balanced diet—whether you have Down syndrome or not."[22]

Another popular argument is that, even allowing that children eat poorly, there is insufficient evidence that Down's is aggravated by poor nutrition, or helped by good nutrition. After all, Down's is a genetically-determined disease. But surely the genes do not operate in a nutrient vacuum. For example, vitamin E has been demonstrated to preferentially protect genetic material in Down's patients' cells. "Vitamin E treatment decreased the basal and G2 chromosomal aberrations both in control and Down Syndrome (DS) lymphocytes. In DS cells, this protective effect, expressed as a decrease in the chromosomal damage, was greater (50%) than in controls (30%). These results suggest that the increment in basal and G2 aberrations yield in DS lymphocytes may be related to the increase in oxidative damage reported in these patients." The results would also suggest that antioxidant vitamin supplements would be an especially good idea for Down's individuals.[23]

Although the greater question may be, can optimum nutrition help compensate for a genetic defect, the essential question must be this: can nutrition help a given Down's child? Dianne Craft, a special-education teacher, comments on Harrell's 1981 research:

> Dr. Harrell noted that one of the observations that they made during this study was that when there was a ten point rise in IQ, the family noticed it. When there was a fifteen point rise in IQ, the teachers noticed it. When there was a twenty point rise in IQ, the neighborhood noticed it.
>
> The story of one child is particularly poignant. This seven-year-old child was still wearing diapers, didn't recognize his parents, and had no speech. His motor skills were relatively unimpaired and he could walk and run fairly well. In forty days, after some of the supplements were increased, his mother telephoned . . . saying, "He's turned on, just like an electric light. He's asking the name of everything. He points and says, 'What zis?' Finally he pointed to his father and said, 'Zis?' I said, 'That's your father and you call him daddy, and he looked at him and said, 'Daddy.' I'm your mother; can you call me mommy?" She went on to say, "I think he saw us for the first time." This little boy went on to do very well in his learning, and eventually tested with an IQ of 90, which is an average IQ."[24] I have seen a beautiful photo in *Medical Tribune*[9] of Dr. Harrell being hugged by one of the study-group children. The kids noticed their own improvement.

Perhaps Harrell's dramatic IQ gains were merely due to the placebo effect. If so, I want every school district on earth to lay in a stock of sugar pills, for gains like this, in only eight months, are astounding. Perhaps success was due to Dr. Harrell's group's expectations or to her bedside manner. But, as Abram Hoffer has said, "I am nice to all my patients. Only the ones on vitamins improve." Harrell colleague Donald Davis writes, "No amount of matching or variable control with Harrell's subjects could change their large IQ gains which are the crucial and so far unexplained difference between the Harrell group and others."[25]

When Dr. Harrell died in 1991, she was far from being alone in reporting success with high-dose nutrition therapy. Dianne Craft writes, "For over forty years, Dr. Henry Turkel[26,27] treated Down's children successfully using orthomolecular methods. He used a combination of vitamins, minerals, and thyroid hormone replacement. His patients improved mentally and they lost the typical Down's syndrome facial appearance. With over 600 children treated, he found an eighty to ninety percent improvement rate."[24]

To date, the orthodox Down's authorities' position may be summed up as follows: there is no evidence that it helps, so do not try it. Dr. Harrell's view would be: there is reason to believe that nutrition might help, so let's see if it does. The first view prevents physician reports. The second generates them.

Theorization can only go so far. The proof is in the pudding, and Ruth Flinn Harrell's approach yielded smarter, happier children. Her results are sufficiently compelling justification for a therapeutic trial of orthomolecular supplementation for every learning-impaired child.

REFERENCES FOR "THE PIONEERING WORK OF RUTH FLINN HARRELL"

1. Harrell RF, Capp RH, Davis DR, et al. Can nutritional supplements help mentally retarded children? An exploratory study. *Proc Natl Acad Sci USA* 1981;78:574–578.

2. Harrell RF. Effect of added thiamine on learning. NY: Bureau of Publications, Teachers College, Columbia University, 1943. Issued in the series: Contributions to education, no. 877. Reprinted: New York, AMS Press, 1972.

3. Harrell RF. Further effects of added thiamine on learning and other processes. NY: Bureau of Publications, Teachers College, Columbia University, 1947. Issued in the series: Contributions to education, no. 928. Reprinted: New York, AMS Press, 1972.

4. Harrell RF. Mental response to added thiamine. *J Nutr* 1946; 31:283–298.

5. Harrell RF, Woodyard E, Gates AI. The effect of mothers' diets on the intelligence of offspring. Also known as: Relation of maternal prenatal diet to intelligence of the offspring. NY: Bureau of Publications, Teachers College, Columbia University, 1956.

6. Dr. Ruth Flinn Harrell: Effect of added thiamine on learning. *The Health Seeker,* p 18–19.

7. Garrison RH, Somer E. *The Nutrition Desk Reference.* New Canaan, CT: Keats, 1990.

8. Novelli P. American kids' poor food choices: fewer than 15 percent eat recommended fruits and vegetables. *EurekAlert.* May 16, 2002. Available at: http://www.eurekalert.org/pub_releases/2002–05/pn-akp051602.php.

9. Winter A. Differential diagnosis of memory dysfunction: Finding the cause when your patient can't remember. http://www.afpafitness.com/articles/Memory.htm (no longer available).

10. Horwitz N. Vitamins, minerals boost IQ in retarded. *Medical Tribune* 1981;22(3):1,19.

11. Bennett FC, McClelland S, Kriegsmann EA, et al. Vitamin and mineral supplementation in Down's syndrome. *Pediatrics* 1983; 72(5):707–713.

12. Bidder RT, Gray P, Newcombe RG, et al. The effects of multivitamins and minerals on children with Down syndrome. *Dev Med Child Neurol* 1989;31(4):532–537.

13. Menolascino FJ, Donaldson JY, Gallagher TF, et al. Vitamin supplements and purported learning enhancement in mentally retarded children. *J Nutr Sci Vitaminol (Tokyo)* 1989;35(3):181–192.

14. Smith GF, Spiker D, Peterson CP, et al. Failure of vitamin/mineral supplementation in Down syndrome. *Lancet* 1983; 2:41.

15. Weathers C. Effects of nutritional supplementation on IQ and certain other variables associated with Down syndrome. *Am J Ment Defic* 1983;88(2):214–217.

16. Pruess JB, Fewell RR, Bennett FC. Vitamin therapy and children with Down syndrome: a review of research. *Except Child* 1989;55(4):336–341.

17. Smith GF, Spiker D, Peterson CP, et al. Use of megadoses of vitamins with minerals in Down syndrome. *J Pediatr* 1984;105(2):228–234.

18. Davis DR, Capp RH. Vitamins and minerals in Down Syndrome. *J Pediatr* 1985;106(3):531.

19. Thiel R.J. Facial effects of the Warner protocol for children with Down syndrome. *J Orthomolecular Med* 2002;17(2):111–116.

20. Warner FJ. Metabolic supplement for correction of raging free radicals in Trisomy 21: A noncomparative open case study. http://www.warnerhouse.com/radicals.htm (no longer available).

21. National Down Syndrome Society. *Position Statement on Vitamin Related Therapies,* 1997. http://www.ndss.org.

22. Sacks B and Buckley F. Multi-nutrient formulas and other substances as therapies for Down syndrome: An overview. *Down Syndrome News and Update* 1998; 1(2): 70–83.

23. Pincheira J, Navarrete MH, de la Torre C, et al. Effect of vitamin E on chromosomal aberrations in lymphocytes from patients with Down syndrome. *Clin Genet* 1999;55(3):192–197.

24. Craft D. Can nutritional supplements help mentally retarded children? 1998. http://www.diannecraft.com/nut-sup1.html (no longer available).

25. Davis DR. The Harrell study and seven follow-up studies: A brief review. *J Orthomolecular Med,* 1987; 2(2):111–115.

26. Turkel H. Medical amelioration of Down's syndrome incorporating the orthomolecular approach. *Journal of Orthomolecular Psychiatry* 1975; 4:102–115.

27. Turkel H. *Medical Treatment of Down's Syndrome and Genetic Diseases.* Southfield, MI: Ubiotica, 1985.

NEGATIVE AND POSITIVE SIDE EFFECTS OF VITAMIN B_3

by Abram Hoffer MD, PhD

From *J Orthomolecular Med* 2003;18(3 & 4):146–160.

Introduction

I think the best way to describe the many properties of vitamin B_3 is to tell the story of my long love affair with this amazing vitamin. It began in 1951, after Humphry Osmond, MD, John Smythies, MD, and I had developed the adrenochrome hypothesis of schizophrenia.[1] I will not refer to this hypothesis further as it is in relatively good shape and has been adequately reviewed in a series of reports.[2–7] We desperately needed a treatment for schizophrenia. Our hypothesis led to the conclusion that large doses (3,000 milligrams [mg] per day) of vitamin B_3, niacin or niacinamide, might be helpful in reversing the reaction that produced excess adrenochrome. In 1951, I obtained 50 pounds of pure niacin and 50 pounds of pure niacinamide from Merck and Co., and our hospital pharmacist made it up into 500 mg capsules. The largest dosage in commercial tablets was 100 mg but the fillers in these tablets, if they took 30 daily, would have made our patients sick. A mental hospital in southern California made a halfhearted attempt to try niacin but was not allowed to use anything stronger than 100 mg. Patients became sick on the 30 tablets daily. Before we could start our pilot trials I had to know something about its toxicity. As I suspected, niacin was non-toxic, but did have some undesirable effects and would have to be used knowing these potential side effects; the same, of course, applies to food and water.

Niacin and niacinamide were available over the counter in very small doses. They had been given in large doses to some patients with chronic pellagra. Acute pellagra patients responded very quickly to these small vitamin doses, but chronic patients often needed up to 600 mg daily. Over 60 years ago, during the height of the Great Depression, this dose of pure niacin was very high and was not encouraged. The literature did not contain very much material about toxicity, chiefly because it was considered safe by all the established medical associations that commented on it. Merck prepared comprehensive bulletins outlining its properties. When we started in 1951, only one physician had given the doses we were going to use (3,000 mg per day). William Kaufman, MD, began to use niacinamide in 1945 for treating diseases of aging, including the arthritides. He gave 500 mg four times daily, but I did not know this until 1957. We were the second group to go above 600 mg daily. We did that because it had been used in much smaller doses for treating patients with depression. A small proportion responded but most did not. We assumed that had it been therapeutic in lower doses for schizophrenia this would have been reported, and our hypothesis called for enough niacin to absorb methyl groups and thus to decrease the formation of adrenaline and therefore of adrenochrome.

Our first pilot studies were successful. The first three patients I treated at the General Hospital in Regina and the first eight patients Dr. Osmond treated at the Saskatchewan Hospital in Weyburn all responded. This was exciting but we did not consider it proof, and therefore we started the first of six prospective, randomized, double-blind, controlled, therapeutic trials. These became the basis for orthomolecular psychiatry. Since then over 50 reports which followed our original protocols have corroborated our findings. A few reports did not corroborate, but neither did they treat the same kind of patients. We used patients early in their diagnoses. Very chronic patients did not respond. Later we discovered that chronic patients will respond, but it will take much more time and much more patience. Most of these corroborative papers were published in the *Journal of Orthomolecular Medicine* beginning about 30 years ago.

Factors That Determine Toxicity and Side Effects

The dose is a main factor in determining side effects and toxicity. With all substances, toxicity and side effects increase as the dose increases. The difference between the toxic dose, as defined by animal studies, and the optimum therapeutic dose is called the "therapeutic range." With vitamins the therapeutic range is very high as the toxic dose is so large. With drugs the therapeutic dose range is much narrower. This is why one should always use the lowest possible effective dose. Any factor that allows one to decrease the effective dose will decrease the toxicity. An example is the effect of antipsychotic drugs in inducing tardive dyskinesia. This was common with the early antipsychotics and still is present, even if to a lesser degree, with modern atypical drugs. When niacin or niacinamide is also used, the dose of the drugs can be reduced markedly, and this decreases the tendency to develop tardive dyskinesia. Many years ago David Hawkins[8] surveyed a number of orthomolecular psychiatrists who between them had at that time treated about 58,000 patients. There were no cases of tardive dyskinesia among them. If every psychiatrist had used the same approach there would have been no reason to search for the new drugs, except of course that the patents on the older drugs had expired. I have had several patients already displaying tardive dyskinesia at their first visit but have not seen any develop this condition after starting on an orthomolecular program.

Vitamins-as-Prevention Paradigm

The optimum dose range varies from a few milligrams daily to many grams daily. It ranges from the usual small vitamin doses as defined by the vitamins-as-prevention paradigm to the large or megadose level as called for by the vitamin-as-treatment paradigm. The term "megadoses" has no scientific meaning and should not be used. The first paradigm is the logical outcome of the search for vitamins, which began over 100 years ago with the first one, the anti-beriberi vitamin, thiamine. The usual pattern of discovery followed the observation that certain diets made people sick. Japanese sailors given polished rice as their main staple food became sick with beriberi, but on whole-grain brown rice this did not happen. This led to the discovery of thiamine. Later the active fraction was isolated and after that the active compounds were synthesized and they became known as vitamins (vital amines), even though later it was found that they are not all amines. Once the pure vitamins became available, large-scale clinical trials were possible, but because these substances were present in such small concentrations, it appeared obvious that they were always required only in small quantities. This became part of the definition of vitamins: they are chemicals needed in tiny amounts to catalyze reactions in the body and their function was to prevent the deficiency diseases from appearing. Thus, thiamine in food prevents beriberi, vitamin C prevents scurvy, vitamin B_3 prevents pellagra, vitamin D prevents rickets, and so on. Niacin should be classified with the amino acids since it is made in the body from tryptophan and by definition vitamins cannot be made in the body; this was not known for a while, and long usage has placed it in the vitamin camp. If it were thought of as an amino acid the large doses so effective in many diseases would be easier to understand. According to the vitamin definition, once the diet contains enough of those substances to prevent the classical deficiency diseases there is no need to give more.

These ideas became the vitamin-as-prevention paradigm, which still holds sway and is defended with relentless vigour. Doctors have lost their licenses to practice because they did not obey these principles. This concept, apparently written in stone, declares that vitamins are needed only in very small doses to prevent deficiency disease. It follows that giving more is useless and even harmful and that giving even small amounts to patients who do not have any deficiency diseases is also not indicated and potentially harmful. The preventive dose ranges in this concept are very narrow even though toxicity does not appear. Doses range from zero, i.e. to depend only on what is present in food, to the recommended daily doses established by government agencies. Those dose ranges only apply to populations of healthy people. They do not include populations under stress, pregnant women, or people who are sick. The recommended doses are not applicable to at least half of any population, yet they are still applied firmly.

Paradigms, or articles of faith, or systems of thought are not easily dislodged. They are usually changed by evolution or revolution. In medicine it has taken over 40 years before major new ideas were accepted. This applies to concepts which are now part of the modern paradigm, such as washing one's hands, using a stethoscope, using electrocardiograms, doing heart catheterizations, and using antibiotics. They do change because with continuing investigation the old concepts fail to account for new observations. This is now occurring with the vitamin-as-prevention paradigm. The seeds of doubt were planted by the work of Evan Shute, MD, and Wilfrid Shute, MD, who reported that large doses of vitamin E were useful in treating heart disease, with the work of Dr. Kaufman[9] in treating arthritis with niacinamide, and with our work in using niacin and niacinamide in treating schizophrenia.[10] We all broke the cardinal rules because we used very large doses of vitamins to treat conditions that were not considered vitamin-deficiency diseases. The Shutes' and Kaufman's work had little impact; it was ignored. The first major break in the vitamins-as-prevention armor was our discovery that niacin in large doses lowered cholesterol levels. We used megadoses, for a condition everyone knew was not a vitamin-deficiency disease. This was easy to confirm, but even then it took many favorable confirmatory reports and several decades before niacin became acceptable as the best compound available for lowering cholesterol levels. Our work is considered the first major onslaught against the vitamin-as-prevention paradigm. We need much more.

Vitamins-as-Treatment Paradigm

This modern paradigm was given a tremendous boost by the report by biochemists Bruce Ames, Elson-Schwab, and Silver.[11] Following Dr. Linus Pauling's[12] seminal report, it provides the explanation of why so many patients do need large doses. Vitamins are converted into coenzymes, which combine with enzymes to carry on essential metabolic functions. If the ability of the enzyme to combine with its coenzyme is impaired, increasing the amount of vitamin will increase the amount of coenzyme, thus overcoming the defect and increasing the reaction toward normal. About 50 genetic diseases affecting vitamin metabolism are already known, perhaps 10 percent of what may eventually be discovered. It is another blow to the original vitamins-as-prevention paradigm and powerful support for the modern paradigm. The basic concepts of the vitamins-as-treatment paradigm are that optimum doses, which may be large or small, may be therapeutic, very helpful, for diseases that are not classical deficiency diseases.

The optimum dose range for the modern paradigm varies with the disease being treated, but often has to be determined by the response of the individual. Thus, the dose range for lowering cholesterol is 1,000 to 9,000 mg of niacin daily in three divided doses. The usual dose for treating schizophrenia is about the same, but a few may need much more. The optimum dose can be determined by the dose that causes nausea—the optimum dose is below the nauseant dose. For vitamin C the dose ranges enormously, from a few thousand milligrams to 100,000 mg taken orally. For cancer, my patients take between 12,000 and 40,000 mg daily. The higher doses are probably best reserved for intravenous administration. The laxative-effect level determines the optimum oral doses. If the dose causes loose stools, dosage should be decreased to below that level. We need a therapeutic dose range for every disease. This will be much higher than the usual vitamin dose range. There are no toxic doses since vitamins do not kill, but the higher the dose, the more apt will be the development of side effects.

How Much Niacin Should I Take?

The answer is: it depends. "Not everyone will need large amounts of niacin. If you have no treatment reason to take niacin, megadosing is not the answer. Are you suffering from depression? Anxiety? High cholesterol? Having trouble quieting your mind so you can fall asleep? If so, your need for niacin may be greater. Certainly, a few hundred milligrams a day can benefit everyone. Those seeking to address a health issue may benefit from more. You may wish to start small: try taking just 25 mg of niacin after each meal. Gradually increase your dose over subsequent days until you achieve a flush. Dr. Saul explains, "As a general rule, the more you hold, the more you need. If you flush early, you don't need much niacin. If flushing doesn't happen until a high level, then your body is obviously using the higher amount of the vitamin." If you cannot tolerate the flush, try taking niacinamide instead. Once again, start small and see how you feel. As research biochemist Richard Passwater, PhD, would recommend, take the smallest dose of a nutrient that gets you the positive health result you seek." (From Case HS. *Vitamin & Pregnancy: The Real Story,* Basic Health Publications, 2016.)

Vitamin B_3 Dependency and Deficiency

Conditions that require large doses of vitamins are due to genetic errors, due to the disease causing the suffering, or have been created by prolonged severe malnutrition and stress. Niacin was shown to be vitamin B_3 in the mid 1930s. Early pellagrologists were able to study it as soon as they were able to obtain some. They reported that early cases of pellagra improved on the usual tiny vitamin doses, but that if they had been sick for a long time they would not; some needed 600 mg daily, an enormous dose at that time. They also found that dogs with black tongue (pellagra), if kept on the diet that made them sick, recovered given tiny vitamin doses, but if they were left on the deficient diet too long they would thereafter need much larger doses. It is clear that prolonged deficiency of vitamin B_3 created a need for a lot more. This is called a vitamin dependency. Whatever happened, those patients could no longer be well with small vitamin doses. A vitamin-deficiency disease is one in which the disease is present because the diet is so poor. On a good diet, the patient would be well. But if they need much more, an amount that no diet can ever provide, they have a dependency.

The response to vitamins depends on the relative condition of the patients. A person with pellagra is severely deficient. They respond to very small amounts rather quickly. I suspect that all patients still in the deficiency area will also respond quickly.

However, once they have been moved into the dependency area the response will be slower and less dramatic. People kept in concentration camps in Europe or in the Far East were subjected to absolutely horrible and severe physical, psychological, and nutritional stress. I shudder to think about all the populations today who are exposed to prolonged malnutrition, disease, and psychological stress. There will be a massive increase in very sick people who will be vitamin B_3 dependent and will be helped by their physicians or governments if they see that they get enough of this important vitamin, perhaps by enriching their flour and/or rice above the modern standards of enrichment.

In the scientific debate that occurs when one paradigm is in the process of replacing an older one, each side uses the weapons at hand. If one side does not like the concept of using large doses, they may maintain that these doses are harmful, in spite of vast evidence that they are not. If one does not like the concept of using vitamins for conditions that are not deficiency diseases, they will deny that they are effective and/or will declare that even if they may be effective, they are toxic. The modern assault on the new paradigm maintains that they are not effective, not needed in large doses, and that they are dangerous.

Negative Side Effects

The word "toxic" does not really apply to vitamin B_3 any more than it does when applied to most of the common substances we use, such as food and water. Nor should the word be used without specifying what the toxic dose range is. To say that something is toxic is meaningless, since theoretically everything is toxic if the dose is pushed high enough. Therapeutic substances theoretically should be free of negative side effects at dose levels that are therapeutic. The lethal quality of the compound, i.e., how much it will take to kill the subject, is first determined. The LD (lethal dose) 50 is that amount of compound which, over a period of time, will kill half the animals being tested. If this number is high, one can proceed to the next step–to determine whether the substance is therapeutic—if the number is very low, the substance will never become therapeutic. The LD 50 of niacin when tested on dogs was about 5,000 mg per kilogram body weight. This would be about 350,000 mg, more than one half a pound, for a 70-kilogram (154 lb.) adult. The real LD 50 for people is not known since no one would run the test, and so far no one has died from a high dose of vitamin B_3. One of my patients, a 16-year-old schizophrenic girl, swallowed the whole bottle of niacin pills I had given her, all at once. She took 200 tablets of the 500 mg size because she was angry with her mother. For the next three days she complained of a stomachache. Another patient, not mine, increased her dose until she was taking 60,000 mg daily. At that level her auditory hallucinations (voices) ceased. Eventually she was maintained on 3,000 mg. No one has ever committed suicide with vitamin B_3.

Another way to determine toxicity is to compare the toxic effect of the substance against the toxic effect of the disease being treated. One of the most toxic drugs is insulin given by injection. A slight overdose can kill by driving the blood sugar down to near zero. Yet it is used safely by millions of patients, and they will continue to use it as the consequences of not taking insulin are so much worse. In the same way all the modern drugs used in treating schizophrenia are very toxic, but the condition being treated is more serious; therefore, these drugs are tolerated.

Toxicity or negative side effects can never be considered in the absence of the therapeutic value of the substances. If there is no therapeutic value it will never be used, whether it is toxic or not. If the therapeutic value is great, as, for example, in the use of insulin for treating diabetes mellitus, even toxic compounds will be used. Doctors are taught how to deal with toxic substances, and only they are permitted to prescribe these to their patients. If doctors think a substance has no therapeutic value they will argue that even the remotest degree of toxicity is too much and that the substance cannot be used. If they consider it valuable, even the greatest degree of toxicity will be tolerated. Thus, the consensus among the psychiatric profession is that vitamins are of no value in the treatment of schizophrenia; therefore they search assiduously for evidence of toxicity and often, when they cannot find any evidence, it is hypothesized or grossly exaggerated. If they consider a drug very valuable, its toxicity is minimized. An example is the drug clozapine, which is very dangerous and has caused death, but if used carefully will be tolerated. Another example is olanzapine, which can cause tremendous weight gain and increases the odds of getting diabetes mellitus but is tolerated. A clinical example is a patient I once saw who was getting on very well with one of the older drugs. Her psychiatrist wanted to experiment with a new one, but on the new one she gained 60 pounds in a few months and this destroyed her life, her self-image. She pleaded with him to change her medication back, and he bluntly told her it was better to be fat than schizophrenic. In fact she was still schizophrenic, but he had given her no choice. Niacin does not cause weight gain, but he would not use niacin, perhaps because he considered it too toxic. Thus, in the discussion of toxicity of vitamins some information must given about their value in treating many conditions.

A good way of comparing toxicity is to count the number of pages in any pharmaceutical compendium for each compound listed. One could count the number of pages listed for therapy and for all the adverse side effects and warnings. Both niacin and Zyprexa are used for treating schizophrenic patients, and niacin and Lipitor are used to bring down blood cholesterol levels. Table 1 (page 328) shows how these three substances compare.

Drugs are described very carefully, and the companies that own the patents vet these descriptions very carefully in order to make sure they are properly described. However, there are no companies that provide the same editorial care for the write-ups of the vitamins, as they are not patented. Over the years I found that these nutrient descriptions tend to be lax and not accurate, usually erring on the side of making them appear more toxic and less useful than is warranted. For many years after niacin was generally recognized as one of the best compounds for lowering cholesterol levels in blood, this was not indicated in the Compendium description.

Each page of the Compendium contains three columns of 80 lines each. The side effects of niacin listed are:

- Gastrointestinal: nausea, vomiting, bloating, and flatulence
- Blood pressure: hypotension
- Skin: hyperpigmentation, dry, and urticaria
- Blood constituent values: elevated glucose, elevated uric acid
- Liver: elevated liver function test results, pathology

Merck Manual, 16th edition (1992), lists the following contraindications for niacin: hepatic dysfunction, active peptic ulcer, diabetes mellitus, severe hypotension, arterial hemorrhage, and hyperuricemia. It discusses briefly the toxicity of vitamin D and vitamin K. None of the other vitamins are discussed.

Many patients given a prescription for a drug will read the information on the medication information sheet that is available and will decide not to take the drug. This has not happened with niacin.

The toxic effects of drugs are potentially much more serious than the side effects of vitamins. There have been no deaths from vitamins in 25 years compared to about 110,000 deaths yearly in the United States from the proper use of drugs in hospitals. That is the real comparison of the relative toxic effects of drugs and vitamins.

Finally, one must recognize that very safe compounds may causes idiosyncratic reactions in a very few patients and cause serious side effects. Even the filler in some tablets may cause these reactions. If peanut oil got into a pill taken by a peanut-sensitive patient, it might cause death.

Positive Side Effects

A positive side effect is any reaction that improves the health of any individual when taking a compound for another purpose. Thus, if a patient taking niacin to lower cholesterol levels also finds a decrease in the pain from his arthritis, this is a positive side effect, because the arthritis was not the indication for taking the niacin. I recommended to a colleague that he give niacin to one of his patients because he was concerned about fat deposits (lipomas) in his skin. I suggested that this would remove them, which it did. In addition, this patient had been paranoid, and that symptom also vanished; this is a positive side effect. The main action of the niacin flush is to increase blood circulation to the tissues, including the brain. Many of my patients complain of what they call brain fog. I do not know anything more effective in removing this brain fog than niacin. I consider this as evidence for improved circulation of blood to the brain.

Drugs usually are targeted to do one thing, to be used for one indication. Therefore drugs to lower cholesterol levels do that and little more. Vitamins are involved in so many different reactions in the body that they have multiple positive side effects. For most patients they produce a feeling of well-being not usually associated with drugs. Vitamins improve energy production and increase the rate of healing. Niacin's vasodilatation properties are very valuable. For many patients the flushing form is much better than the nonflush or slow-release preparations. In some patients with diseases such as chronic fatigue syndrome or multiple sclerosis, the red blood cells are too large[13] and have difficulty traversing the capillaries. Increasing the lumen of these vessels permits more blood to flow through the capillaries and thus oxygenates the tissues more efficiently. In addition, it disperses aggregated red blood cells, called sludging, according to Ed Boyle (personal communication). Finally, many patients, especially those with arthritis, like the flush and will often take a niacin "holiday" for a few days in order to reactivate the flush.

Here are a few positive side effects:

1. a feeling of well-being and improved energy; not needing as much sleep and rest
2. longer life[14]
3. relief from arthritic pain[15]
4. a slowing down of the aging process[16]

McCracken[17] provides a more complete list of positive side effects.

The important therapeutic effect of niacin on blood lipid levels is one of its most important side effects because it was discovered as a result of studying niacin to treat schizophrenic patients. This arose from the collegial relationship I had with Rudl Altschul, professor of anatomy, University of Saskatchewan Medical School, in Saskatoon. He had also been my teacher in histology. He was exploring the connection between arteriosclerosis and diet using cooked egg yoke to elevate cholesterol levels in his rabbits and using ultraviolet radiation to decrease it. I had observed that my gums, which had been bleeding for a long time in spite of good dental care, stopped bleeding two weeks after I started to take niacin. I was taking it because I wanted to experience the flush so I would understand better what patients would experience. I had hypothesized that the niacin had improved the ability of my gums to repair themselves after the trauma of chewing with maloccluded teeth. Altschul believed that rate of repair of the intima, the inner lining of blood vessels, was a key factor in the pathology of arteriosclerosis. As soon as I heard that, I made the association between the rate of repair of my gums and rate of repair of the intima in arteries. I suggested that he try niacin. Altschul did not know anything about niacin, so I described it and gave him a pound of pure niacin. A few months later he called me. He had given niacin to his rabbits, and their cholesterol levels promptly went back to normal. We then collaborated on a human study and found that niacin, even after a few days, was very effective.[18] Since then it has become the gold standard for lowering cholesterol because it does even more. It lowers triglycerides, elevates HDL, and lowers lipoprotein(a). Of course if the indication for niacin use is high blood cholesterol levels, then this beneficial effect is not a side effect, it is the main effect. Niacin was the first vitamin to be released by the FDA to be used in large doses. They would have to consider that niacin's effect on schizophrenia, if they ever believe this, is a positive side effect.

The excessive weight gain in schizophrenic patients given olanzapine is one of the major toxic side effects.[19] This antipsychotic markedly increases serum leptin and triglycerides in schizophrenic patients.[20] Leptin increases appetite, driving patients to eat too much, especially of the carbohydrates. The elevated triglycerides are very dangerous, increasing the risk of heart disease. Niacin is one of the best compounds for lowering triglyceride levels. This may be considered another positive side effect. Perhaps if olanzapine is to be saved as a useful antipsychotic it will have to be combined with niacin. The therapeutic effect on schizophrenic patients will of course be very much better, since niacin is a major antipsychotic and not as much olanzapine will be needed.

I will discuss the side effects in the order in which we had to meet them as our therapeutic trials continued.

Vasodilatation and the Niacin Flush

Niacin is a potent vasodilator, but not a very good one for chronic use since the body adapts to it and the flush eventually ceases or occurs only intermittently. No one should ever take niacin without knowing about this flush because the reaction can be very dramatic and frightening. In Detroit, one of my colleagues forgot to warn his patient. This patient took the niacin, flushed, and in fear called the closest poison control center. The person who took the call probably had never heard of it, advised the patient that he had taken a lethal dose, and sent the ambulance for him. By the time he arrived at the hospital, he was feeling fine. The flush usually starts in the anterior part of the body, in one's forehead, and moves posterially. It first appears as a reddening in the forehead and then slowly or quickly travels down the body, occasionally involving even the toes, but usually only travels as far as the abdomen. The skin is red, itchy, and the patient feels warm, but there is no sweating. If the reaction comes on very quickly, the person may feel faint; a few subjects have fainted. One subject who fainted was given the pills by her friend or neighbor and was not told about the flush. The anxiety and fear probably aggravated this reaction. The flush may last up to three hours. The first flush is the most striking, and after that with each dose there is less and less flushing, and in most people it is minor or gone in a few weeks. A few never get adjusted to it, and of course they will be able to take very small amounts or may have to use the nonflushing forms of niacin.

Factors in the Flush Intensity

1. The amount of niacin taken in one dose. There will be very little flush with 50 mg or less, while most patients will flush with 100 mg or more. The relationship is not linear. There is a threshold effect, and the flush does not appear until that threshold is reached. This can be used to introduce niacin gradually. I also use it to decrease the reactivity of patients with severe allergies. I start with 25 mg after each meal, at the same time giving 1,000 mg of vitamin C. As the flush moderates, the dose is very slowly increased by 25 mg per week. The niacin releases histamine, which is partially responsible for the flush, and the ascorbic acid destroys the histamine dumped into the blood. In this way it is possible to increase the dose to its full therapeutic value.
2. The amount of food in one's stomach and whether niacin is taken with a hot drink or cold drink. The rate of absorption is important, and heat accelerates this. If the vitamin is taken right after a meal the flush is minimal; taken on an empty stomach it is maximal. The greatest flush is experienced when niacin is injected intravenously. I suspect that, dissolved in hot tea and swallowed immediately on an empty stomach, niacin would produce the kind of flush seen after IV administration.
3. Time elapsed between dosages. Most patients tend to flush more in the morning after their first daily dose because they have gone all night without taking any. This can often be remedied by taking the last dose just before bed.
4. Aspirin. An aspirin tablet taken once a day, beginning two days before starting on niacin, can minimize the flush. Once the first flush has occurred, aspirin is no longer needed, as niacin itself is the best antiflush preparation if it is taken regularly. Some antihistamines can also minimize the flush, and the early tranquilizers such as chlorpromazine were very effective in preventing excessive flushing. Schizophrenic patients flush much less than do patients who are not schizophrenic or have other diseases. David Horrobin[21] developed this into a diagnostic test. It is based upon the observations I reported in 1962 that schizophrenic patients are usually less disturbed by the flush. A patch with four pockets, each containing different amounts of methyl nicotinate, is applied to the forearm, left on for five minutes, and then stripped off. In most schizophrenic patients the areas in contact with the nicotinate do not turn red. There is very little overlap.[22] Many schizophrenic patients do not flush after starting to take 3,000 mg of niacin daily. This inability to flush may well be related to their disease, as an appreciable number of schizophrenic patients

begin to flush after several years of medication. This is a good prognostic sign and usually coincides with complete recovery.[23]

5. Age. Usually patients over age 50 flush less than young people do.
6. Skin color. Dark-skinned people will flush less, but the reaction may be just as uncomfortable. Patients who tan very poorly may have more severe reactions.
7. Patients' need for the vitamin. I have observed that patients who need it the most, such as patients with high blood cholesterol levels, or patients with arthritis or schizophrenia, flush much less than other patients.
8. Motivation. Patients motivated by the disease that they have and the explanation given to them by their doctors find the flush much more tolerable.
9. Physicians' comfort with niacin. Parsons[24] in his excellent book makes the point that physicians must know niacin before they work with it. For many patients, the flushing form is much better than the nonflush or slow-release preparations, particularly patients with chronic fatigue syndrome and multiple sclerosis, as mentioned earlier, and many patients do like the flush.

Mechanism of the Flush

The niacin flush may be due to the release of histamine and/or interference with prostaglandins. The niacin-induced flush is very similar to the flush induced by the injection of histamine, with one major exception: histamine injections will lower blood pressure below normal levels, while the niacin flush does not, with few exceptions.

A colleague of mine with high blood pressure discovered that if he took a flushing dose of niacin his blood pressure would fall markedly and then would start to go up again so that in three days it was high again. Then he would repeat the procedure. If he had another flush it would go down again. The amount of decrease is related to the intensity of the flush. He has been doing this for several months. When he took the niacin regularly, the blood pressure went back up to its initial high level and remained there.

Dr. Ed Boyle observed many years ago that the vesicles storing histamine in the mast blood cells were emptied after taking niacin. He also found that guinea pigs pretreated with niacin for one week did not die from anaphylactic shock. I have used it for many patients for many years to decrease the response to foods and insect bites in combination with ascorbic acid to destroy the histamine released into the bloodstream.

Horrobin postulated that the vasodilation was related to prostaglandin D2. He assumed that this was due to reduced membrane arachidonic acid levels in schizophrenics. Aspirin decreases the intensity of the flush, again pointing to the prostaglandins. I think it is most likely that both histamine and the prostaglandins are involved.

Gastrointestinal Side Effects: Nausea, Vomiting, Pain from Peptic Ulcer

In 1962, I reported that occasionally niacin caused nausea and vomiting. This reaction is dose related. Everyone will react if the dose taken is high enough, and this level varies from 3,000 to 30,000 mg daily. I use this nauseant dose as an indicator of how much is needed. Patients who respond best include schizophrenic patients, patients with elevated cholesterol levels, and arthritics. Elderly patients and these patients can usually tolerate much more than younger patients. Niacinamide also has a narrower threshold level than niacin. If the tolerance level is too low, I use a combination of both. If the tolerance level is 1,500 mg daily for each, using them both will provide the patient with 3,000 mg without nausea. Nausea must be dealt with immediately as it may lead to vomiting. Most patients will stop taking their medication when they develop nausea, but a few are very determined and will not. In one study, reputed to be replicating our treatment, the dose of niacin was set at 8,000 mg daily. Not only were the wrong patients used, as they were all chronic and the study was to determine the effect on early cases, but the dose was too high. Many of these patients were very nauseated, but the protocol was followed regardless. I cannot imagine patients getting better when they are continually nauseated.

Children may not complain of nausea but will lose their appetite. When that happens, one should suspect that they are nauseated and stop the niacin or decrease the dose. If vomiting is not stopped it will of course lead to dehydration. Niacin increases the secretion of hydrochloric acid, but this is not the explanation since niacinamide also causes nausea when the dose is too high and it has no effect on HCl secretion. It must be due to some central effect. Inositol hexanicotinate does not cause nausea, and the slow-release preparations seldom do.

When I first began to use niacin I recommended that it not be given to patients with peptic ulcer. Parsons also avoided giving it to peptic ulcer patients, but as he became more familiar with it realized that it could be given safely to people with ulcers. It must be given after meals, with food in the stomach. The Coronary Drug Project[14] found that 13.9 percent of the niacin patients complained of stomach pain, compared to 7.9 percent of the placebo group. Nausea was found in 8.5 percent compared to 6.2 percent, and decreased appetite in 4.1 percent compared to 1.5 percent for the placebo group.

Parsons has been using niacin to lower cholesterol levels since 1955. He was the first physician outside of Canada to become interested and has retained his interest. His book is a must-read. His description of niacin and the gastrointestinal system is excellent. After reviewing the few reports about the effect of niacin on peptic ulcers, he wrote, "To me the most significant fact is that my 37 years of further experience (since my 1960 paper) and the Coronary Drug Project experience failed to demonstrate any cases in which the drug activated peptic ulcer. My 1960 report regarding activation of peptic ulcers by niacin was wrong."

Niacinamide can also cause nausea and vomiting at lower doses than is the case with niacin.

Effect of Niacin on Liver Function Tests

In 1950, doctors' awareness was greatly raised about the disease-producing effects of methyl deficiency. This caused fatty livers in animals. Niacin and niacinamide combine with methyl groups and are two of the few methyl acceptors. Thus it made sense to think that a large dose of this vitamin would cause a methyl deficiency. Another methyl acceptor is noradrenalin; methylation of noradrenalin produces adrenalin. We hoped to decrease the production of adrenochrome by inhibiting the product of adrenalin from noradrenalin. This was one of many factors that pointed in the direction of this vitamin in the treatment of schizophrenia. But we were concerned about the possible danger of producing fatty livers. In 1942, a study on animals suggested that niacin did injure the liver. Altschul repeated this animal study and, on the contrary, found no evidence of any liver toxicity; their livers were normal when examined histologically and chemically. We tested a small series of patients being treated with niacin and again found no evidence of liver damage. Rarely a patient would develop an obstructive jaundice. I would routinely stop the niacin until the jaundice cleared because of the possibility of a reaction. One of my patients became very psychotic again and I resumed the niacin but his jaundice did not recur. The incidence of jaundice was very rare and I have seen no cases in the past 20 years.

However, when the modern liver-function tests came into use, some of the patients on niacin and niacinamide showed elevated liver-function tests. Most physicians assumed that this indicated underlying liver pathology and warned against the use of niacin. Parsons was also concerned but eventually, with his long and extensive experience with niacin, concluded that elevated liver-function tests did not mean that there was underlying liver pathology. He concluded that niacin is not liver toxic. His opinion was reinforced by the results of the Coronary Drug Project conducted between 1966 and 1974. This followed 1,100 men receiving niacin for five to eight years. The lead investigator, Dr. Paul Canner, told Parsons that there were no abnormalities that could be attributed to niacin. Parsons concluded that the elevated tests were not evidence of liver pathology and that they indicated an abnormality only if the liver function tests were elevated two to three times the upper limit: "Minor elevations in enzyme tests reflecting liver function are a normal part of niacin therapy and are not a reason to discontinue treatment." Elevated tests will return to normal in patients while they are still taking niacin; however, Parsons pointed out that the slow-release preparations were much more apt to increase liver-function tests. Nevertheless I do not give this vitamin in large doses to anyone with hepatitis, not because I think it will be harmful but because I know the niacin will be blamed even if it is not responsible if something does happen.

Capuzzi[25] has been studying niacin for several decades. He found that giving patients lecithin, 1,200 mg twice daily, prevents any elevations of liver-function tests. McCarty[26] suggested that high demand for methyl groups created by niacin could reduce levels of S-adenosylmethionine, which could lead to an increase in production of homocysteine. This, he suggested, could be avoided by using betaine supplements with the niacin. But lecithin is much cheaper and more readily available. Both lecithin and betaine are methyl donors.

The effect of niacinamide on liver-function tests has not been studied.

Effect of Niacin on Carbohydrate Metabolism

Before 1960, I found that in a few patients, niacin increased the glucose tolerance. In one-third of the diabetic patients it increased the need for insulin slightly, in one-third there was no change, and in the last one-third the need for insulin was decreased. Siblings of diabetics were more apt to show abnormal glucose tolerance tests. Parsons found no difficulty in using niacin in diabetics taking oral hypoglycemics, but recommended against giving it to patients with diabetes type 1. I have given it to type 1 diabetics in order to lower cholesterol levels and to protect them against the sequelae of diabetes, and it has been very effective. Elam and colleagues[27] concluded, "[L]ipid modifying dosages of niacin can be safely used in patients with diabetes and niacin therapy may be considered as an alternative to statin drugs or fibrates for patients with diabetes in whom these agents are not tolerated or fail to sufficiently correct hypertriglyceridemia or low HDL-C levels."

Effect of Niacin on Gout

Parsons found that niacin increased blood uric acid levels slightly but concluded that this should not interfere with niacin therapy. In the Coronary Drug Project the average blood uric acid levels before entering the project was 6.75 and after five years on niacin 6.80. Men on niacin had uric acid levels above 8.0. However, this was insignificant because there was no increase in any of the symptoms of gout ,including increase in uric acid stones or acute gouty arthritis. This has been my conclusion as well. I do not consider niacin a risk factor for gout. My father-in-law suffered from both arthritis and gout, and they were independent of each other. While taking niacin his arthritis disappeared, but he continued to suffer recurrent short episodes of gout in the same pattern as before. Niacin neither increased nor decreased these episodes.

The slight increase in blood uric acid levels may be a positive side effect. According to McCracken, uric acid is a central stimulant and the increase in uric acid activity, a genetic change from about 20 million years ago, was beneficial for this reason. College professors were found to have higher blood uric acid levels than their equivalent noncollege controls. Uric acid is also an antioxidant, and this is, of course, very helpful.

Thus the threat of gout should not deter anyone from using niacin if they need it. If gout does develop it is very readily treated.

Effect of Niacin on Skin

There are three negative side effects in the skin and two positive side effects. The side effects are generalized skin dryness, which Parsons suggests is due to the decreased cholesterol levels, a nonspecific rash which is rare, and increased pigmentation. The first side effect is seldom a problem. I think that adding omega-three essential fatty acids—present in flaxseed, in flaxseed oil, and in fish oils (not the liver oils)—will help remove this dryness. The nonspecific rash may lead to scratching, and if it remains a problem the niacin will have to be stopped.

The third side effect is never a problem except to patients whose doctors are not familiar with it and make them fearful by suggesting that it is dangerous. It consists of an increased brown or dark pigmentation of the skin, usually in the flexor surfaces of the body as in the armpits. This is more common in schizophrenic patients but can occur to a slight degree in anyone. It has been erroneously called acanthosis nigricans, which is dangerous, but it is not this condition. Parsons called it a skin change which resembles acanthosis nigricans. It does resemble it but only in color not in pathology. Usually after a while the dark skin wears away as does an old tan. It can be rubbed off when the skin is wet and leaves healthy skin behind. I think it is due to the accumulation of melanin pigments, which the body is excreting via the skin. Skin is one of the major excretory organs.

One of my patients turned almost black, and it was very embarrassing, but after a while it disappeared completely. I saw the same pigments in one of my schizophrenic patients. All the nails on her fingers and toes became dirty brown. After being on niacin for many months the pigment deposition ceased and her nails grew out clean. It was the first time I saw the schizophrenic pigment, perhaps from adrenochrome. This female patient had been catatonic and mute, but three months after her nails began to grow clean she began to talk again. This pigmentation can also occur in many patients and in normal people on niacin who are not schizophrenic, and it has no diagnostic value. Once it has cleared it never comes back.

Another very positive side effect of niacin is that it clears xanthoma tuberosum. These are due to deposits of cholesterol in patients with high blood cholesterol. They never recur as long as the patients remain on the niacin. Xanthoma tendinosum, cholesterol deposits in the tendons, and xanthelasmata, deposits in the eyelids, also clear slowly on niacin therapy.

Niacin has a remarkable effect on the health of the skin. My skin at 85 years of age is normal. A fold of skin when pulled from the back of my hand will return to normal in three seconds. Most people over age 60 require much more time before this happens.

Atrial Fibrillation

There was a slight increase in atrial fibrillation reported in the Coronary Drug Project study. It was diagnosed in 4.7 percent in the niacin group and in 2.9 percent in the placebo group. Parsons pointed out that since these patients had already had one or more heart attacks before entering the study, the elevated level in the niacin group is not surprising. Again I agree. I have given niacin to several thousand patients since 1955 and I cannot recall anyone that had any atrial fibrillation.

Homocysteine (Hcy)

Elevated homocysteine levels are associated with increased risk of ischemic heart disease (IHD) and stroke.[28] But according to this study these elevated levels are at most a modest independent predictor of IHD and stroke in healthy populations. Garg and colleagues[29] found that niacin increased homocysteine levels by about 55 percent in a series of 52 patients given 3,000 mg of niacin daily. These two sets of findings have suggested that niacin might also increase this risk. However I cannot take this very seriously since the Coronary Drug Project showed that niacin decreased mortality 11 percent and increased longevity nearly two years in a large group of men already having suffered one stroke. Even if there is a small risk that niacin will increase the risk for IHD and stroke, how will this ever be established in view of the large-scale Coronary Drug Project? Assuming that there is a risk, it is easily removed by having each patient take a B-complex tablet containing pyridoxine, folic acid, and vitamin B_{12}. Parsons wrote, "I always advise my patients not to lose any sleep over this. We are a long way from establishing that reducing homocysteine will reduce coronary events or other artery troubles so homocysteine shouldn't yet be considered a correctable risk factor. I would not want something they might read about Hcy to distract anyone from concentrating on controlling the established risk factors: smoking, high blood pressure, abnormal cholesterol profile, diabetes, obesity and lack of exercise." It is interesting that even though niacin elevates homocysteine levels, the negative risk effect of elevated homocysteine does not come into play; the effect in lowering cholesterol and in elevating HDL cholesterol compensates for this. Another factor is that niacin modifies abnormal coagulation factors that accompany peripheral arterial disease (PAD). Patients with PAD have high rates of cardiovascular pathology and morbidity.[30]

Vitamin B_3 and Cancer

Oncologists are generally opposed to their patients taking vitamins during chemotherapy or radiation. This is based upon conjecture, not upon data. Vitamin B_3 may be very important in preventing radiation- and chemotherapy-induced cancers.[31] Chemotherapy causes DNA damage in bone marrow, and it is more severe in niacin-deficient rats. This brings on new treatment-related cancers such as leukemia and cancer of the bone marrow. Patients undergoing chemotherapy are ten to 100 times more likely to develop such cancers, and three to ten times more likely than cancer patients undergoing radiation. Niacin deficiency leads to chromosomal instability. Pellagra is not common anymore in developed nations, but many people still suffer from subclinical deficiency, including women and the elderly. About 40 percent of cancer patients are deficient in niacin. Kirkland and Spronck[31] suggest that these deficiencies increase the risk of developing secondary treatment-related cancers. Skin cancer also may be invoked. In animals, skin cancer is highly influenced by niacin status. Professor James Kirkland, of the Department of Human Biology and Nutritional Sciences, University of Guelph, Ontario, released a press statement on March 25, 2003, with the lead sentence, "Extra niacin could help prevent treatment related cancers, study finds."

Other Negative Side Effects

Other side effects have been reported, but they are so rare it is impossible to draw any conclusions. As with any chemical idiosyncrasies, allergenic reactions to either the active tablet ingredient or to the fillers are possible. The best advice is for patients who start or have been on niacin to tell their doctor as soon as they note any adverse side effect.

Conclusion

Niacin and niacinamide are both important therapeutic compounds with a very wide range of activity, including lowering cholesterol, treating arthritis, decreasing the ravages of aging, and treating schizophrenia. They have no toxic effects and must be considered non-toxic; they have very few minor side effects. However, as with any substances, they must be used with care. Parsons makes the point repeatedly that physicians who are familiar with niacin and its properties are very pleased with the results.

Editor's Note: Dr. Hoffer further discusses niacin in these books: Niacin: The Real Story; Orthomolecular Medicine for Everyone; How to Live with Schizophrenia; The Orthomolecular Treatment for Schizophrenia; and *Feel Better, Live Longer with Vitamin B_3.*

Table 1. Comparison of Side Effects of Niacin, Lipitor, and Zyprexa.*

	Niacin	Lipitor	Zyprexa
Total pages	<1	2	3
Indications	6 lines	96 lines	6 lines
Contraindications	5 lines	3 lines	2 lines
Precautions & Warnings	12 lines	240 lines	240 lines
Drug interactions	17 lines	—	—
Adverse effects	25 lines	49 lines	240 lines

*Taken from the Compendium of Pharmaceuticals and Specialties, Canada 2003

REFERENCES FOR "NEGATIVE AND POSITIVE SIDE EFFECTS OF VITAMIN B_3"

1. Hoffer A, Osmond H, Smythies J. Schizophrenia: a new approach. II. Results of a year's research. *J Ment Sci* 1954; 100: 29–45.

2. Hoffer A. The adrenochrome hypothesis of schizophrenia revisited. *J Orthomolecular Psychiat* 1981; 10: 98–118.

3. Hoffer, A. Dopamine, noradrenalin and adrenalin metabolism to methylated or chrome indole derivatives: two pathways or one? *J Orthomolecular Psychiat,* 1985; 14: 262–272.

4. Smythies JR. Oxidative reactions and schizophrenia: a review-discussion. *Schizophren Res* 1997; 24: 357–364.

5. Smythies J, Galzigna L. The oxidative metabolism of catecholamines in the brain: a review. *Biochimica Et Biophysica Acta* 1998; 1380: 159–162.

6. Smythies J. Recent advances in the neurobiology of schizophrenia. *German J Psych* 1998; 1: 24–40.

7. Smythies J. The adrenochrome hypothesis of schizophrenia revisited. *Neurotox Res* 2002; 4: 147–150.

8. Hawkins DR. The prevention of tardive dyskinesia with high dosage vitamins: a study of 58,000 patients. *J Orthomolecular Med,* 1986; 1: 24–26.

9. Shute WE: *The Complete Updated Vitamin E Book.* New Canaan, CT: Keats Publishing, 1975.

10. Hoffer A, Osmond H, Callbeck MJ, et al. Treatment of schizophrenia with nicotinic acid and nicotinamide. *J Clin Exper Psychopathol* 1957; 18: 131–158.

11. Ames BN, Elson-Schwab I, Silver EA. High-dose vitamin therapy stimulates variant enzymes with decreased coenzyme binding affinity (increased Km): relevance to genetic disease and polymorphisms. *Am J Clin Nutr* 2002; 75: 616–658.

12. Pauling L. Orthomolecular Psychiatry. *Science,* 1968; 160: 265–271.

13. Simpson, LO. Myalgic encephalomyelitis (ME): A haemorrheological disorder manifested as Impaired Capillary Blood Flow. *J Orthomolecular Med* 1997; 12: 69–76.

14. Canner PL, Berge KG, Wenger NK, et al. Fifteen year mortality in coronary drug project patients: Long term benefit with niacin. *J Amer Coll Cardiol* 1986; 8: 1245–1255.

15. Kaufman W. *The Common Form of Niacinamide Deficiency Disease: Aniacinamidosis* New Haven, CT: Yale University Press, 1943.

16. Hoffer A. Hong Kong veterans study. *J Orthomolecular Psychiat* 1974; 3: 34–36.

17. McCracken RD. *Niacin and Human Health Disorders.* Fort Collins, CO: Hygea Publishing Co, 1994.

18. Altschul R, Hoffer A, Stephen JD. Influence of nicotinic acid on serum cholesterol in man. *Arch Biochem Biophys* 1955; 54: 558–559.

19. Soholm B, Lublin H. Long-term effectiveness of risperidone and olanzapine resistant or intolerant schizophrenic patients. A mirror study. *Acta Psychiatric Scand* 2003; 107: 344–350.

20. Atmaca M, Kuloglu M, Tezcan E, Ustundag B. Serum peptin and triglyceride levels in patients on treatment with atypical antipsychotics. *J Clin Psychiatry* 2003; 64: 598–604.

21. Horrobin DF. Schizophrenia: a biochemical disorder? *Biomedicine* 1980; 32:54–55.

22. Craig PE, Sutherland J, Glen EM, et al. Niacin skin flush in schizophrenia: a preliminary report. *Schizophren Res* 1998; 29: 269–274.

23. Hoffer A. *Niacin Therapy in Psychiatry.* Springfield, IL: CC Thomas,1962.

24. Parsons EB Jr. *Cholesterol Control Without Diet. The Niacin Solution.* Scottsdale, AZ: Lilac Press, 1998. Revised 2003.

25. Capuzzi D. Personal communication 2002.

26. McCarty MF. Co-administration of equimolar doses of betaine may alleviate the hepatotoxic risk associated with niacin therapy. *Med Hypoth* 1999; 55: 189–194.

27. Elam MB, Hunninghake DB, Davis KB, et al. Effect of niacin on lipid and lipoprotein levels and glycemic control in patients with diabetes and peripheral arterial disease. The ADMIT study: a randomized trial. *J Am Med Assoc* 2000; 284: 1263–1270.

28. Clarke R, et al. The homocysteine studies collaboration. Homocysteine and risk of ischemic heart disease and stroke. A meta-analysis. *J Am Med Assoc.* 2002; 288: 2015–2043.

29. Garg et al. Niacin treatment increases plasma homocysteine levels. *Am Heart J* 1999; 138: 1082–1087.

30. Chesney CM, Elam MB, Herd JA, et al. Effect of niacin, warfarin and antioxidant therapy on coagulation parameters in patients with peripheral arterial disease in the arterial disease multiple intervention trial. *Am Heart J* 40: 631–636, 2000.

31. Kirkland JB, Spronck JC. Niacin status, poly(ADP-ribose) metabolism and genomic instability. Molecular Nutrition. *CCAB Intl* Ed Zempleni J & Daniel H. 27–291, 2003.

VITAMINS FIGHT MULTIPLE SCLEROSIS

From the *Orthomolecular Medicine News Service,* October 4, 2006.

Research confirms that niacinamide, also known as vitamin B_3, is a key to the successful treatment of multiple sclerosis and other nerve diseases.[1] Niacinamide, say researchers at Harvard Medical School, "profoundly prevents the degeneration of demyelinated axons and improves the behavioral deficits."

This is very good news, but it is not at all new news. Over 60 years ago, Canadian physician H. T. Mount began treating multiple sclerosis patients with intravenous B_1 (thiamine) plus intramuscular liver extract, which provides other B vitamins. He followed the progress of these patients for up to 27 years. The results were excellent and were described in a paper published in the *Canadian Medical Association Journal* in 1973.[2]

Mount was not alone. Forty years ago, Frederick Robert Klenner, MD, of North Carolina, was using vitamins B_3 and B_1, along with the rest of the B-complex vitamins, vitamins C and E, and other nutrients, including magnesium, calcium, and zinc, to arrest and reverse multiple sclerosis.[3,4] Klenner's complete treatment program was originally published as "Treating Multiple Sclerosis Nutritionally" in *Cancer Control Journal* 2(3), pages 16–20.

Drs. Mount and Klenner were persuaded by their clinical observations that multiple sclerosis, myasthenia gravis, and many other neurological disorders were primarily due to nerve cells being starved of nutrients. Each physician tested this theory by giving his patients large, orthomolecular quantities of nutrients. Mount's and Klenner's successful cures over decades of medical practice proved their theory was correct. B-complex vitamins, including thiamine as well as niacinamide, are absolutely vital for nerve cell health. Where pathology already exists, unusually large quantities of vitamins are needed to repair damaged nerve cells.

Nutritional therapy is inexpensive, effective, and, most important, safe. There is not even one death per year from vitamins.[5]

Vitamin supplementation is not the problem. It is undernutrition that is the problem. Vitamins are the solution.

Restoring health must be done nutritionally, not pharmacologically. All cells in all persons are made exclusively from what we drink and eat. Not one cell is made out of drugs.

REFERENCES FOR "VITAMINS FIGHT MULTIPLE SCLEROSIS"

1. Kaneko S, Wang J, Kaneko M, et al. Protecting axonal degeneration by increasing nicotinamide adenine dinucleotide levels in experimental autoimmune encephalomyelitis models. *J Neurosci* 2006;26(38):9794–9804.

2. Mount HT. Multiple sclerosis and other demyelinating diseases. *Can Med Assoc J* 1973;108(11):1356–1358.

3. Klenner FR. Response of peripheral and central nerve pathology to mega-doses of the vitamin B-complex and other metabolites. *J Appl Nutr* 1973.

4. Dr. Klenner's "Clinical Guide to the Use of Vitamin C" (which discusses orthomolecular therapy with all vitamins, not just vitamin C) is now posted in its entirety at http://www.seanet.com/~alexs/ascorbate/198x/smith-lh-clinical_guide_1988.htm It includes a multiple sclerosis protocol, which takes up about five pages. See also: http://www.doctoryourself.com/klennerpaper.html.

5. Watson WA, et al. 2003 annual report of the American Association of Poison Control Centers Toxic Exposure Surveillance System. *Am J Emerg Med* 2004;22(5):335–404. Available at: http://www.aapcc.org/annual-reports/.

Why Niacin Will Always Be the Good One

by W. Todd Penberthy, PhD

From the *Orthomolecular Medicine News Service,* July 25, 2014.

Niacin has been used for over 60 years in tens of thousands of patients with tremendously favorable therapeutic benefit.[1] In the first-person *NY Times* best seller *8 Weeks to a Cure for Cholesterol,* the author describes his journey from being a walking heart attack time bomb to a becoming a healthy individual. He hails high-dose niacin as the one treatment that did more to correct his poor lipid profile than any other.[2] Many clinical studies have shown that high doses of niacin (3,000–5,000 milligrams [mg] of plain old immediate-release niacin taken in divided doses spread out over the course of a day) cause dramatic reductions in total mortality in patients who experienced previous strokes.[3] High-dose niacin has also been clinically proven to provide positive transformational relief to many schizophrenics in studies involving administration of immediate-release niacin in multi-thousand-milligram quantities to greater than 10,000 patients.[4,5] Most importantly, after 60 years of use, niacin (especially immediate-release niacin) remains far safer than the safest drug.[6]

Bad Reporting

So why has the media suddenly presented the following niacin-alarmist headlines in response to the study in the *New England Journal of Medicine*?[7]

"Niacin drug causes serious side effects, study says"—*Boston Globe,* 7/16/14

"Niacin safety, effectiveness questioned in new heart study"—*Healthday News,* 7/17/14

"Doctors say cholesterol drug risky to take"—*Times Daily,* 7/16/14

"Niacin risks may present health risks claim scientists"—*Viral Global News,* 7/17/14

"Studies reveal new niacin risks"—*Drug Discovery and Development,* 7/17/14

"No love for niacin"—*Medpage Today,* 7/17/14

"Niacin could be more harmful than helpful"—*Telemanagement,* 7/18/14

The truth of the matter is that the study quoted used laropiprant (trade names: Cordaptive and Tredaptive). Laropiprant is a questionable drug, and the results say next to nothing about niacin. The study compared over 25,000 patients treated with either niacin along with laropiprant, or placebo. The patients in this study had previous history of myocardial infarction, cerebrovascular disease, peripheral arterial disease, or diabetes mellitus with evidence of symptomatic coronary disease. The side effects observed in those who took the laropiprant-niacin combination were serious and included an increase in total mortality as well as significant increases in the risk for developing diabetes.

For responsible reporters, this should have raised the question of which compound, the drug laropiprant, or the vitamin niacin, is the culprit.

Such side effects have not been seen in over ten major clinical trials of niacin involving tens of thousands of patients, not in over 60 years of regular usage of niacin in clinics across the country. However, niacin causes a warm flush on the skin. Some people find the warm niacin flush uncomfortable, although many people enjoy this temporary sensation. In this study, niacin was given in combination with laropiprant, a drug that prevents the niacin flush. By including a dose of laropiprant along with the niacin to eliminate the flush, the thought was that more patients could benefit from niacin without complaint. But in fact the niacin flush is healthy. A reduced flush response to niacin is a diagnostic for increased incidence of schizophrenia, and this assay is now widely available.[8–11]

Problems with Laropiprant

So what about the other half of the combo, the drug laropiprant?

- Laropiprant has never been approved by the FDA for use in the USA and when taken alone has been shown to increase gastrointestinal bleeding.
- Laropiprant interferes with a basic prostaglandin receptor pathway that is important for good health.
- Last year Merck announced it would withdraw laropiprant worldwide due to complaints from continental Europe. Therefore the clinical trials in this study could only be performed in the UK, Scandinavia, and China.

So why did so many media outlets and even some MDs conclude that niacin was the problem? Simple: none of the headlines mentioned laropiprant, which is quite clearly the real culprit that caused the side effects reported. The simplest way to put it is to say that sensational stories promulgated by the media are quite often completely wrong. This suggests a hidden agenda.

Confusing and fantastical headlines can increase readership for hysteria-based business models. Which headline is likely to garner the greatest attention: "Laropiprant Is a Dangerous Medication That Has Not Been Approved by the FDA" or "Niacin Causes Serious Side Effects"? The correct headline would be, "Niacin doesn't cause serious side effects; drugs do."

Why the B Vitamins Are So Important

The B vitamins were discovered due to terrible nutritional epidemics: pellagra (niacin/vitamin B_3 deficiency) and beriberi (thiamine/vitamin B_1 deficiency). We are very sensitive to a deficiency of niacin. Over 100,000 people died in the American south in the first two decades of the 20th century due to a lack of niacin in their diet. It was perhaps the worst nutritional epidemic ever observed in modern times, and was a ghastly testimony to how vulnerable the human animal is to niacin deficiency. The pellagra and beriberi epidemics took off shortly after the introduction of processed foods such as white rice and white flour. Poor diets, mental and physical stresses, and certain disease conditions have all been proven to actively deplete nicotinamide adenine dinucleotide (NAD) levels, causing patients to respond favorably to greater than average niacin dosing.

How is it possible that niacin can be useful for many different conditions? It seems too good to be true. The reason is that niacin is necessary for more biochemical reactions than any other vitamin-derived molecule: over 450 different gene-encoded enzymatic reactions.[12] That is more reactions than any other vitamin-derived cofactor! Niacin is involved in just about every major biochemical pathway. Some individuals, who have a genetically encoded amino acid polymorphism within the NAD-binding domain of an enzyme protein, will have a lower binding affinity for NAD that can only be treated by administering higher amounts of niacin to make the amount of NAD required for normal health. Genetic differences such as these are why many individuals require higher amounts of niacin in order for their enzymes to function correctly.[13]

It is a deadly shame that the media so often ignores this information. Fortunately, many physicians will see through the headlines that give misinformation about niacin, having already personally witnessed how effective high-dose niacin therapy is for preventing cardiovascular disease.

Nutrients Are the Solution, Not the Problem

So what is the solution? At the end of the day the data on patients with problem cholesterol/LDL levels still support 3,000 to 5,000 mg of immediate-release niacin as the best clinically proven approach to maintaining a healthy lipid profile. Niacin in 250 mg to 1,000 mg doses can be purchased inexpensively from many sources. Extended-release niacin is the form of niacin that is most frequently sold by prescription, but it has more side effects than immediate-release (plain old) niacin . . . and it costs much more.

Tangential to niacin but pointed to cardiovascular disease, conventional medicine is finally beginning to respect chelation therapy as an approach owing to the unparalleled positive clinical results for cardiovascular disease patients with diabetes—up to 50 percent prevention of recurrent heart attacks and 43 percent reduction in death rate from all causes.[14] Sometimes chelation therapy can be expensive. However, there are other inexpensive approaches, including high-dose IP6 therapy, that are yet to be conventionally appreciated. Other supplements desirable for any ideal cardiovascular disease: a nutritional regimen include additional vitamin C, magnesium, coenzyme Q, fat-soluble vitamins (A, D, E, and K2), and grass-fed organic butter. Your ideal intake varies with your individuality.

Nutrients such as niacin you need. Media misinformation you don't.

REFERENCES FOR "WHY NIACIN WILL ALWAYS BE THE GOOD ONE"

1. Carlson LA. Nicotinic acid: the broad-spectrum lipid drug. A 50th anniversary review. *J Intern Med* 2005;258(2):94–114.

2. Kowalski RA. *The New 8-Week Cholesterol Cure: The Ultimate Program for Preventing Heart Disease.* Harper Collins, 2001.

3. Creider JC, Hegele RA, Joy TR. Niacin: another look at an underutilized lipid-lowering medication. *Nat Rev Endocrinol* 2012;8(9):517–528.

4. Hoffer A, Osmond H. Treatment of schizophrenia with nicotinic acid. A ten year follow-up. *Acta Psychiatr Scand* 1964;40:171–189.

5. Osmond H, Hoffer A. Massive niacin treatment in schizophrenia. Review of a nine-year study. *Lancet* 1962;1:316–319.

6. Guyton JR, Bays HE. Safety considerations with niacin therapy. *Am J Cardiol* 2007;99(6A):22C-31C.

7. Group HTC, Landray MJ, Haynes R, et al. Effects of extended-release niacin with laropiprant in high-risk patients. *N Engl J Med* 2014;371(3):203–212.

8. Horrobin DF. Schizophrenia: a biochemical disorder? *Biomedicine* 1980;32(2):54–55.

9. Messamore E, Hoffman WF, Janowsky A. The niacin skin flush abnormality in schizophrenia: a quantitative dose-response study. *Schizophr Res* 2003;62(3):251–258.

10. Liu CM, Chang SS, Liao SC, et al. Absent response to niacin skin patch is specific to schizophrenia and independent of smoking. *Psychiatry Res* 2007;152(2–3):181–187.

11. Smesny S, Klemm S, Stockebrand M, et al. Endophenotype properties of niacin sensitivity as marker of impaired prostaglandin signalling in schizophrenia. *Prostaglandins Leukot Essent Fatty Acids* 2007;77(2):79–85.

12. Penberthy WT. Niacin, Riboflavin, and Thiamine. In: Stipanuk MH, Caudill MA, eds. *Biochemical, physiological, and molecular aspects of human nutrition.* 3rd ed. St. Louis, Mo.: Elsevier/Saunders; 2013:p.540–564.

13. Ames BN, Elson-Schwab I, Silver EA. High-dose vitamin therapy stimulates variant enzymes with decreased coenzyme binding affinity (increased K(m)): relevance to genetic disease and polymorphisms. *Am J Clin Nutr* 2002;75(4):616–658.

14. Avila MD, Escolar E, Lamas GA. Chelation therapy after the Trial to Assess Chelation Therapy (TACT): results of a unique trial. *Curr Opin Cardiol* 2014;29(5):481–488.

"SAFE UPPER LEVELS" OF FOLIC ACID, B_6, AND B_{12}

by Eddie Vos

From *J Orthomolecular Med* 2003;18(3 & 4):166–167.

Homocysteine (Hcy) is an amino acid and a "natural blood toxin" linked to about 100 illnesses. This brief review concerns the three main players that jointly lower blood homocysteine as seen by the Expert Group on Vitamins and Minerals (EVM).[1] The group concerns itself with "Safe Upper Levels" (SULs) and produces an exhaustive review with many references. Their mandate clearly excluded considerations of "optimal" levels that may well be higher than SULs for therapeutic reasons or to obtain optimal (minimal) levels of homocysteine. Other players in homocysteine metabolism (reduction) include vitamin B_2, zinc, magnesium, betaine, and fish oil omega-3.

Folic Acid

In the U.S.A., 30,000 milligram (mg) tablets of folic acid can be obtained by mail order; in the U.K., doses over 5 mg (5,000 micrograms [mcg]) require a prescription. Doses of 1 to 20 mg (1,000 to 20,000 mcg) per day would be considered safe (p. 44) if it were not for a vitamin B_{12} deficiency–masking problem, and for some anti-folate drugs, such as methotrexate. Recommended daily intakes are 0.2 mg (200 mcg) per day in the U.K. and double that in the U.S.A. Actual mean intakes are near those amounts in these countries respectively.

There is no argument by the EVM of proven or potential benefits regarding Hcy, neural tube defects, and other therapies. "The main concern" about folic acid is its potential for masking a vitamin B_{12} deficiency at over 5 mg (5,000 mcg) per day and thus a "guidance level" of 1 mg (1,000 mcg) per day supplemental was concluded. Later in the report a SUL for B_{12} is given of 2 mg (2,000 mcg) per day, a massive amount of about 1,300 times recommended daily intakes. One must wonder why then the EVM did not issue a much higher SUL for folic acid in B_{12}-replete individuals, especially in light of the statement that "no likely mechanisms for toxicity have been hypothesized" for folic acid.

Pyridoxine—Vitamin B_6

Recommended daily intakes are about 1.3 mg per day. Deficiency is "unusual" in humans and mean intakes are ~2 mg per day. Therapeutic doses, for example, in carpal tunnel syndrome, may be well in excess of 100 mg per day, and side effects (neuropathy) are "generally" reversible. Dr. K. S. McCully, discoverer of the deleterious effects of Hcy, expressed concern (private communication) about the low recommended intake level. He recommends that it be about double, or 3 mg per day, making most people deficient by their actual intakes. Doses of 50 to 300 mg per day have been taken for as long as 20 years without neurotoxicity and with reduced myocardial infarction (heart attack) and extended life span.[2]

The EVM bases its SUL on a single-dose Lowest Observed Adverse Effect Level (LOAEL), in dogs, of 30 grams (30,000 mg), and then applies an arbitrary safety factor of 300 to arrive at a SUL of 10 mg per day. This is a low dose but one that is about five times that of common intakes and one that would be expected to help lower Hcy in most individuals. The EVM laments the lack of long-term safety data below 200 mg per day but suggests risk below this level "may well be minimal" in the short-term.

B_6 Safety

Editor's Note: Deficiency of B_6 is not common but insufficiency is. The RDA is very low, not even 2 mg per day. Higher doses would be safe and beneficial for many people. Very high doses of B_6 (thousands of milligrams) taken by itself can cause temporary neurological symptoms such as numbness or tingling of the limbs. These symptoms go away once dosages are reduced. Persons taking B-complex with B_6 very rarely report any side effects.

Cobalamin—Vitamin B_{12}

Recommended intakes are about 1.5 mcg per day. Best sources are meats; in a 100 gram (3.5 ounce) serving, chicken contains ~0.5 mcg, beef ~3 mcg, and liver ~20+ mcg. Deficiencies are more common in vegans and in the elderly, the latter primarily due to (common) absorption problems.

The EVM settled on a SUL of 2 mg (2,000 mcg) per day, a level well in excess of any level for common benefit. Supplements may contain amounts around 0.1 mg (100 mcg), which should circumvent absorption problems in nearly everyone, but not necessarily all.

Safe Upper Level of Homocysteine

The proposed SULs or guidance levels are, except in the case of B_{12}, well above those commonly obtained from foods. Considering the virtually certain and preventable detrimental effects in about 100 illnesses of higher than minimal amounts of Hcy, the question of a SUL for Hcy itself becomes important. This is especially true because of very common genetic disorders that require higher than minimal amounts of nutrients, and the fact that anything one does to a food (refining, canning, freezing, and storing) reduces specifically folic acid and B_6 (B_{12} is little affected).

One can argue that a SUL for Hcy in blood plasma is about 8 micromoles per liter (micromol/L) and that supplementation is not necessarily warranted below that level.[3] For people at "mild risk" (in poor diet or age greater than 60 and Hcy 8 to 12 millimoles per liter [mmol/L]), supplemental amounts of 3 mg per day B_6, 0.1 mg (100 mcg) B_{12}, and 0.4 mg (400 mcg) folic acid are suggested. These amounts increase at "very high risk" (in angina, ischemic attacks, kidney failure, diabetes, and Hcy 16–30 mmol/L) to 100 mg B_6, 1 mg (1,000 mcg) B_{12} and 5 mg (5,000 mcg) folic acid.

Based on the EVM report, these amounts are safe with some remaining uncertainty regarding vitamin B_6. Higher than minimal Hcy (which de facto means: low folic acid, B_6, and B_{12}) is firmly linked to some of the most devastating illnesses, from heart and vascular diseases, to cancers and Alzheimer's disease. In the next few years important and possibly conclusive randomized controlled trial data should become available. One thing is certain: there is no benefit from higher than minimal blood Hcy levels, which, incidentally, is the best marker for sub-optimal nutrition in people and populations.

The Expert Group should revisit their data considering the universal unsafe levels of Hcy in the Western world and elsewhere, and increase the SUL or guidance levels of folic acid and B_6. If there is merit in establishing SULs for the B vitamins, it is at least as important to now do so for homocysteine.

REFERENCES "'SAFE UPPER LEVELS' OF FOLIC ACID, B_6, AND B_{12}"

1. Expert Group on Vitamins and Minerals. Safe upper levels for vitamins and minerals. May 2003. Available at: https://cot.food.gov.uk/sites/default/files/vitmin2003.pdf.

2. Ellis JM, McCully KS. Prevention of myocardial infarction by vitamin B_6. *Res Commun Mol Pathol Pharmacol* 1995; 89(2): 208–220.

3. McCully KS, McCully M. *The Heart Revolution* (chap. 5). HarperCollins, 2002.

WHAT ABOUT THE REST OF THE B VITAMINS?

"B vitamins can protect you from depression, anxiety, stress, confusion, fatigue, mental dullness, and emotional fragility and can even boost IQ."

—HYLA CASS, MD

Riboflavin (B_2)

Very few people are riboflavin deficient. Your diet probably provides plenty. Riboflavin (B_2) is found in dairy products, eggs, nuts, mushrooms, and green vegetables like peas, broccoli, and spinach. B_2 is extremely safe. Zero toxic side effects—none—have ever been reported in humans.[3]

Pantothenic Acid (B_5)

Roger J. Williams, PhD, discovered pantothenic acid (B_5) back in 1933. "Pantothen" means "from everywhere." True to its name, pantothenic acid is present in all cells in all forms of life. This makes it easy to obtain, and therefore it is extremely rare for anyone to be deficient. Eat a good diet and you will be all set. Stress increases your need for many nutrients, and more B_5 may be helpful. "Pantothenic acid, along with the whole vitamin B complex, is calming for the nervous system but especially the adrenals," says Carolyn Dean, MD. To help deal with the stresses of a busy life, Dr. Dean personally takes B complex and an additional 1,000 mg of pantothenic acid.[4]

B_6 for Carpel Tunnel Syndrome

Nancy Watson Dean (age 90-plus) of Rochester, NY, writes:

"I have just experienced such an amazing relief from this condition, which came upon me about a year ago, in the shape of hands tingling and hurting more often as time went on. I presently realized it was carpal tunnel, when shooting pains hit both hands.

"I knew vitamin B_6 would help, and it did, but only a little. So remembering a paper by the Texas doctor, John Marion Ellis, MD, who said that large amounts didn't seem to bother him in any way, I pulled out all the stops and increased it to 200 milligrams four times daily. I also stopped eating salt. The carpal tunnel

disappeared. I am thrilled, out of pain, and the hands are growing stronger by the hour.

"This is a very widespread ailment. Perhaps the maintenance and attacks of the condition are entirely individual: just find the amount that 'cures' you. Wouldn't the medics hate that idea!"

"Vitamin B_6 (pyridoxine) has been successfully used for years to treat carpal tunnel syndrome and related problems," says Andrew W. Saul. "Dr. John M. Ellis, a physician in Texas, published an entire book on vitamin B_6 (pyridoxine) in 1983 titled *Free of Pain.* Linus Pauling reports in *How to Live Longer and Feel Better* that Ellis found that 'B_6 shrinks the synovial membranes that line the weight-bearing surfaces of the joints. It thus helps to control pain and to restore mobility in the elbows, shoulders, knees, and other joints.' While very large doses of B_6 alone may cause transient neurological side effects, relatively modest doses of around 75 to 300 mg daily are very safe. The safety of one B vitamin is magnified by giving it with the rest of the B complex."[5]

Cobalamin (B_{12})

B_{12} can't kill you unless you don't get any. It is safe and essential. B_{12} is found primarily in animal-based products like eggs, cheese, yogurt, meat, fish, and milk. If you do not eat any animal products, you rely solely on your body's ability to synthesize B_{12} from your friendly colon bacteria. Vegans: it is a good idea to get your B_{12} levels tested regularly by your doctor. If you are in good health, you may find you have exceptional B_{12} status. But not everyone's gut flora is in good shape. Avoid antibiotics whenever possible, and eat fermented and probiotic foods to help boost beneficial bacteria. If your B_{12} is low, supplementation is important. Oral B_{12} supplements are not easy to absorb. Some, however, are better than others. Seek out sublingual tablets (the kind that dissolve under your tongue) in the form of methylcobalamin.

Some people may have pernicious (harmful and destructive) anemia or the inability to absorb B_{12} through what they eat. In the old days, this condition could literally kill you. Nowadays, B_{12} can be administered directly via patches, creams, oral tablets, nasal sprays, nasal gel, or a shot from the doctor. For cases of pernicious anemia, about 1 percent of oral vitamin B_{12} can still be absorbed.[6] However, to bypass your gut's faulty absorption system, your doctor may also administer intramuscular shots. In healthy folks, oral B_{12} can be as effective as an intramuscular shot.[7]

At early onset of a headache, B_{12} may help. "Vitamin B_{12} inhibits nitric oxide and can lower the inflammation and blood vessel dilation that occurs in a migraine," says Dr. Steve Hickey.[8] A lack of B_{12} can cause feelings of depression, and supplementation may be helpful, especially if deficient.[9] High-dose B_{12} may also help relieve tinnitus.

The RDA is low: just over 2 *micrograms* per day.[10] Therapeutic doses are higher and could range from about 1,000 mcg daily to 3,000 to 5,000 mcg weekly.[11]

Biotin

Thanks to your friendly neighborhood gut bacteria, biotin is made in your large intestine. This, among other reasons, makes it a very good idea to keep your gut flora as healthy as possible. Eat lots of vegetables and consume probiotics or fermented foods. Avoid antibiotics whenever possible. While biotin deficiency is rare, if you develop brittle nails, hair loss, or skin rashes, investigate your biotin intake. Biotin is very safe at the doses available in supplements.[12] Typically, they range from 50 mcg to 5,000 mcg. Food sources of biotin include eggs, salmon, and avocados.

Choline

Choline is an honorary B vitamin: it is an essential nutrient, but not strictly speaking a vitamin. In animal studies, choline has been found to improve brain function.[13] It may also help you stay asleep. Another benefit of choline is simply feeling better. Your body knows how to make its own acetylcholine from choline. "Acetylcholine is the end neurotransmitter of your parasympathetic nerve system. This means that, among other things, it facilitates good digestion, deeper breathing, and slower heart rate. You may perceive its effect as 'relaxation,'" says Andrew W. Saul.[14] The trick is to get enough choline so your body can do this. Choline is found in wheat germ, eggs, soy, meat, quinoa, broccoli, nuts, milk, seeds, lentils, seafood, and cauliflower. It is also in lecithin. Lecithin granules have a nutty flavor and can be added to smoothies or yogurt or simply taken with water. Carolyn Dean, MD, recommends taking 2 tablespoons of lecithin per day.[15] If you don't want to eat lecithin granules, you can try lecithin supplements. You have to take quite a few of them to get the same amount of choline contained in a couple tablespoons of lecithin. That being said, lecithin is cheaper in the granular form, but capsules have the added advantage of being convenient and taste-free. It is available in the form of soy or sunflower lecithin.

CHAPTER 10 REFERENCES

1. Pauling, L. *How to Live Longer and Feel Better.* Corvallis, OR: Oregon State University Press, 2006.

2. Hoffer, A., A. W. Saul. *Orthomolecular Medicine for Everyone: Megavitamin Therapeutics for Families and Physicians.* Laguna Beach, CA: Basic Health Publications, 2008.

3. Linus Pauling Institute. Micronutrient Information Center. Oregon State University-."Riboflavin." http://lpi.oregonstate.edu/infocenter/vitamins/riboflavin/ (accessed May 2016).

4. Dean, C. *Hormone Balance.* Avon, MA: Adams Media, 2005.

5. Saul, A.W. *The Doctor Yourself Newsletter*, 1(23): Sept 24, 2001.

6. Office of Dietary Supplements. National Institutes of Health. "Vitamin B12: Fact Sheet for Health Professionals." http://ods.od.nih.gov/factsheets/VitaminB12-HealthProfessional/#en5 (accessed May 2016). Johnson, M.A. "If High Folic Acid Aggravates Vitamin B12 Deficiency What Should Be Done About It?" *Nutr Rev* 65(10) (Oct 2007):451–8.

7. Vidal-Alaball, J., C.C. Butler, R. Cannings-John, et al. "Oral Vitamin B12 versus Intramuscular Vitamin B12 for Vitamin B12 Deficiency." *Cochrane Database Syst Rev 3* (Jul 20, 2005): CD004655. Butler, C.C., J. Vidal-Alaball, R. Cannings-John, et al. "Oral vitamin B12 Versus Intramuscular Vitamin B12 for Vitamin B12 Deficiency: A Systematic Review of Randomized Controlled Trials." *Fam Pract* 23(3) (Jun 2006):279–85.

8. Hickey, S. *The Vitamin Cure for Migraines.* Laguna Beach, CA: Basic Health Publications, Inc. 2010.

9. Jonsson, B.H., A.W. Saul. *The Vitamin Cure for Depression.* Laguna Beach, CA: Basic Health Publications, 2012.

10. Linus Pauling Institute. Micronutrient Information Center. Oregon State University. Vitamin B12. http://lpi.oregonstate.edu/mic/vitamins/vitamin-B12 (accessed June 2016).

11. Gaby, Alan R. *Nutritional Medicine*, Concord, NH: Fritz Perlberg Publishing, 2011.

12. Gaby, Alan R. *Nutritional Medicine*, Concord, NH: Fritz Perlberg Publishing, 2011.

13. Challem, J. *The Food Mood Solution.* Hoboken, NJ: John Wiley & Sons, 2007.

14. Saul, A.W. *Doctor Yourself.* Laguna Beach, CA: Basic Health Publications, 2012.

15. Dean, C. *The Magnesium Miracle.* Updated Edition. New York: Ballantine Books, 2007.

CHAPTER 11

Other Nutrients, Including Vitamin K and Minerals

"You cannot heal selectively. When you truly heal, you don't heal only one disease. The whole body heals."

—CHARLOTTE GERSON

VITAMIN K

Getting enough vitamin K may mean less heart disease, less cancer, and fewer bone fractures.[1] If you eat green leafy vegetables, eat fermented foods, and avoid antibiotics, you are absolutely on the right track: between what you eat (K_1 is found in plants like green veggies) and what your friendly gastrointestinal bacteria manufacture (K_2), your levels of the fat-soluble vitamin K are likely OK. If you have a really bad diet, a health condition that prevents you from absorbing nutrients, or you take (or have taken) antibiotics, a supplement may be needed.[2] Still, the Adequate Intake (AI) is considered to be 90 to 120 micrograms (mcg) per day.[3] This is a very small amount. You can obtain this, and more, from your diet. Eating just one *ounce* of cooked kale per day would provide enough. Eat and drink green leafy vegetables and save yourself from another supplement to buy. Vitamin K is very safe. According to the Linus Pauling Institute, "[T]here is no known toxicity associated with high doses (dietary or supplemental) of the phylloquinone (vitamin K_1) or menaquinone (vitamin K_2) forms of vitamin K."[4] Remember: K is for kale. Eat kale. Just a little is all you need. Kase klosed.

MINERALS

Most multivitamins also contain a variety of essential minerals, but you may find your body requires more of certain minerals and that additional supplementation is necessary. Eating a diet rich in fruits and vegetables is a great way to get a variety of nutrients, especially trace or micro minerals, minerals of which you only need a small amount. Keep in mind, the quality of soil your food is grown in matters: better soil means better vitamin, mineral, enzyme, and micronutrient content in your food. Among other reasons, this makes buying organic produce a good idea. Think about it: if vegetables are high in minerals, where did they get them from? The soil. That's why you buy organic. That's why you grow a vegetable garden yourself. Eat a plant-based diet. This is the best way to get your trace minerals. For the macro minerals, supplementation may be necessary. For magnesium, I think supplementation is essential. Getting the larger doses we require is singularly difficult to obtain from food alone.

Mineral Measurements

Trace or micro minerals, like iodine, selenium, and chromium, are usually measured in micrograms (mcg). We only need a little bit. Macro minerals, like magnesium and calcium, are usually measured in milligrams (mg). We require relatively more of the macro minerals as compared to the trace minerals.

A microgram is a thousandth of a milligram (mg). A milligram is a thousandth of a gram (g). A gram is about a quarter teaspoon. Therefore, a milligram is about a thousandth of a quarter teaspoon, and a microgram is about a millionth of a quarter teaspoon.

Boron

Boron is for bones. This trace mineral keeps bones strong. "Calcium deficient rats had vertebrae that contained higher calcium content and required more force to break than the vertebrae of rats fed a low boron diet," says Andrew W. Saul, author of *Doctor Yourself.* "Urinary excretion of calcium and magnesium is higher when either rats or humans are boron deficient." The good news is you only need a small amount. Fruits and vegetables will be the main source of boron in your diet. This should be sufficient for most people as long as you actually eat them. Getting somewhere between 1 mg and 3 mg per day is about right.[5]

Calcium

Everybody knows calcium is essential for good health. Among other vital functions, it is required for bone growth, which is of special concern for growing children and for pregnant women who are growing children, and, subsequently, their bones. Getting the right amount is important. A good diet can do this. Along with calcium, it is *equally* important to get adequate vitamin D and magnesium.[6] Calcium will not work properly without them. Current recommendations for calcium for adults are between 1,000 and 1,200 mg per day.[7] According to Thomas Levy, MD, this amount is far too high. In his book *Death by Calcium,* he says, "[T]he average person has a small need (for calcium) that is more than adequately met when a balanced diet that includes meat, eggs, and vegetables is coupled with the maintenance of normal vitamin D levels."[8] Carolyn Dean, MD, recommends that you match your intake of calcium with supplemental magnesium.[9]

Chromium

Chromium, a trace mineral, works with insulin to help glucose metabolism.[10] This can come in very handy. Here's why: chromium can help even out the highs and lows of blood sugar. By helping to curb carbohydrate cravings[11] and reduce overeating, chromium can help keep us from raiding our cupboards for a quick carbohydrate fix when our blood sugar crashes. Adequate chromium can also reverse the feeling of depression.[12] Malcolm N. McLeod, MD, recommends taking anywhere from 400 to 1,000 mcg of chromium picolinate daily, or about 4 mcg per pound of body weight, to help treat depression.[13] For overall good health Abram Hoffer, MD, supports taking 200 mcg a day,[14] an amount most of us are not getting in our diet. Chromium is safe. Dr. McLeod says, "It is far safer to take chromium than not to take it."

Copper

You only need a little copper: just under 1 mg per day.[15] With copper pipes still running through many homes, it is unlikely that you will need to supplement this one. Your countertop water filter may remove some copper for you. Copper supplements are not necessary since excess copper is far more common than copper deficiency.[16] Elevated copper can be addressed with the intake of other essential nutrients. "In combination with ascorbic acid (vitamin C), zinc is used to reduce high serum copper levels," says Dr. Hoffer. Taking vitamin C, a combination of zinc and manganese (in a 20:1 ratio), and eating a high-fiber diet is recommended for excess copper.[17]

Iodine

Here's one we should all be paying some attention to, and your thyroid will thank you for it. You don't need much iodine, but it is very important that you get the small amount you need, and many of us are not.[18] The US Recommended Dietary Allowance (RDA) is 150 mcg per day for adults, with a "safe upper limit" set at 1,100 mcg per day.[19] Dr. David Brownstein recommends between 6,000 and 50,000 mcg a day.[20] Clearly, that is a lot of iodine. Perhaps you don't need that much, but note how low the RDA is. The right amount of iodine for you is probably somewhere in the middle, but likely far more than the RDA. If iodine is not available in your multivitamin and -mineral supplement, you can try this: smear a small amount of tincture of iodine on your skin every few weeks or so, and your body will decide how much to absorb. According to Guy E. Abraham, MD, "[S]kin application of iodine is an effective if not efficient and practical way for supplementation of iodine with an expected bioavailability of 6 to 12 percent of the total iodine applied to the skin."[21] Dairy, eggs, poultry, and especially seafood all provide a measure of iodine. Iodine is also in "iodized" salt, but not very much.

Iron

Iron will be found in your diet in red meat and turkey. Eat grass-fed, free-range, organic if you can. You don't have to eat meat. Ounce for ounce, dark *chocolate* contains more iron than beef. Iron is also found in plant foods in large quantity. Beans, lentils, spinach, and fortified cereals all contain iron. Do you cook your food in a cast iron pan? You'll get a little iron that way, too. However, a large number of us remain deficient. According to the Linus Pauling Institute, iron deficiency is "the most common nutrient deficiency in the US and the world."[22] It's easy to get your iron levels tested by your doctor. Absorption of too much iron, or hemochromatosis, affects one million Americans. This is a genetic disease you should ask your doctor about.

Your daily requirement for iron is somewhere between 5 and 20 mg. Women, who lose iron during menstruation, need about 15 to 20 mg a day; men need about 10 mg.[23] Taking vitamin C will help you absorb the iron you get in your diet and from supplements. Vitamin E, calcium, and zinc may interfere with iron absorption, so take your iron at a different time of day. Avoid ferrous sulfate (it may make you feel sick to your stomach).

Magnesium

Magnesium is a major mineral and we need far more than the minor amount we typically get. Magnesium is present in peas, broccoli, spinach, almonds, cashews, oatmeal, and more.[24] However, only about half is absorbed.[25] If you have ever suffered from leg cramps, twitches, anxiety, insomnia, or migraines, more magnesium should be on the menu. The US RDA for magnesium is 320 to 420 mg a day,[26] an amount that should probably be seen as a minimum.[27] Magnesium expert Dr. Carolyn Dean has come to the conclusion that "everyone could benefit from extra supplementation."[28] There are a variety of ways in which to do this: there are magnesium pills, powders, salts, and oils. Taking an Epsom salt bath is a great way to get additional magnesium transdermally, that is, through the skin. (I do this once a week.) Magnesium supplements come in many forms, including magnesium taurate, magnesium glycinate, magnesium citrate, magnesium malate, magnesium orotate, and magnesium chloride. However, "weight for weight dollar for dollar, magnesium citrate may be the best buy for general use," says Dr. Dean, as it is inexpensive and easily absorbed. Make a point to avoid magnesium oxide. Why? Because it absorbs very poorly. You only absorb about 4 percent, and what isn't absorbed tends to act as a laxative. Speaking of which: taking too much magnesium results in loose stools, which is the way our bodies excrete excess. If this happens, try taking magnesium on an empty stomach (in the morning or at night), and divide your dose. Or just take less.[29] It is not a contest to see how much you can hold. It is a matter of getting the right amount. The US RDA is the absolute bare minimum.

Manganese

While deficiency of manganese is rare, it is important to get a small amount (about 2 mg per day) of this essential trace mineral.[30] If you are eating the right foods, like whole grains, beans, nuts, and seeds, it is likely that you are getting sufficient manganese.[31] However, manganese-deficient soils, processing, and cooking decrease the amount of manganese present in what you eat, and only a very small amount is absorbed from your diet.[32] Exposure to high levels of industrial manganese can be toxic but, says the Linus Pauling Institute, "[m]anganese toxicity resulting from foods alone has not been reported in humans, even though certain vegetarian diets could provide up to 20 mg/day. . . . There is presently no evidence that the consumption of a manganese-rich plant-based diet results in manganese toxicity."[33]

Selenium

Selenium is a trace mineral that reduces inflammation and stimulates your immune system to fight infection.[34] Selenium "is antagonistic to (and so protective against) arsenic, mercury, and cadmium,"[35] and it may also have anticancer properties.[36] Selenium is important for DNA production, reproduction, and proper thyroid gland function.[37] The RDA for selenium is 55 mcg a day with a "tolerable upper limit" set at 400 mcg a day. Nutrients work best together, and selenium is no exception. It works with vitamin E, and therefore these nutrients should be taken together.[38] Just one Brazil nut provides about 80 mcg of selenium.

How Selenium Fights Viral Illness, Including AIDS

Harold D. Foster, PhD reports:

"Dr. Will Taylor and colleagues at the University of Georgia, Athens, have shown that there is a group of viruses that encode for glutathione peroxidase. This means that as they are replicated, they remove the four key nutrients that lie at the core of this enzyme (selenium, cysteine, glutamine, and tryptophan) from the human body. Eventually they can cause severe deficiencies of these nutrients and kill their hosts. Included in this group of viruses are hepatitis B and C, Coxsackie B, and HIV-1 and HIV-2. Anyone infected by one or more of these viruses needs elevated selenium, cysteine, tryptophan, and glutamine to remain healthy. Think tapeworm! That is, a parasite-induced functional deficiency.

"What needs to be done with HIV/AIDS patients is to raise their selenium, cysteine, tryptophan, and glutamine levels back to normal. The ideal treatment then depends on what they previously have been eating. In sub-Saharan Africa, most patients are very selenium deficient and are given 600 micrograms of this trace element daily for the first month. This then drops down to 400 micrograms daily. They also tend to eat too much maize (corn) and are, therefore, very tryptophan deficient. They get 540 mg 5-HTP each day to deal with the tryptophan deficiency."

Comment from Dr. Abram Hoffer:

"While HIV plays an important role in the causation of AIDS, it is only one factor, and perhaps least important, since it only attacks in the absence of the essential components of glutathione peroxidase, especially selenium, the key variable.

Much as the addition of niacinamide in 1942 to white flour by the US government eradicated pellagra from the southeast United States, so will the addition of selenium to our staple foods lead to the eradication of AIDS. The virus may still spread and attack, but in the presence of ample amounts of selenium and three amino acids in the body it will do little harm. Dr. Foster's work must be taken very seriously and followed up."

For the full text of Andrew W. Saul's interview with the late Dr. Foster please see: http://www.doctoryourself.com/fosterinterview.html.

Zinc

Zinc also helps your body defend against infection.[39] Zinc plays an important role in growth and development, brain function, and reproduction. Men need more zinc than women because they lose zinc in seminal fluid. Zinc deficiency is common, suggesting that supplementation would be wise for most people. The US RDA is only 8 mg per day for women and 11 mg a day for men.[40] Dr. Hoffer maintains that adults need 15 mg per day, and most diets provide less. Zinc absorption from supplements is good but not perfect.[41] Zinc gluconate is readily available, relatively well-absorbed, and inexpensive. Zinc citrate and zinc picolinate are also good choices.

Minerals: Which Ones and How Much?

Your optimal dose of minerals may differ from the next person's. However, the following list may meet the needs of many adults.[42] A daily mineral supplement program could include the following:

- Magnesium: 500 to 600 milligrams (mg)
- Calcium: 500 mg
- Iron: 10 to 15 mg
- Zinc: 15 to 25 mg
- Boron: 0.5 to 3 mg
- Copper: 1 to 3 mg
- Manganese: 5 mg
- Chromium: 200 to 400 micrograms (mcg)
- Iodine: 150 mcg
- Selenium: 200 mcg

OTHER NUTRIENTS

They are not vitamins or minerals, but these other nutrients are important, too.

Coenzyme Q_{10}

Coenzyme Q_{10} (CoQ_{10}) is important and that's why it is found in virtually every cell in our body. "In addition to being a potent antioxidant, CoQ_{10} helps maintain healthy blood pressure and cholesterol levels, promotes arterial health, and supports a strong heartbeat," says Julian Whitaker, MD. "It also has proven health benefits for your gums, brain, and skin, and studies suggest that it may help prevent migraines and slow hearing loss."[43] CoQ_{10} is safe; our bodies literally make it. It can be found in small amounts in many foods, but particularly in meat, nuts, and fish. Even then, our daily intake is typically less than 10 mg per day. As some physicians recommend 300 mg per day, supplementation makes a lot of sense. Aging may warrant the addition of a CoQ_{10} supplement.[44] For migraine headache sufferers, 100 mg per day of CoQ_{10} may be helpful.[45]

In mild to moderate depression, drug treatment works no better than placebo, an inert, inactive pill.[46] Here's what does work: nutrition and exercise. "[R]egular exercise can improve mood in people with mild to moderate depression"[47] and "nutrition can play a key role in the onset as well as severity and duration of depression."[48]

Essential Fatty Acids

We tend to get a lot of omega-6 fatty acids in our diets. It's those other fatty acids we have to worry about: the omega-3s. Adequate intake of omega-3s can reduce your risk for cardiovascular disease, heart attack, and help alleviate depression.[49] Your body converts omega-3s into docosahexaenoic acid (DHA) and eicosapentaenoic acid (EPA). For healthy individuals, getting 250 to 500 mg of DHA and EPA is about right.[50] Higher doses may be beneficial for those suffering with depression, anxiety, and memory deficits.[51] Sources of omega-3s include fish, seeds, and, of course, supplements. Eating fatty fish, like salmon, is a great way to get a dose of essential fatty acids. Eat "wild caught" fish or organic options to reduce your exposure to heavy metals. For those who do not eat animal foods, walnuts, winter squash, leafy greens, broccoli, cabbage, berries, and even mangoes are all excellent sources of omega-3s. Just five walnuts a day provides the RDA. Fish oil or krill oil supplements provide a safe, virtually mercury-free dose of omega-3s.[52] Concerns about purity should be directed to the supplement manufacturer.

CHAPTER 11 REFERENCES

1. Linus Pauling Institute. Micronutrient Information Center. Oregon State University. "Vitamin K." http://lpi.oregonstate.edu/infocenter/vitamins/vitaminK/ (accessed May 2016). Mercola, J. "10 Important Facts about Vitamin K That You Need to Know." Mar 24, 2004. http://articles.mercola.com/sites/articles/archive/2004/03/24/vitamin-k-part-two.aspx (accessed May 2016).

2. Mercola, J. "10 Important Facts about Vitamin K That You Need to Know." Mar 24, 2004. http://articles.mercola.com/sites/articles/archive/2004/03/24/vitamin-k-part-two.aspx (accessed May 2016).

3. Linus Pauling Institute. Micronutrient Information Center. Oregon State University. "Vitamin K." http://lpi.oregonstate.edu/infocenter/vitamins/vitaminK/ (accessed May 2016).

4. Ibid.

5. Hoffer, A., A.W. Saul. *Orthomolecular Medicine for Everyone: Megavitamin Therapeutics for Families and Physicians.* Laguna Beach, CA: Basic Health Publications, 2008.

6. Dean, C. *The Magnesium Miracle,* Updated edition. New York: Ballantine Books, 2006. See also: Linus Pauling Institute. Micronutrient Information Center. Oregon State University. "Calcium." http://lpi.oregonstate.edu/mic/minerals/calcium (accessed May 2016).

7. Linus Pauling Institute. Micronutrient Information Center. Oregon State University. "Calcium." http://lpi.oregonstate.edu/mic/minerals/calcium (accessed May 2016).

8. Levy, T. E. *Death by Calcium.* Henderson, NV: MedFox Publishing, 2013.

9. Dean, C. *The Magnesium Miracle,* Updated edition. New York: Ballantine Books, 2006.

10. Linus Pauling Institute. Micronutrient Information Center. Oregon State University. "Chromium." http://lpi.oregonstate.edu/infocenter/minerals/chromium/ (accessed May 2016).

11. Docherty, J.P., D.A. Sack, M. Roffman, et al. "A Double-Blind, Placebo-Controlled, Exploratory Trial of Chromium Picolinate in Atypical Depression: Effect on Carbohydrate Craving." J Psychiatr Pract 11(5) (Sep 2005):302–314.

12. Challem, J. *The Food Mood Solution.* Hoboken, NJ: John Wiley & Sons, 2007.

McLeod, M.N. *Lifting Depression: The Chromium Connection.* Laguna Beach, CA: Basic Health Publications, 2005.

13. McLeod, M.N. *Lifting Depression: The Chromium Connection.* Laguna Beach, CA: Basic Health Publications, 2005.

14. Hoffer, A., A.W. Saul. *Orthomolecular Medicine for Everyone: Megavitamin Therapeutics for Families and Physicians.* Laguna Beach, CA: Basic Health Publications, 2008.

15. Linus Pauling Institute. Micronutrient Information Center. Oregon State University. "Copper." http://lpi.oregonstate.edu/mic/minerals/copper (accessed May 2016).

16. Hoffer, A., A.W. Saul. *Orthomolecular Medicine for Everyone: Megavitamin Therapeutics for Families and Physicians.* Laguna Beach, CA: Basic Health Publications, 2008.

17. Ibid.

18. Linus Pauling Institute. Micronutrient Information Center. Oregon State University. "Iodine." http://lpi.oregonstate.edu/mic/minerals/iodine (accessed May 2016).

19. Ibid.

20. Trentini, D. "Busting the Iodine Myths." Hypothyroid Mom, May 28, 2014. http://hypothyroidmom.com/busting-the-iodine-myths/ (accessed May 2016).

21. Abraham, G.E. "The Bioavailability of Iodine Applied to the Skin." www.optimox.com/pics/Iodine/updates/UNIOD-02/UNIOD_02.htm (accessed May 2016).

22. Linus Pauling Institute. Micronutrient Information Center. Oregon State University. "Iron." http://lpi.oregonstate.edu/mic/minerals/iron (accessed May 2016).

23. Hoffer, A., A.W. Saul. *Orthomolecular Medicine for Everyone: Megavitamin Therapeutics for Families and Physicians.* Laguna Beach, CA: Basic Health Publications, 2008. Cass, H. *8 Weeks to Vibrant Health.* New York: McGraw Hill, 2005.

24. Linus Pauling Institute. Micronutrient Information Center. Oregon State University. "Magnesium." http://lpi.oregonstate.edu/mic/minerals/magnesium (accessed May 2016).

25. Dean, C. *The Magnesium Miracle,* Updated edition. New York: Ballantine Books, 2006.

26. Linus Pauling Institute. Micronutrient Information Center. Oregon State University. "Magnesium." http://lpi.oregonstate.edu/mic/minerals/magnesium (accessed May 2016).

27. Hoffer, A., A.W. Saul. *Orthomolecular Medicine for Everyone: Megavitamin Therapeutics for Families and Physicians.* Laguna Beach, CA: Basic Health Publications, 2008.

28. Dean, C. *The Magnesium Miracle,* Updated edition. New York: Ballantine Books, 2006.

29. Ibid.

30. Linus Pauling Institute. Micronutrient Information Center. Oregon State University. “Manganese.” http://lpi.oregonstate.edu/infocenter/minerals/manganese/ (accessed May 2016).

31. Ibid.

32. Tuormaa, T.E. “The Adverse Effects of Manganese Deficiency on Reproduction and Health: A Literature Review Deficiency.” *J Orthomolecular Med* 11(2nd Q) (1996): http://orthomolecular.org/library/jom/1996/articles/1996-v11n02-p069.shtml (accessed May 2016).

33. Linus Pauling Institute. Micronutrient Information Center. Oregon State University. “Manganese.” http://lpi.oregonstate.edu/infocenter/minerals/manganese/ (accessed Oct 2014).

34. National Institutes of Health. Office of Dietary Supplements. “Selenium: Fact Sheet for Consumers.” http://ods.od.nih.gov/factsheets/Selenium-Consumer/ (accessed May 2016).

35. *Orthomolecular Medicine News Service.* “Vitamin Supplements Help Protect Children from Heavy Metals, Reduce Behavioral Disorders.” (Oct 8, 2007): www.orthomolecular.org/resources/omns/v03n07.shtml (accessed May 2016).

36. Hoffer, A., A.W. Saul. *Orthomolecular Medicine for Everyone: Megavitamin Therapeutics for Families and Physicians.* Laguna Beach, CA: Basic Health Publications, 2008.

37. National Institutes of Health. Office of Dietary Supplements. “Selenium: Fact Sheet for Consumers.” http://ods.od.nih.gov/factsheets/Selenium-Consumer/ (accessed May 2016).

38. Linus Pauling Institute. Micronutrient Information Center. Oregon State University. “Selenium.” http://lpi.oregonstate.edu/mic/minerals/selenium (accessed May 2016).

39. Linus Pauling Institute. Micronutrient Information Center. Oregon State University. “Zinc.” http://lpi.oregonstate.edu/mic/minerals/zinc (accessed May 2016).

40. Ibid.

41. Hoffer, A., A.W. Saul. *Orthomolecular Medicine for Everyone: Megavitamin Therapeutics for Families and Physicians.* Laguna Beach, CA: Basic Health Publications, 2008.

42. Dean, C. *The Magnesium Miracle,* Updated edition. New York: Ballantine Books, 2006. Cass, H. *8 Weeks to Vibrant Health.* New York: McGraw Hill, 2005. Hoffer, A., A.W. Saul. *Orthomolecular Medicine for Everyone: Megavitamin Therapeutics for Families and Physicians.* Laguna Beach, CA: Basic Health Publications, 2008. Levy, T. E. *Death by Calcium.* Henderson, NV: MedFox Publishing, 2013.

43. Whitaker, J. “The Benefits of CoQ10.” http://www.drwhitaker.com/benefits-of-coq10/ (accessed May 2016).

44. Linus Pauling Institute. Micronutrient Information Center. Oregon State University. "Coenzyme Q10." http://lpi.oregonstate.edu/mic/dietary-factors/coenzyme-Q10 (accessed May 2016).

45. Sandor, P.S., L. Di Clemente, G. Coppola, et al. "Efficacy of Coenzyme Q10 in Migraine Prophylaxis: A Randomized Controlled Trial." *Neurology* 64(4) (Feb 22, 2005): 713–15.

46. Fournier, J.C., R. J. DeRubeis, S. D. Hollon, et al. "Antidepressant Drug Effects and Depression Severity: A Patient-Level Meta-analysis." *JAMA* 303(1) (Jan 2010):47–53. doi:10.1001/jama.2009.1943.

47. Harvard Health Publications. Harvard Medical School. "Exercise and Depression." http://www.health.harvard.edu/mind-and-mood/exercise-and-depression-report-excerpt (accessed May 2016).

48. Sathyanarayana Rao, T. S., M. R. Asha, B. N. Ramesh, et al. "Understanding Nutrition, Depression and Mental Illnesses." *Indian J Psychiatry* 50(2) (Apr-Jun 2008): 77–82. doi: 10.4103/0019–5545.42391.

49. Linus Pauling Institute. Micronutrient Information Center. Oregon State University. "Essential Fatty Acids." http://lpi.oregonstate.edu/mic/other-nutrients/essential-fatty-acids (accessed May 2016).

50. Linus Pauling Institute. Micronutrient Information Center. Oregon State University. "Essential Fatty Acids." http://lpi.oregonstate.edu/mic/other-nutrients/essential-fatty-acids (accessed May 2016). Mercola, J. "How Much Omega-3 Is Right for You and What Are the Best Sources?" Jan 4, 2016. http://articles.mercola.com/sites/articles/archive/2016/01/04/how-much-omega-3.aspx.

51. Ibid.

52. Melanson, S.F., E.L. Lewandrowski, J.G. Flood, et al. "Measurement of Organochlorines in Commercial Over-the-Counter Fish Oil Preparations: Implications for Dietary and Therapeutic Recommendations for Omega-3 Fatty Acids and a Review of the Literature." *Arch Pathol Lab Med* 129(1) (Jan 2005): 74–7.

CHAPTER 12

Nutrient News You Haven't Heard

"The news media by their own words are the very personification of ignorance. They warn people off supplements when supplementation is the very thing people need to be healthier, or at the very least, less sick."

—ANDREW W. SAUL, PHD

Vitamin C may cure Ebola? *And* shingles? Vitamins D and C can treat tuberculosis? Vitamin C prevents heart disease? Magnesium can prevent kidney stones? Vitamin C *doesn't* cause kidney stones? Niacin (B_3) is the safest and best way to lower "bad" cholesterol? *Don't* get a flu shot and take vitamin D instead? Come now. We haven't heard *any* of this on TV.

"First they ignore you, then they laugh at you, then they fight you, then you win."

—ATTRIBUTED TO MAHATMA GANDHI

If there were recognition, there could at least be debate. But there is none. Vitamin therapy is marginalized at best and vilified at worst. Vitamin and mineral supplements are proclaimed "useless" and "harmful" when they are neither. Decades of real results with nutritional therapy, obtained by real doctors, are dismissed out of hand. Practically no positive press about vitamins ever reaches large audiences. Instead, the public is inundated with pharmaceutical ads and the periodic (but far-reaching) article about vitamin "dangers" plastered on the "news."

"Attacks on vitamin safety are really attacks on vitamin efficacy," says Abram Hoffer, MD. "It is an indirect method of downgrading the value of orthomolecular medicine." Nutritional therapeutics continues to be disregarded as if it simply has no place in modern medicine. Millions of people who could benefit from optimal nutrition are left with the faulty belief system that current medical practice has all the answers, and that no answers can be found in giving the body "excess" nutrients.

Until you see the news discuss niacin as treatment for mood disorders, those suffering from mental illness are being criminally neglected. Failure to ensure that all children receive high-dose vitamin C with every vaccination is institutionalized child abuse.

Vitamin Bias

"The test to determine whether a treatment has become popular within the medical profession is to measure the relative strength of the positive and negative assertions made about the treatment. The use of antibiotics is so well entrenched in medicine that side effects and toxicities are recognized but are accepted as the price one must pay for their positive therapeutic properties. In sharp contrast, vitamins, which are safe even in large doses, have not been acceptable to the profession, and their negative side effects have been consistently exaggerated and overemphasized, to the point that many of these so-called toxicities have been invented, without there being any scientific evidence that these side effects are real. This pervasive negative attitude has spilled over to the news media, who have consistently followed the official line and have ignored all the claims made about the benefits of vitamins used in optimum amounts."

—ABRAM HOFFER, MD, PhD

Niacin and Schizophrenia

by Nick Fortino, PhD

From the *Orthomolecular Med News Service*, October 27, 2014.

Schizophrenia is usually treated with prescription antipsychotic drugs, many of which produce severe adverse effects,[1–6] are linked to an incentive for monetary profit benefiting pharmaceutical corporations,[7–13] lack sufficient evidence for safety and efficacy,[9,14] and have been grossly misused.[15–20] Orthomolecular (nutritional) medicine provides another approach to treating schizophrenia, which involves the optimal doses of vitamin B_3: also known as niacin, niacinamide, nicotinamide, or nicotinic acid—in conjunction with an individualized protocol of multiple vitamins. The orthomolecular approach involves treating "mental disease by the provision of the optimum molecular environment for the mind, especially the optimum concentrations of substances normally present in the human body."[21]

Evidence for the Niacin Treatment of Schizophrenia

Vitamin B_3 as a treatment for schizophrenia is typically overlooked, which is disconcerting considering that historical evidence suggests it effectively reduces symptoms of schizophrenia and has the added advantage, in contrast to pharmaceuticals, of mild to no adverse effects.[22–35] After successful preliminary trials treating schizophrenia patients with niacin, pilot trials of larger samples commenced in 1952 and were reported in 1957 by Hoffer, Osmond, Callbeck, and Kahan. Dr. Abram Hoffer began an experiment involving 30 patients who had been diagnosed with acute schizophrenia. Participants were given a series of physiological and psychological tests to measure baseline status and were subsequently assigned randomly to treatment groups. Nine subjects received a placebo, ten received nicotinic acid, and 11 received nicotinamide (the latter two are forms of vitamin B_3). All participants received treatment for 42 days, were in the same hospital, and received psychotherapy from the same group of clinicians. The two experimental groups were administered 3 grams of vitamin B_3 per day. Each of the three treatment groups improved, but the two vitamin B_3 groups improved more than the placebo group as compared to baseline measures. At one year follow up, 33 percent of patients in the placebo group remained well, and *88 percent of patients in the B_3 groups remained well.* These results inspired many subsequent trials, and those that replicated the original method produced similarly positive results.

Antipsychotic Drugs

That schizophrenia may be caused or aggravated by a deficiency of essential nutrients appears to have eluded the majority of the health care providers serving the schizophrenic population, as evidenced by the fact that "antipsychotic medications represent the cornerstone of pharmacological treatment for patients with schizophrenia."[36] Waves of different antipsychotic drugs have been developed throughout the last 60 years, which have not decreased the prevalence of schizophrenia; in fact it has increased.[15,37]

Although dangerous when taken in high doses and for a long period of time, the value of antipsychotics appears to be that in the short term they can help to bring some control to schizophrenic symptoms, not by curing the condition but by inducing a neurological effect that is qualitatively different from the schizophrenic state. Dr. Hoffer acknowledged their value and in his private practice he would introduce antipsychotics and vitamins simultaneously because antipsychotics work rapidly and vitamins work more slowly, so a person could benefit from the short-term relief from symptoms that antipsychotics provide while the vitamins slowly, but surely, healed the deficiency causing the schizophrenic symptoms. This also allowed for a much easier process of tapering from the drugs.

> *"For schizophrenia, the recovery rate with drug therapy is under 15 percent. With nutritional therapy, the recovery rate is 80 percent."*
>
> —ABRAM HOFFER, MD, PHD

REFERENCES FOR "NIACIN AND SCHIZOPHRENIA"

1. Arana GW. An overview of side effects caused by typical antipsychotics. *J Clin Psychiatry* 2000; 61(8): 5–11.

2. Ciranni MA, Kearney TE, Olson KR. Comparing acute toxicity of first- and second-generation antipsychotic drugs: A 10-year, retrospective cohort study. *J Clin Psychiatry* 2009;70(1): 122–129.

3. Ho BC, Andreasen NC, Ziebell S, et al. Long-term antipsychotic treatment and brain volumes: A longitudinal study of first-episode schizophrenia. *Arch Gen Psychiatry* 2011; 68(2): 128.

4. Pope HG, Keck PE, McElroy SL. Frequency and presentation of neuroleptic malignant syndrome in a large psychiatric hospital. *Am J Psychiatry* 1986; 143(10): 1227–1233.

5. Saddichha S, Manjunatha N, Ameen S, et al. Diabetes and schizophrenia—effect of disease or drug? Results from a randomized, double blind, controlled prospective study in first-episode schizophrenia. *Acta Psychiatrica Scandinavica* 2008;117: 342–347.

6. Woods SW, Morgenstern H, Saksa JR, et al. Incidence of tardive dyskinesia with atypical and conventional antipsychotic medications: Prospective cohort study. *J Clin Psychiatry* 2010:71(4): 463–475.

7. Angell M. *The truth about the drug companies: How they deceive us and what to do about it.* New York, NY: Random House LLC, 2004.

8. Berenson A. Lilly settles with 18,000 over zyprexa. *The New York Times,* 2007. Available at: http://www.nytimes.com/2007/01/05/business/05drug.html?_r=0.

9. Kendall T. The rise and fall of atypical antipsychotics. *Br J Psychiatry,* 2011;199(4): 266–268. doi:10.1192/bjp.bp.110.083766.

10. Moynihan R, Alan C. *Selling sickness: How the world's biggest pharmaceutical companies are turning us all into patients.* New York, NY: Nation Books, 2005.

11. Moynihan R, Heath I, Henry D. Selling sickness: the pharmaceutical industry and disease mongering. *Br Med J,* 2002;324(7342): 886.

12. Scherer FM. Pricing, profits, and technological progress in the pharmaceutical industry. *The Journal of Economic Perspectives* 1993;7(3): 97–115.

13. Spielmans GI, Parry PI. From evidence-based medicine to marketing-based medicine: Evidence from internal industry documents. *Journal of Bioethical Inquiry* 2009;7(1): 13–29. doi:10.1007/s11673–010–9208–8.

14. Lieberman JA, Stroup TS, McEvoy JP, et al. Effectiveness of antipsychotic drugs in patients with chronic schizophrenia. *N Engl J Med,* 2005;353(12): 1209–1223.

15. Whitaker R. *Anatomy of an epidemic: Magic bullets, psychiatric drugs, and the astonishing rise of mental illness in America.* New York, NY: Crown Publishers, 2010.

16. Kuehn BM. Questionable antipsychotic prescribing remains common, despite serious risks. *JAMA* 2010; 303(16): 1582–1584.

17. Moran M. Misuse of antipsychotics widespread in nursing homes. *Psychiatric News* 2011;46(11): 2.

18. Ray WA, Federspiel CF, Schaffner W. A study of antipsychotic drug use in nursing homes: Epidemiologic evidence suggesting misuse. *Am J Public Health* 1980;70(5): 485–491.

19. Stevenson DG, Decker SL, Dwyer LL, et al. Antipsychotic and benzodiazepine use among nursing home residents: Findings from the 2004 National Nursing Home Survey. *Am J Geriatr Psychiatry* 2010;18(12): 1078–1092.

20. Szaz T. *The myth of mental illness: Foundations of a theory of personal conduct.* New York, NY: Harper Perennial, 1974.

21. Pauling L. Orthomolecular psychiatry. Varying the concentrations of substances normally present in the human body may control mental disease. *Orthomolecular Psychiatry Science* 1968; 160: 265–271.

22. Cleckley HM, Sydenstricker VP, Geeslin LE. Nicotinic acid in the treatment of atypical psychotic states. *JAMA* 1939;112(21): 2107–2110.

23. Hoffer A. *Niacin Therapy in Psychiatry.* Springfield, IL: CC Thomas, 1962.

24. Hoffer A. Nicotinic acid: An adjunct in the treatment of schizophrenia. *Am J Psychiatry* 1963;120: 171–173.

25. Hoffer A. The effect of nicotinic acid on the frequency and duration of re-hospitalization of schizophrenic patients: A controlled comparison study. *Int J Neuropsychiatry* 1966;2(3): 234–240.

26. Hoffer A. Childhood schizophrenia: A case treated with nicotinic acid and nicotinamide. *Schizophrenia* 1970a; 2: 43–53.

27. Hoffer A. A neurological form of schizophrenia. *Can Med Assoc J* 1973;108, 186–194.

28. Hoffer A. Chronic schizophrenic patients treated ten years or more. *J Orthomolecular Med* 1994;9(1): 7–37.

29. Hoffer A. Inside schizophrenia: Before and after treatment. *J Orthomolecular Med* 1996;11(1): 45–48.

30. Hoffer A., Fuller F. Orthomolecular treatment of schizophrenia. *J Orthomolecular Med* 2009;24(3,4): 151–159.

31. Hoffer A, Osmond H. Treatment of schizophrenia with nicotinic acid: A ten year follow up. *Acta Psychiatrica Scandinavica* 1964;40: 171–189. doi:10.1111/j.1600–0447.1964.tb05744.x.

32. Hoffer A, Osmond H. Schizophrenia: Another long term follow-up in Canada. *Orthomolecular Psychiatry* 1980;9(2): 107–113.

33. Hoffer A, Osmond H, Callbeck MJ, Kahan I. Treatment of schizophrenia with nicotinic acid and nicotinamide. *J Clin Exp Psychopathol* 1957;18(2): 131–157.

34. Tung-Yep T. The use of orthomolecular therapy in the control of schizophrenia-a study preview. *The Australian Journal of Clinical Hypnotherapy,* 1981;2(2): 111–116.

35. Verzosa PL. A report on a twelve-month period of treating metabolic diseases using mainly vitamins and minerals on the schizophrenias. *Orthomolecular Psychiatry* 1976;5(4): 253–260.

36. Gilmer TP, Dolder CR, Lacro JP, et al. Adherence to treatment with antipsychotic medication and health care costs among Medicaid beneficiaries with schizophrenia. *Am J Psychiatry* 2004;161(4): 692–699.

37. McGrath J, Saha S, Chant D, Welham J. Schizophrenia: A concise overview of incidence, prevalence, and mortality. *Epidemiol Rev* 2008;30: 67–76.

38. Saha S, Chant D, McGrath J. A systematic review of mortality in schizophrenia. *Arch Gen Psychiatry* 2007;64(10): 1123–1131.

VITAMIN C PREVENTS VACCINATION SIDE EFFECTS, INCREASES EFFECTIVENESS

by Thomas E. Levy, MD, JD

From the *Orthomolecular Med News Service,* February 14, 2012.

The routine administration of vaccinations continues to be a subject of controversy in the United States, as well as throughout the world. Parents who want the best for their babies and children continue to be faced with decisions that they fear could harm their children if made incorrectly. The controversy over the potential harm of vaccinating, or of not vaccinating, will not be resolved to the satisfaction of all parties anytime soon, if ever. This brief report aims to offer some practical information to pediatricians and parents alike who want the best long-term health for their patients and children, regardless of their sentiments on the topic of vaccination in general.

While there seems to be a great deal of controversy over how frequently a vaccination might result in a negative outcome, there is little controversy that at least some of the time vaccines do cause damage. The question that then emerges is whether something can be done to minimize, if not eliminate, the infliction of such damage, however infrequently it may occur.

Causes of Vaccination Side Effects

When vaccines do have side effects and adverse reactions, these outcomes are often categorized as resulting from allergic reactions or the result of a negative interaction with compromised immune systems. While either of these types of reactions can be avoided subsequently when there is a history of a bad reaction having occurred at least once in the past as a result of a vaccination, it is vital to try to avoid encountering a negative outcome from occurring the first time vaccines are administered.

Due to the fact that all toxins, toxic effects, substantial allergic reactions, and induced immune compromise have the final common denominator of causing and/or resulting in the oxidation of vital biomolecules, the antioxidant vitamin C has proven to be the ultimate nonspecific antidote to whatever toxin or excess oxidative stress might be present. While there is also a great deal of dispute over the inherent toxicity of the antigens that many vaccines present to the immune systems of those vaccinated, there is no question, for example, that thimerosal, a mercury-containing preservative, is highly toxic when present in significant amounts. This then begs the question: rather than argue whether there is an infinitesimal, minimal, moderate, or significant amount of toxicity associated with the amounts of thimerosal or other potentially toxic components presently being used in vaccines, why not just neutralize whatever toxicity is present as completely and definitively as possible?

Vitamin C Is a Potent Antitoxin

In addition to its general antitoxin properties,[1] vitamin C has been demonstrated to be highly effective in neutralizing the toxic nature of mercury in all of its chemical forms. In animal studies, vitamin C can prevent the death of animals given otherwise fatal doses of mercury chloride.[2] Having vitamin C on board prior to mercury exposure was able to prevent the kidney damage the mercury otherwise typically caused.[3] Vitamin C also blocked the fatal effect of mercury cyanide.[4] Even the very highly toxic organic forms of mercury have been shown to be effectively detoxified by vitamin C.[5]

Vitamin C Improves Vaccine Effectiveness

By potential toxicity considerations alone, then, there would seem to be no good reason not to pre- and postmedicate an infant or child with some amount of vitamin C to minimize or block the toxicity that might significantly affect a few. However, there is another compelling reason to make vitamin C an integral part of any vaccination protocol: vitamin C has been documented to augment the antibody response of the immune system.[6–14] As the goal of any vaccination is to stimulate a maximal antibody response to the antigens of the vaccine while causing minimal to no toxic damage to the most sensitive of vaccine recipients, there would appear to be no medically sound reason not to make vitamin C a part of all vaccination protocols. Except in individuals with established, significant renal insufficiency, vitamin C is arguably the safest of all nutrients that can be given, especially in the amounts discussed below. Unlike virtually all prescription drugs and some supplements, vitamin C has never been found to have any dosage level above which it can be expected to demonstrate any toxicity.

Vitamin C Reduces Mortality in Vaccinated Infants and Children

Archie Kalokerinos, MD,[15] demonstrated repeatedly and quite conclusively that Aboriginal infants and children, a group with an unusually high death rate after vaccinations, were almost completely protected from this outcome by dosing them with vitamin C before and after vaccinations. The reason articulated for the high death rate was the exceptionally poor and near-scurvy-inducing (vitamin C–depleted) diet that was common in the Aboriginal culture. This also demonstrates that with the better nutrition in the United States and elsewhere in the world, the suggested doses of vitamin C should give an absolute protection against death (essentially a toxin-induced acute scurvy) and almost absolute protection against lesser toxic outcomes from any vaccinations administered. Certainly, there appears to be no logical reason not to give a nontoxic substance known to neutralize toxicity and stimulate antibody production, which is the whole point of vaccine administration.

Dosage Information for Pediatricians and Parents

Practically speaking, then, how should the pediatrician or parent proceed? For optimal antibody stimulation and toxin protection, it would be best to dose for three to five days before the shot(s) and to continue for at least two to three days following the shot. When dealing with infants and very young children, administering a 1,000 milligram (mg) dose of liposome-encapsulated vitamin C would be both easiest and best, as the gel-like nature of this form of vitamin C allows a ready mixture into yogurt or any other palatable food, and the complete proximal absorption of the liposomes would avoid any possible loose stools or other possible undesirable bowel effects.

Vitamin C as sodium ascorbate powder will also work well. Infants under ten pounds can take 500 mg daily in some fruit juice, while babies between ten and 20 pounds could take anywhere from 500 mg to 1,000 mg total per day, in divided doses. Older children can take 1,000 mg daily per year of life (5,000 mg for a five-year-old child, for example, in divided doses). If sodium must be avoided, calcium ascorbate is well-tolerated and, like sodium ascorbate, is non-acidic. Some but not all children's chewable vitamins are made with calcium ascorbate. Be sure to read the label. Giving vitamin C in divided doses, all through the day, improves absorption and improves tolerance. As children get older, they can more easily handle the ascorbic acid form of vitamin C, especially if given with meals. For any child showing significant bowel sensitivity, either use liposome-encapsulated vitamin C, or the amount of regular vitamin C can just be appropriately decreased to an easily tolerated amount.

Very similar considerations exist for older individuals receiving any of a number of vaccinations for preventing infection, such as the yearly flu shots. When there is really no urgency, and there rarely is, such individuals should supplement with vitamin C for several weeks before and several weeks after, if at all possible.

Even taking a one-time dose of vitamin C in the dosage range suggested above directly before the injections can still have a significant toxin-neutralizing and antibody-stimulating effect. It's just that an even better likelihood of having a positive outcome results from extending the pre- and postdose periods of time.

REFERENCES FOR "VITAMIN C PREVENTS VACCINATION SIDE EFFECTS"

1. Levy T. *Curing the Incurable. Vitamin C, Infectious Diseases, and Toxins*. Henderson, NV: MedFox Publishing, 2004.

2. Mokranjac M, Petrovic C. Vitamin C as an antidote in poisoning by fatal doses of mercury. *C R Hebd Seances Acad Sci 1964;258:1341–1342.*

3. Carroll R, Kovacs K, Tapp E. Protection against mercuric chloride poisoning of the rat kidney. *Arzneimittelforschung* 1965;15:1361–1363.

4. Vauthey M. Protective effect of vitamin C against poisons. *Praxis* (Bern) 1951;40:284–286.

5. Gage J. Mechanisms for the biodegradation of organic mercury compounds: the actions of ascorbate and of soluble proteins. *Toxicol Appl Pharmacol* 1975;32(2):225–238.

6. Prinz W, Bortz R, Bregin B, et al. The effect of ascorbic acid supplementation on some parameters of the human immunological defence system. *Int J Vitam Nutr Res* 1977;47(3):2248–2257.

7. Vallance S. Relationships between ascorbic acid and serum proteins of the immune system. *Br Med J* 1977;2(6084):437–438.

8. Prinz W, Bloch J, Gilich G, et al. A systematic study of the effect of vitamin C supplementation on the humoral immune response in ascorbate-dependent mammals. I. The antibody response to sheep red blood cells (a T-dependent antigen) in guinea pigs. *Int J Vitam Nutr Res* 1980;50(3):294–300.

9. Feigen GA, Smith BH, Dix CE, et al. Enhancement of antibody production and protection against systemic anaphylaxis by large doses of vitamin C. *Res Commun Chem Pathol Pharmacol* 1982;38(2):313–333.

10. Li Y, Lovell R. Elevated levels of dietary ascorbic acid increase immune responses in channel catfish. *J Nutr* 1985;115(1):123–131.

11. Amakye-Anim J, Lin T, Hester P, et al. Ascorbic acid supplementation improved antibody response to infectious bursal disease vaccination in chickens. *Poult Sci* 2000;79(5):680–688.

12. Wu C, Dorairajan T, Lin T. Effect of ascorbic acid supplementation on the immune response of chickens vaccinated and challenged with infectious bursal disease virus. *Vet Immunol Immunopathol* 2000;74 (1–2):145–152.

13. Lauridsen C, Jensen SK. Influence of supplementation of all-rac-alpha-tocopheryl acetate preweaning and vitamin C postweaning on alpha-tocopherol and immune responses in piglets. *J Anim Sci* 2005;83(6): 1274–1286.

14. Azad I, Dayal J, Poornima M, et al. Supra dietary levels of vitamins C and E enhance antibody production and immune memory in juvenile milkfish. Chanos chanos (Forsskal) to formalin-killed *Vibrio vulnificus. Fish Shellfish Immunol* 2007;23(1):154–163.

15. Kalokerinos A. *Every Second Child.* New Canaan, CT: Keats Publishing, 1974.

SHINGLES TREATMENT THAT WORKS

From the *Orthomolecular Medicine News Service,* June 15, 2005.

Shingles (herpes zoster) can be cleared up by using a safe, convenient, inexpensive, nonprescription treatment of vitamin C. Vitamin C is antiviral and antitoxin and inactivates the virus that causes shingles. If you have shingles and want relief, you can try this:

Go to a discount store and buy a large bottle of 1,000 milligram (mg) vitamin C tablets. The cost should be less than $15.

Begin when you wake in the morning by taking 3,000 mg of vitamin C every 30 minutes and continue until you have a single episode of loose stool (not quite diarrhea). If you haven't had loose stool after 15 hours on this dosage, increase the vitamin C to 4,000 mg every 30 minutes.

After you have a loose bowel movement, reduce the dosage to 2,000 mg of vitamin C taken every hour. You will quickly find the dosage that is right for you. Adjust the dosage of vitamin C downward to stay below the dosage that will cause loose stool, and adjust it upward to relieve shingles symptoms. Continue the oral vitamin C therapy until the shingles disappear. It sounds too simple to be true, doesn't it? But it works in the majority of cases, as recently reconfirmed by Thomas E. Levy, MD, JD.[1]

Sometimes it's necessary to take vitamin C intravenously (IV) for massive shingles outbreaks.[2] Much higher concentrations of vitamin C in the blood can be achieved intravenously than when taken orally. As early as 1950, the medical literature reported that one physician had confirmed that intravenous vitamin C cured shingles in 327 patients within 72 hours.[3] Ask your doctor if he or she offers vitamin C IV and, if not, ask friends or search the Internet to find a doctor or facility that does offer this treatment.

Vitamin C blood serum levels of individuals fall during periods of high stress and they develop sub-clinical scurvy (depleted vitamin C levels). This situation can set the stage for a shingles attack.

Remember, a vitamin can act as a drug, but a drug can never act as a vitamin.

With vitamin therapy, at any given quantity, frequently divided doses are more effective than a large single dose.

The reason one nutrient can cure so many different illnesses is because a deficiency of one nutrient can cause many different illnesses.

REFERENCES FOR "SHINGLES TREATMENT THAT WORKS"

1. Levy TE. *Vitamin C, Infectious Diseases, and Toxins: Curing the Incurable [Kindle Edition]*. Xlibris, 2002.

2. Klenner FR. Observations on the dose and administration of ascorbic acid when employed beyond the range of a vitamin in human pathology. *J Appl Nutr* 1971; 23(3 & 4): 61–88.

3. Zureick M. Therapy of herpes and herpes zoster with intravenous vitamin C. *J Prat Rev Gen Clin Ther* 1950;64(48):586.

VITAMINS D AND C AND TREATING TB

by Steve Hickey, PhD, and William B. Grant, PhD

From "Progress with TB or a Return to the Dark Ages?" *Orthomolecular Medicine News Service,* Jun 17, 2013.

Tuberculosis (TB) was formerly one of the most devastating scourges of mankind and remains a leading cause of death. The disease has been with humans over recorded history, and likely throughout the evolution of our species. Through the industrial revolution and into the 20th century, TB became a long-term medical emergency, particularly with the poor. Roughly one person in four was dying of the disease in England, and similar death rates were observed in other modernizing countries. One solution was to isolate the afflicted in sanatoria. The "fresh air and sunlight" solution practiced in those times may have been at least partly effective.

Sunlight and vitamin D played an early role in preventing and treating TB. In the early 20th century, TB patients were often sent to sanatoria in the mountains where they were exposed to solar radiation. Dr. Auguste Rollier set up such facilities in the Swiss Alps.[1] Sun exposure is associated with a lower incidence of TB six months later.[2] It wasn't until 2006-7 that researchers at UCLA determined how sunlight increased vitamin D levels and helps the body's immune system prevent bacterial infections.[3]. Higher blood levels of 25-hydroxyvitamin D can reduce the time required to control TB during treatment.[4,5] Recent research suggests the sanatoria approach to treatment could have been at least partly effective.

The modern myth about conquering infectious diseases such as TB is that vaccination and antibiotics came to the rescue, saving humanity from the earlier suffering. However, TB like the other major life threatening infections had already declined to a low level before these interventions were introduced. The tubercle bacillus was identified by Robert Koch in 1882,[6] by which time the death rates in England and Wales had already dropped to about half the earlier levels. The introduction of the drug isoniazid in the early 1950s was a breakthrough in antibiotic treatment but had little effect on overall mortality. Similarly, BCG vaccination was first tried in people in the early 1920s, but its widespread introduction was delayed until well after World War II. A chart of mortality (on page 366) from TB shows its historical decline in England and Wales, for which the most extensive historical statistics are available.[7] The decline of TB was similar to the reduction in mortality for the other major infectious diseases. This graph illustrates the relative contribution of vaccination and antibiotic chemotherapy. By the time these interventions had been introduced, the major infections had already been largely defeated.

The question raised by this graph is what really caused the decline in death rates from TB and other infections. We can answer this easily and directly. Firstly, TB did not go away. There is a reasonable chance that a reader is harboring the disease. Roughly one person in every three in the world (two to three billion) has the infection. However, only ten to 20 million have the active disease. So only one person in every 100 or so infected will have any symptoms. The rest will happily coexist with their "infection" without concern.

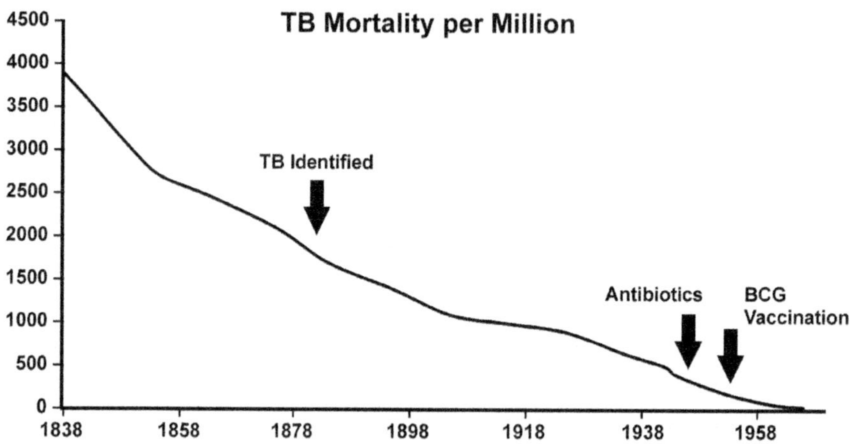

People who come down with TB have poor or compromised immune systems. The disadvantaged were living in crowded and damp slum conditions. Although such conditions facilitate spread of the infection, this explanation is insufficient. Poor nutrition provides a more direct explanation of why only some of the infected go on to succumb to the illness.

TB and Vitamin C

Despite the data strongly suggesting the impact of nutrition, corporate medicine has consistently decried the use of supplements. However, there has been a long overdue development. Catherine Vilchèze and colleagues have returned to testing the extraordinary antibiotic properties of vitamin C for TB.[8] They found that "*M. tuberculosis* is highly susceptible to killing by vitamin C,"[3] which is consistent with previous data.[9] Notably, the mechanism of action is similar to vitamin C's anticancer role in generating hydrogen peroxide locally, which kills the unwanted cells.[10] We have been using antibiotic treatment of TB as a model for the role of vitamin C–based redox therapy for cancer. The same mechanism is used to protect the body against both microorganisms and abnormal cancer cells.

Supplementation with vitamin C may prevent TB infection from becoming overt. Furthermore, vitamin C could provide an effective biological treatment for TB with the advantage of a mechanism refined by millions of years of evolution. As scientific history demonstrates, good nutrition, particularly vitamins C and D, are likely to be far more effective than antibiotics and vaccination in preventing this and other dangerous infective diseases.

Vilcheze's research suggests that drugs with a similar mechanism of action to vitamin C might be developed (presumably with great commercial advantage). However, such drugs are an unnatural intervention and are likely to have unnecessary side effects while vitamin C is safe. The rather obvious implication of providing high-dose nutritional supplements is once again ignored. If supplementation were to be widely applied, our society may find controlling TB is unexpectedly easy.

The recent history of antibiotics is one of misuse leading to microbial resistance. Following Multiple Drug Resistant TB (MDRTB) and eXtensively Drug Resistant forms (XDRTB), we are now faced with Totally Drug Resistant forms (TDRTB). The increasingly ineffective antibiotics have helped promote the return to study vitamin C as a potential treatment. However, we may be faced with something far more threatening. The history of antibiotic abuse is not reassuring. It may be possible to generate more virulent forms despite Vilcheze's confirmation that resistance to vitamin C is exceptionally difficult to induce. The use of drugs with a similar mechanism to vitamin C may lead to resistance to our basic biological defense mechanisms. In other words, corporate misuse of this latest development could return us to the dark days of uncontrolled infections when TB was killing one in four people in the developed nations.

Conclusion

Much of the recent freedom from deadly infectious disease reflects historical improvements in nutrition. Over time the mechanisms by which nutrients help people be more resistant to infections are being elucidated. Increased levels of vitamin D may have provided a lower risk of TB and other infections as well as the deficiency disease rickets. It now appears that vitamin C is "extraordinarily" effective in killing the TB microorganism. Importantly vitamin C kills TB in essentially the same way as it destroys cancer cells. Linus Pauling, PhD, Robert Cathcart, MD, and others may have been prescient in suggesting vitamin C provides a unique way of maintaining good health.

REFERENCES FOR "VITAMINS D AND C AND TREATING TB"

1. Hobday RA. Sunlight therapy and solar architecture. *Med Hist* 1997; 41(4): 455–472.

2. Koh GC, Hawthorne G, Turner AM, et al. Tuberculosis incidence correlates with sunshine: an ecological 28-year time series study. *PLoS One* 2012; 8(3): e57752.

3. Liu PT, Stenger S, Tang DH, et al. Cutting edge: vitamin D-mediated human antimicrobial activity against *Mycobacterium tuberculosis* is dependent on the induction of cathelicidin. *J Immunol* 2007; 179(4): 2060–2063.

4. Sato S, Tanino Y, Saito J, et al. The relationship between 25-hydroxyvitamin D levels and treatment course of pulmonary tuberculosis. *Respir Investig* 2012; 50(2): 40–45.

5. Coussens AK, Wilkinson RJ, Hanifa Y, et al. Vitamin D accelerates resolution of inflammatory responses during tuberculosis treatment. *Proc Natl Acad Sci U S A* 2012; 109(38):15449–15454.

6. Mörner KAH. Nobel Prize in Physiology or Medicine 1905, Presentation Speech, 2005.

7. McKeown T. *The Role of Medicine,* Blackwell, 1979.

8. Vilchèze C, Hartman T, Weinrick B, et al. *Mycobacterium tuberculosis* is extraordinarily sensitive to killing by a vitamin C-induced Fenton reaction. *Nature Communications* 2013; doi:10.1038/ncomms2898.

9. Hickey S, Saul AW. *Vitamin C: The Real Story: The Remarkable and Controversial Healing Factor.* Laguna Beach, CA: Basic Health Publications, 2008.

10. Hickey S, Roberts H. Vitamin C and cancer: is there a role for oral vitamin C? *J Orthomolecular Med* 2013; 28(1): 33–46.

WHAT REALLY CAUSES KIDNEY STONES (AND WHY VITAMIN C DOES NOT)

From the *Orthomolecular Medicine News Service,* February 11, 2013.

A widely-publicized study claimed that vitamin C supplements increased the risk of developing kidney stones by nearly a factor of two.[1] The study stated that the stones were most likely formed from calcium oxalate, which can be formed in the presence of vitamin C (ascorbate), but it did not analyze the kidney stones of participants. Instead, it relied on a different study of kidney stones in which ascorbate was not tested. This type of poorly organized study does not help the medical profession or the public, but instead causes confusion.

The study followed 23,355 Swedish men for a decade. They were divided into two groups, one that did not take any supplements (n=22,448), and another that took supplements of vitamin C (n=907). The average diet for each group was tabulated, but not in much detail. Then the participants who got kidney stones in each group were tabulated, and the group that took vitamin C appeared to have a greater risk of kidney stones. The extra risk of kidney stones from ascorbate presented in the study is very low, 147 per 100,000 person-years, or only 0.15 percent per year.

Key points the media missed:

- The number of kidney stones in the study participants who took ascorbate was very low (31 stones in over a decade), so the odds for statistical error in the study are fairly high.
- The study was observational. It simply tabulated the intake of vitamin C and the number of kidney stones to try to find an association between them.

- This method does not imply a causative factor because it was not a randomized controlled study; that is, vitamin C was not given to a group selected at random.
- This type of observational study is fraught with limitations that make its conclusion unreliable.
- It contradicts previous studies that have clearly shown that high-dose ascorbate does not cause kidney stones.[2–6]
- The study authors' conclusion that ascorbate caused the low rate of stones is likely due to a correlation between the choice of taking a vitamin C supplement with some other aspect of the participants' diet.
- The study could not determine the nature of this type of correlation, because it lacked a detailed study of each patient's diet and a chemical analysis of each stone to provide a hint about the probable cause.

So we have a poorly designed study that did not determine what kind of stone was formed, or what caused the stones that were formed. These are serious flaws. Drawing conclusions from such a study can hardly be a good example of "evidence-based medicine."

Different Types of Kidney Stones (Renal Calculi)

There is a considerable variety of kidney stones. Here are five well-known ones:

1. *Calcium phosphate stones* are common and easily dissolve in urine acidified by vitamin C.
2. *Calcium oxalate stones* are also common but they do not dissolve in acid urine. We will discuss this type further below.
3. *Magnesium ammonium phosphate (struvite) stones* are much less common, often appearing after an infection. They dissolve in urine acidified by vitamin C.
4. *Uric acid stones* result from a problem metabolizing purines (the chemical base of adenine, xanthine, theobromine [in chocolate], and uric acid). They may form in a condition such as gout.
5. *Cystine stones* result from a hereditary inability to reabsorb cystine. Most children's stones are this type, and these are rare.

The Oxalate Oxymoron

The oxalate/vitamin C issue appears contradictory. Oxalate is in oxalate stones and oxalate stones are common. Ascorbate (the active ion in vitamin C) may slightly increase the body's production of oxalate. Yet, in practice, vitamin C does not increase oxalate stone formation. Emanuel Cheraskin, MD, DMD, professor of oral medicine at the University of Alabama, explains why: "Vitamin C in the urine tends to bind calcium and decrease its free form. This means less chance of calcium's separating out as calcium oxalate (stones)."[7] Also, the diuretic effect of vitamin C reduces urine concentration of oxalate. Fast-moving rivers deposit little silt. If on a consultation, a doctor advises that you are especially prone to forming oxalate stones, read the suggestions below before abandoning the benefits of vitamin C. Once again: vitamin C increases oxalate but inhibits the union of calcium and oxalate.

Oxalate is generated by many foods in the diet, including spinach (100–200 milligrams [mg] oxalate per ounce of spinach), rhubarb, and beets. Tea and coffee are thought to be the largest source of oxalate in the diet of many people, up to 150–300 mg per day.[8–11] This is considerably more than would likely be generated by an ascorbate dose of 1,000 mg per day.[5,12]

The study we are discussing didn't tabulate the participants' intake of oxalate, but on average they had relatively high intakes (several cups) of tea and coffee. It is possible that those who had kidney stones had them before the study started, or got them during the study, due to a particularly high intake of oxalate. For example, the participants that took vitamin C may have been trying to stay healthy, but the subset of those who got kidney stones might also have been trying to stay healthy by drinking a lot of tea or coffee, or eating green leafy vegetables such as spinach. Or they may have been older people who got dehydrated, which is also very common among men who are active outside during the summer. Among the most important factors in kidney stones is dehydration, especially among the elderly.[13]

To summarize:

- Ascorbate in low or high doses generally does not cause significant increase in urinary oxalate.[2–6]
- Ascorbate tends to *prevent* formation of calcium oxalate kidney stones.[3,4]
- Risk factors for kidney stones include a history of hypertension, obesity, chronic dehydration, poor diet, and a low dietary intake of magnesium.

Magnesium

Kidney stones and magnesium deficiency share the same list of causes, including a diet high in sugar, alcohol, oxalates, and coffee. Magnesium has an important role in the prevention of kidney stone formation.[14] Magnesium stimulates production of calcitonin, which draws calcium out of the blood and soft tissues back into the bones, preventing some forms of arthritis and kidney stones. Magnesium suppresses parathyroid hormone, preventing it from breaking down bone. Magnesium converts vitamin D into its active form so that it can assist in calcium absorption. Magnesium is required to activate an enzyme that is necessary to form new bone. Magnesium regulates active calcium transport. All these factors help place calcium where it needs to be, and not in kidney stones.

One of magnesium's many jobs is to keep calcium in solution to prevent it from solidifying into crystals; even at times of dehydration, if there is sufficient magnesium, calcium will stay in solution. Magnesium is a pivotal treatment for kidney stones. If you don't have enough magnesium to help dissolve calcium, you will end up with various forms of calcification. This translates into stones, muscle spasms, fibrositis, fibromyalgia, and atherosclerosis (as in calcification of the arteries). Dr. George Bunce has clinically demonstrated the relationship between kidney stones and magnesium deficiency. As early as 1964, Bunce reported the benefits of administering a 420 mg dose of magnesium oxide per day to patients who had a history of frequent stone formation.[14,15] If poorly absorbed magnesium oxide works, other forms of better-absorbed magnesium will work better.

Calcium oxalate stones can effectively be prevented by getting an adequate amount of magnesium, through either foods high in magnesium (buckwheat, green vegetables, beans, nuts), or magnesium supplements. Take a magnesium supplement of *at least* the US RDA of 300 to 400 mg per day (more may be desirable in order to maintain an ideal 1:1 balance of magnesium to calcium). To prevent a laxative effect, take a supplement that is readily absorbable, such as magnesium citrate, chelate, malate, or chloride. Magnesium oxide, mentioned above, is cheap and widely available. However, magnesium oxide is only about 5 percent absorbed and thus acts mostly as a laxative.[14] Milk of magnesia (magnesium hydroxide) is even more of a laxative, and unsuitable for supplementation. Magnesium citrate is a good choice: easy to find, relatively inexpensive, and well absorbed.

The Role of Vitamin C in Preventing and Dissolving Kidney Stones

The calcium phosphate kidney stone can only exist in a urinary tract that is not acidic. Ascorbic acid (vitamin C's most common form) acidifies the urine, thereby dissolving phosphate stones and preventing their formation.

Acidic urine will also dissolve magnesium ammonium phosphate stones, which would otherwise require surgical removal. These are the same struvite stones associated with urinary tract infections. Both the infection and the stone are easily cured with vitamin C in large doses. Both are virtually 100 percent preventable with daily consumption of much-greater-than-RDA amounts of ascorbic acid. A gorilla gets about 4,000 mg of vitamin C a day in its natural diet. The US RDA for humans is only 90 mg. The gorillas are unlikely to all be wrong.

The common calcium oxalate stone can form in an acidic urine whether one takes vitamin C or not. However, this type of stone can be prevented by adequate quantities of B-complex vitamins and magnesium. Any common B-complex supplement, twice daily, plus about 400 mg of magnesium, is usually adequate.

A Dozen Ways to Reduce Your Risk of Kidney Stones

1. Maximize fluid intake.[13] Especially drink fruit and vegetable juices. Orange, grape, and carrot juices are high in citrates, which both inhibit a buildup of uric acid and also stop calcium salts from forming.[16]
2. Control urine pH. Slightly acidic urine helps prevent urinary tract infections, dissolves both phosphate and struvite stones, and will not cause oxalate stones. And of course one way to make urine slightly acidic is to take vitamin C.
3. Avoid excessive oxalates by not eating (much) rhubarb, spinach, chocolate, or dark tea or coffee.
4. Lose weight. Being overweight is associated with substantially increased risk of kidney stones.[17]
5. Calcium is probably not the real culprit. Low calcium may itself cause calcium stones.[18]
6. Most kidney stones are compounds of calcium, and yet many Americans are calcium deficient. Instead of lowering calcium intake, reduce excess dietary phosphorous by avoiding carbonated soft drinks, especially colas. Cola soft drinks contain excessive quantities of phosphorous as phosphoric acid. This is the same acid that is used by dentists to dissolve tooth enamel before applying bonding resins.
7. Take a magnesium supplement of *at least* the US RDA of 300 to 400 mg per day. More may be desirable in order to maintain an ideal 1:1 balance of magnesium to calcium. Many people eating "modern" processed-food diets do not consume optimal quantities of magnesium.
8. Take a good B-complex vitamin supplement twice daily; make sure it contains pyridoxine (vitamin B_6). A deficiency of vitamin B_6 produces kidney stones in experimental animals. Vitamin B_6 deficiency is very common in humans. A vitamin B_1 (thiamine) deficiency also is associated with stones.[19]
9. For uric acid/purine stones (gout), stop eating meat. Nutrition tables and textbooks indicate meat as the major dietary purine source. Natural treatment adds juice fasts and eating sour cherries. Increased vitamin C consumption helps by improving the urinary excretion of uric acid.[12] For these stones, use buffered ascorbate "C."
10. Persons with cystine stones (only 1 percent of all kidney stones) should follow a low-methionine diet and use buffered vitamin C.
11. Kidney stones are associated with high sugar intake, so eat less (or no) added sugar.[20]
12. Infections can cause conditions that favor stone formation, such as overly concentrated urine (from fever sweating, vomiting, or diarrhea). Practice good preventive health care, and it will pay you back with interest.

REFERENCES FOR "WHAT REALLY CAUSES KIDNEY STONES"

1. Thomas LDK, Elinder CG, Tiselius HG, et al. Ascorbic acid supplements and kidney stone incidence among men: A prospective study. *JAMA Intern Med* 2013;173(5):386–388. doi:10.1001/jamainternmed.2013.2296.

2. Wandzilak TR, D'Andre SD, Davis PA, et al. Effect of high dose vitamin C on urinary oxalate levels. *J Urology* 1994;151:834–837.

3. Hickey S, Saul AW. *Vitamin C: The Real Story, the Remarkable and Controversial Healing Factor.* Laguna Beach, CA: Basic Health Publications, 2008.

4. Hickey S, Roberts H. Vitamin C does not cause kidney stones. *Orthomolecular Medicine News Service,* Jul 5, 2005. Available at: http://orthomolecular.org/resources/omns/v01n07.shtml.

5. Robitaille L, Mamer OA, Miller WH Jr, et al. Oxalic acid excretion after intravenous ascorbic acid administration. *Metabolism* 2009;58(2):263–269. doi: 10.1016/j.metabol.2008.09.023.

6. Padayatty SJ, Sun AY, Chen Q, et al. Vitamin C: intravenous use by complementary and alternative medicine practitioners and adverse effects. *PLoS One* 2010;5(7):e11414. doi: 10.1371/journal.pone.0011414.

7. Cheraskin E, Ringsdorf M Jr, Sisley E. *The Vitamin C Connection.* York: Harper & Row, 1983.

8. Noonan SC, Savage GP. Oxalate content of foods and its effect on humans. *Asia Pacific Journal of Clinical Nutrition* 1999; 8:64–74.

9. Kawazua Y, Okimurab M, Ishiic T, et al. Varietal and seasonal differences in oxalate content of spinach. *Scientia Horticulturae* 2003;97:203–210

10. Proietti S, Moscatello S, Famiani F, et al. Increase of ascorbic acid content and nutritional quality in spinach leaves during physiological acclimation to low temperature. *Plant Physiol Biochem* 2009;47(8):717–23.

11. Gasinska A, Gajewska D. Tea and coffee as the main sources of oxalate in diets of patients with kidney oxalate stones. *ROCZN PZH* 2008;58(1):61–67.

12. Pauling L. *How to Live Longer and Feel Better.* Corvallis, Oregon: Oregon State University Press, 2006.

13. Manz F, Wentz A. The importance of good hydration for the prevention of chronic diseases. *Nutr Rev* 2005;63(6 Pt 2):S2-S5.

14. Dean C. *The Magnesium Miracle.* New York: Ballantine Books, 2007.

15. Bunce GE, Li BW, Price NO, et al. Distribution of calcium and magnesium in rat kidney homogenate fractions accompanying magnesium deficiency induced nephrocalcinosis. *Exp Mol Pathol* 1974; 21(1):16–28.

16. Carper J. Orange juice may prevent kidney stones, Lancaster *Intelligencer-Journal,* Jan 5, 1994.

17. Bagga HS, Chi T, Miller J, et al. New insights into the pathogenesis of renal calculi. *Urol Clin North Am* 2013;40(1):1–12. doi: 10.1016/j.ucl.2012.09.006.

18. Smith LH, et al. Medical evaluation of urolithiasis. *Urol Clin North Am* 1974;1(2): 241–260.

19. Hagler L, Herman RH. Oxalate metabolism, II. *Am J Clin Nutr* 1973;26(8): 882–889.

20. Thom JA, Morris JE, Bishop A, et al. The influence of refined carbohydrate on urinary calcium excretion. *Br J Urol* 1978;50(7): 459–464.

How Doctors Use Vitamin C Against Lead Poisoning

by Andrew W. Saul, PhD

From the *Orthomolecular Medicine News Service,* January 26, 2016.

We hear about the hazards of lead. We know that lead poisoning can cause severe mental retardation. Lead has been clearly linked with Alzheimer's disease. We have been told to avoid lead in our homes and in our water, and to clean up lead pollution in our environment. But we have not been told how to remove it from our bodies. Vitamin C megadoses may be the answer.

Dr. Erik Paterson, of British Columbia, reports, "When I was a consulting physician for a center for the mentally challenged, a patient showing behavioral changes was found to have blood lead levels some ten times higher than the acceptable levels. I administered vitamin C at a dose of 4,000 milligrams (mg) per day. I anticipated a slow response. The following year I rechecked his blood lead level. It had gone up, much to my initial dismay. But then I thought that perhaps what was happening was that the vitamin C was mobilizing the lead from his tissues. So we persisted. The next year, on rechecking, the lead levels had markedly dropped to well below the initial result. As the years went by, the levels became almost undetectable, and his behavior was markedly improved."

How Much Vitamin C?

Frederick Robert Klenner, MD, insisted that large amounts of vitamin C are needed to do the job. One old (1940) paper got it wrong, and Dr. Klenner comments: "The report by Dannenberg that high doses of ascorbic acid were without effect in treating lead intoxication in a child must be ignored, since his extremely high dose was 25 mg by mouth four times a day and one single daily injection of 250 mg of C. Had he administered 350 mg per kilogram (kg) body weight every two hours, he would have seen the other side of the coin."

Here is what 350 mg of vitamin C per kilogram body weight works out to in pounds, approximately:

Milligrams Vitamin C	Body Weight
35,000 mg	220 pounds
18,000	110 lb
9,000	55 lb
4,500	28 lb
2,300	14–15 lb
1,200	7–8 lb

Although these quantities may seem high, it must be pointed out that Dr. Klenner administered such amounts every two hours.

Vitamin C may be given intravenously if necessary. Oral vitamin C may be given as liquid, powder, tablet, or chewable tablet. Toddlers often accept powdered, naturally sweetened chewable tablets, which may be crushed between two spoons and added to a favorite food. Infants do well with liquid vitamin C. You can make this yourself by daily dissolving ascorbic acid powder in a small dropper bottle and adding it to fruit juice. Dr. Klenner recommended daily preventive doses, which he described as 1,000 mg of vitamin C per year of a child's age, plateauing at 10,000 mg per day for teens and adults.

"Vitamin C? But . . ."

Common questions from readers are likely to include the following, to which we have provided the briefest of answers.

"Why so much?" Because too little will not be effective. Dr. Klenner, as well as Robert F. Cathcart, MD, Hugh D. Riordan, MD, Abram Hoffer, MD, and many other highly experienced nutritional physicians have all emphasized this.

"Is it safe?" Year after year, decade after decade, national data shows no deaths at all from vitamin C. Vitamin C does not cause kidney stones, either. Read up so you know what you are doing. Work with your doctor. And make sure your doctor has read what you've read.

"Is ascorbic acid really vitamin C?" Yes. Linus Pauling, double Nobel prize–winning chemist, said so. He ought to know. Almost all successful medical research on vitamin C therapy has used plain, cheap, you-can-buy-it-anywhere ascorbic acid. Other forms of C will also work well.

"That's it?" Certainly not. All sources of lead contamination must be addressed and eliminated. Vitamin C has an important role to play in so doing, and should be publicly advocated by the medical professions, government, and the media.

Immediately.

VITAMIN C SAVES LIVES

From the *Orthomolecular Medicine News Service,* April 22, 2005.

Millions die each year from heart disease and stroke, and the overwhelming evidence is that vitamin C supplementation would save many lives.

Two-time Nobel Prize winner Dr. Linus Pauling estimated that the rate of heart disease would be reduced by 80 percent if adults in the US supplemented with 2,000 to 3,000 milligrams (mg) of vitamin C each day. According to Dr. Pauling, "Since vitamin C deficiency is the common cause of human heart disease, vitamin C supplementation is the universal treatment for this disease."[1] Heart disease is the number-one killer in the US. For those with existing heart disease, Dr. Pauling said that blockage of heart arteries could actually be reversed by supplementing with 6,000 mg of vitamin C and 6,000 mg of lysine (a common amino acid), taken in divided doses throughout the day. Vitamin C supplementation both lowers serum cholesterol levels and repairs lesions of arterial walls. Nobel Prize winner Dr. Louis J. Ignarro (1998) found that supplementing with vitamin C and vitamin E significantly reduces the risk of developing arteriosclerosis.[2]

A study examined vitamin E and vitamin C supplement use in relation to mortality risk in 11,178 persons aged 67 to 105 who participated in the Established Populations for Epidemiologic Studies of the Elderly over a nine-year period.[3] Simultaneous use of vitamins E and C was associated with a lower risk of total mortality and coronary mortality after adjusting for alcohol use, smoking history, aspirin use, and medical conditions.

A landmark study following more than 85,000 nurses over a 16-year period for a total of 1,240,000 person-years found that vitamin C supplementation significantly reduced the risk of heart disease.[4] Intake of vitamin C from foods alone was insufficient to significantly affect the rate of heart disease. High quantities of vitamin C from supplements was essential to provide the protective effects. The study adjusted for age, smoking, and a variety of other coronary risk factors.

An international team pooled data from nine prospective studies of 293,000 people that included information on intakes of vitamin E, carotenoids, and vitamin C, with a ten-year follow-up to check for major-incident coronary heart disease events in people without disease when the study began. Dietary intake of antioxidant vitamins was only weakly related to a reduced coronary heart disease risk. However, subjects who took as little as 700 mg of vitamin C daily in supplement form reduced their risk of heart disease events by 25 per cent compared to those who took no supplements.[5]

Researchers in Finland measured serum vitamin C levels in 2,419 middle-aged male participants of the ongoing Kuopio Ischemic Heart Disease Risk Factor Study. Men with a history of stroke were excluded from this analysis. Participants were followed for up to ten years; the outcome of interest was development of stroke. During the follow-up period 120 participants suffered a stroke. After controlling for potential confounders—including age, body mass index (BMI), smoking, blood pressure, and serum cholesterol—the researchers found that men with a low vitamin C level in their blood were more than twice as likely as those with a higher vitamin C blood level to experience a stroke.[6]

A stroke commonly occurs when a blood clot or thrombus blocks the blood flow to parts of the brain. A thrombus may form in an artery affected by arteriosclerosis. A study in *Stroke* has shown how low plasma vitamin C was associated with increased risk of stroke, especially among hypertensive and overweight men.[7]

Vitamin C preserves the integrity of the artery walls and strengthens cardiovascular tissue. Research indicates a reduced incidence of major coronary heart disease events at high supplemental vitamin C intakes.[8] Studies have shown that vitamin C appears to reduce levels of C-reactive protein (CRP), a marker of inflammation, and there is a growing body of evidence that chronic inflammation is linked to an increased risk of heart disease.[9]

Most Americans fail to eat the US Recommended Dietary Allowance (RDA) for several vitamins and minerals. Supplements are not the problem; they are the solution. Malnutrition is the problem.

REFERENCES FOR "VITAMIN C SAVES LIVES"

1. Rath M, Pauling L. A unified theory of human cardiovascular disease leading the way to the abolition of this disease as a cause for human mortality *J Orthomolecular Med* 1992; 7(1): 5–15.

2. Napoli C, Williams-Ignarro S, De Nigris F, et al. Long-term combined beneficial effects of physical training and metabolic treatment on arterioscleroses in hypercholesterolemic mice *Proc Natl Acad Sci U S A* 2004;101(23):8797–802

3. Losonczy KG, Harris TB, Havlik RJ. Vitamin E and vitamin C supplement use and risk of all-cause and coronary heart disease mortality in older persons: the Established Populations for Epidemiologic Studies of the Elderly. *Am J Clin Nutr* 1996;64(2):190–6.

4. Neale RJ, Lim H, Turner J, et al. The excretion of large vitamin C loads in young and elderly subjects: an ascorbic acid tolerance test. *Age Ageing* 1988; 17(1):35–41.

5. Knekt P, Ritz J, Pereira MA, et al. Antioxidant vitamins and coronary heart disease risk: a pooled analysis of 9 cohorts. *Am J of Clin Nutr* 2004; 80(6):1508–1520.

6. Kurl S, Tuomaninen TP, Laukkenen JA, et al. Plasma vitamin C modifies the association between hypertension and risk of stroke. *Stroke* 2002; 33(6):1568–1573.

7. Ibid.

8. Knekt P, Ritz J, Pereira MA, et al. Antioxidant vitamins and coronary heart disease risk: a pooled analysis of 9 cohorts. *Am J of Clin Nutr* 2004; 80(6):1508–1520.

9. Block G, Jensen C, Dietrich M, et al. Plasma C-reactive protein concentrations in active and passive smokers: influence of antioxidant supplementation. *J Am Coll of Nutr* 23(2):141–147.

ORTHOMOLECULAR TREATMENT FOR ADVERSE EFFECTS OF HUMAN PAPILLOMA VIRUS (HPV) VACCINE

by Atsuo Yanagisawa, MD, PhD

From the *Orthomolecular Medicine News Service,* May 7, 2015.

Immunization of adolescent girls with the human papilloma virus (HPV) vaccine was initiated with the intention to prevent uterine and cervical cancer. The first HPV vaccine, called Gardasil (Merck), was approved in 2006, and a second vaccine, called Cervarix (GSK), was introduced in 2007. By the end of 2013, approximately 130 million doses of Gardasil and 44 million doses of Cervarix had been distributed worldwide. In 2010, both vaccines were widely given to Japanese girls. In April 2013, Japan added both HPV vaccines to their government-recommended vaccination schedule.

High Incidence of Side Effects

In June 2013, only two months after the law was issued, the Japanese government suspended the recommendation for these vaccines. A new study reported that the adverse events of Gardasil and Cervarix were 1.7 to 3.6 times higher than those for other vaccines. The government task force analyzed reports of HPV vaccine injuries. They examined 2,500 cases and found 617 (25 percent) cases to be "serious."

Amazingly, the official task force then issued this statement: "We find no physical cause for the alleged and presumed adverse reactions in those vaccinated girls, so we cannot recommend any specific therapy. We conclude that their so-called adverse reactions are psychosomatic. The government should provide counseling to the girls so that they may be freed from their psychosomatic reactions."

Severity of Side Effects

When other health experts reevaluated those cases, they determined 1,112 (44 percent) to be serious. The initial onset of symptoms occurred several weeks to a year after the HPV vaccine was given. They included: headache, dizziness, muscle weakness and pain, nausea, hypersomnia, learning difficulty, impaired writing, photophobia, tremors of arms, feet, and fingers, joint pain, irregular menstruation, gait disturbance, memory loss, skin eczema, and acne.

Girls who had adverse effects from the HPV vaccine were variously diagnosed with:

1. Higher brain dysfunction
2. Guillain-Barré syndrome
3. Multiple sclerosis

4. ADEM: acute disseminated encephalomyelitis
5. SSPE: subacute sclerosing panencephalitis
6. CRPS: Complex regional pain syndrome
7. POTS: Postural orthostatic tachycardia syndrome
8. Anti-phospholipid antibody syndrome
9. SLE: systemic lupus erythematosus
10. Rheumatoid arthritis
11. Chronic fatigue syndrome
12. Fibromyalgia
13. Cushing's syndrome (exposure to high level of cortisol)
14. Hashimoto's disease (immune system attacks the thyroid)
15. Hyperprolactinemia (high prolactin, induces breast development and lactation)

Laboratory findings included:

1. Normal blood chemistry
2. No inflammatory finding in the blood
3. Increased pro-inflammatory cytokines in the spinal fluid (IL-2, IL-10, TNF-à)
4. Reduced brain blood flow by perfusion scintigraphy
5. High leukocyte sensitivity against aluminum

HPV Vaccine Contains Toxic Aluminum

Vaccines often contain an adjuvant, which is an additional chemical added to provoke the body's immune response to the vaccine. The HPV vaccines contained an adjuvant that consisted of an aluminum compound, amorphous aluminum hydroxyphosphate sulfate (AAHS).

Current research strongly implicates aluminum adjuvants in various inflammatory neurological and autoimmune disorders in both humans and animals. For example, one paper explained that nanomaterials such as this aluminum adjuvant can be transported by immune system cells first into the blood, lymph nodes, and spleen, and in some cases may penetrate into the brain.[1] This type of access throughout the body is potentially life-threatening. The brain symptoms are often the most delayed because of the time the aluminum takes to travel from the blood through the blood-brain barrier into the brain.

Aluminum accumulates in neurons in the brain, and it is toxic to neurons, causing a variety of pathological conditions. It inhibits uptake of dopamine and serotonin, which are important neurotransmitters in the brain. Aluminum toxicity is a known factor in Alzheimer's disease, and may contribute to symptoms of Parkinson's disease. Dementia resulting from kidney dialysis is related to aluminum and results in memory loss, loss of coordination, confusion, and disorientation. In animal experiments, rabbits given aluminum showed difficulty in memory retention and difficulty in learning.

Effective Treatments for the Adverse Reactions from the HPV Vaccine

Protocol 1:
Vitamin C, Glutathione Cocktail, given by IV (Dr. Yanagisawa)

- Sterile water, 250 milliliters (ml)
- Vitamin C, 12.5 grams (g)–25 g (12,500–25,000 milligrams [mg])
- Glutathione, 800–1,200 mg
- 0.5 M Magnesium sulfate, 10–20 ml
- 8.5 percent Calcium gluconate, 2 ml
- Vitamin B complex (B_1, B_2, B_3, B_5, B_6, B_{12})

Case History: 17 yrs, female.

May 23, 2014. When she visited the clinic, she could not walk without assistance. She complained of general fatigue, joint pain, and frequent involuntary movement. The patient was treated with intravenous Myers' cocktail containing VCG (vitamin C 12.5 g and glutathione 1,200 mg) and oral nutritious supplements (vitamin C, vitamin B, curcumin, SAMe, etc.). After ten days of vitamin C and glutathione therapy, she could walk without an assistant. By December 2014, she could play tennis. Frequency and duration of involuntary movements were decreased, and fatigue and pain dramatically decreased.

Protocol 2:
Vitamin C, Glutathione & EDTA, given by IV (Dr. Claus Hancke, Denmark)

- 5 percent Glucose, 250 ml
- Vitamin C (500 mg/ml), 50 ml (25,000 mg)
- Na2-EDTA (150 mg/ml), 10 ml (1.5 g)
- 8.4 percent Na Bicarbonate, 10 ml
- MgSO4 (2 millimoles (mmol) per ml), 4 ml
- When the infusion almost done, add glutathione 150 mg/ml, 4 ml (600 mg)

Protocol 3:
Phospholipid Exchange Therapy and Glutathione, given IV (Dr. Damien Downing, UK)

This membrane-stabilizing protocol is a closely-monitored version of the lipid rescue that anesthetists use in toxic emergencies. As with all IV treatments, this should only be done by someone with full training.

- Phosphatidylcholine (as Intralipid or Essentiale only) 1,250 mg plus
- Leucovorin (folinic acid) 10 mg plus
- Glutathione 1,000 mg

Protocol 4:
Oral supplements (Dr. Claus Hancke and Dr. Atsuo Yanagisawa)

Multiple vitamin/mineral	2, 3x per day (Increased slowly from 1 per day to 6 per day)
EPA/DHA/GLA	2 x 3 doses per day
Vitamin D, 1,500 IU	1 x 3
Magnesium citrate	1 x 2
Vitamin C, 750 mg	2 x 2
B complex	1 x 2
Thiamine (B_1), 300 mg	1 x 1
Probiotic	1 x 2
Turmeric	1 x 2
Lipoic acid, 300 mg	1 x 2
CoQ_{10}, 100 mg	1 x 1
S-adenosylmethionine (SAMe)	400 mg per day
5-MTHF methyltetrahydrofolate	5 mg per day

Protocol 5:
Dietary principles (Dr. Claus Hancke)

- Alkaline foods with no fish, sugar, wheat, or milk
- No chemicals or aluminum in the food (e.g. aluminum in table salt)
- More greens, nuts, and berries
- Use healthy fats: olive oil, coconut oil, and organic butter

- Choose tea rather than coffee
- No alcohol or tobacco. To make the body more alkaline, take a glass of water with a teaspoon bicarbonate and the juice from a lemon 3 or 4 times a day

Other treatment options:

1. Ferulic acid from rice bran for memory loss, learning disturbance
2. Low-dose theophylline for headache, 50–100 mg in the morning (excellent improvement in some patients)
3. Low-dose naltrexone (LDN) for hypersomnia, headache, 3 mg before sleep
4. Supplements for joint pain, gait disturbance, and to improve stem cell release

Summary

The timing and appearance of adverse effects and symptoms of the HPV vaccines vary for each patient. These symptoms differ from anything that we have previously experienced. Unfortunately, governments and medical professions have not faced the problem proactively. Although treatment with orthomolecular medicine has been helpful in many cases, it is not always adequate to return the patient to normal. In order to establish an effective protocol, scientists and clinicians must work together.

The onset of adverse effects from HPV vaccines arrives several months to a year or more after the injection. This delay makes it very difficult to link the symptoms with the HPV vaccine. In Japan, more than 1,200 girls have been registered as "severe cases" and more patients are registered every day. We estimate more than 100,000 unrecognized cases of mild to moderate adverse effects in girls vaccinated with HPV. The symptoms are commonly seen as fatigue, muscle pain, headache, learning disturbance, difficulty in awakening, hypersomnia, irregular menstruation, among others.

Doctors should be made aware of HPV vaccine adverse effects. Unfortunately, there is no evidence about the effectiveness of cervical cancer prevention by the HPV vaccines. Therefore, in my opinion as a concerned physician, we should discontinue this harmful HPV vaccine as soon as possible.

REFERENCES FOR "ORTHOMOLECULAR TREATMENT FOR ADVERSE EFFECTS OF HPV VACCINE"

1. Khan Z, Combadière C, Authier F-J, et al. Slow CCL2-dependent translocation of biopersistent particles from muscle to brain. *BMC Medicine* 2013; 11:99. doi: 10.1186/1741–7015–11–99.

Video providing case history: https://www.youtube.com/watch?v=G02i-r39hok.

FLU VACCINE: NO GOOD EVIDENCE

by Damien Downing, MD

From the *Orthomolecular Medicine News Service,* January 14, 2012.

Is it wise to have the flu vaccine, or Tamiflu, or would you get better protection just from taking vitamin D? Having a vaccine should be a matter of personal choice; we don't think that government or insurance companies or medical societies should be telling you what to do. If you're bothering to read this, then you're clearly smart enough to make your own decisions about your own health. While you are deciding, here is a second opinion.

So What About Vaccines?

A major review appeared in the journal *Lancet Infectious Diseases*[1] in October (principal author Prof. Michael Osterholm, a respected researcher into infectious diseases). The paper, which found only 31 studies worthy of inclusion out of a massive 5,700 screened, concluded that there was only good evidence for moderate flu-vaccine efficacy in healthy adults, and no real evidence of protection in those over 65 years, or for that matter in children. Of course it is the elderly, and particularly the frail elderly, that doctors are more concerned about—and in whom 90 percent of flu cases occur—and there was no evidence that flu vaccine prevents flu infection in this group.

Let's do that again; after nearly 6,000 studies of all sorts, there is no good evidence that flu vaccine prevents flu in its main target population.

The pooled effect in those healthy adults aged 18 to 65 is reported as 57 percent, which means the vaccine roughly halves your chances of getting flu. What is well known about placebo effects can account for most of that 57 percent effect. If you know you've had a shot for the flu you think you're invincible. But since the chance of getting flu in that age group was less than 3 percent to begin with, that's really only about a 1 1/2 percent reduction. Rounding the figures off, if you're a healthy adult, the flu vaccine will reduce your risk of actually getting the flu from 1 in 36 to 1 in 83. These are figures that are not offered in any of these studies.

Then of course, this all happens at a price. Whatever you may have heard, there is no such thing as a medication without the risk of side effects. In vaccines that risk can also come from the adjuvants. A vaccine is a small dose of an organism plus adjuvants—chemicals that are irritants to the immune system and trigger it to react to the organism part. Without adjuvants vaccines generally won't work. Popular adjuvants include the antibiotic gentamicin (too much of which can make you deaf), aluminum compounds (which probably contribute to Alzheimer's and other neurological diseases),[2] and the mercury antiseptic thiomersal/thimerosal (long known to be toxic and more recently suspected in autism)—after all, they have to be toxic to work as adjuvants. Fluarix, one of the main brands of flu vaccine in the USA and UK, is stated by the manufacturers to contain both gentamicin and thimerosal.

We also used to think that flu vaccine prevented deaths from flu to a significant extent, even if it didn't prevent overt infection—until we realized there was a major artifact at work. This is known as the *healthy vaccine recipient effect,* and the clue is in the name; a frail elderly person is much less likely to get down to their GP to have the vaccine than is a fit elderly person, who by the way is more likely to eat and live well, take vitamins, and so on, and so has better resistance to viruses anyway.

What Osterholm and colleagues concluded, citing a couple of Californian studies, is that flu vaccine reduced all-cause mortality in those over 65 by a mere 4.6 percent. Is that worth the risk of adverse effects? That's the choice you have to make, but now you can make it knowing these facts.

Tamiflu

So if the vaccine can't prevent you from getting the flu, how about Tamiflu (oseltamivir)? Well, it reduces the duration of flu symptoms by 1 to 1 1/2 days, and can give you other unpleasant symptoms, such as nausea and vomiting, and serious brain fog ("I couldn't think past a comma"), even according to the official website.[3] We also became aware of another problem with Tamiflu; basically, the whole planet is starting to become resistant to it—already.[4] Here's how it works: Tamiflu is excreted largely unchanged by patients, and is barely affected by sewage treatment. So the drug enters the waterways, as was shown during a flu outbreak in Japan, where ducks, the natural reservoir for the virus, can pick it up. And when this happens, the virus can probably (which means that so far it has happened in a lab experiment) develop resistance to Tamiflu.

So Tamiflu, which governments were stockpiling and then handing out like candy in the last big flu outbreak, may already be on the fast track past its sell by date. We've been here before, with overuse of antibiotics leading to seriously resistant hospital bugs like MRSA. But that took decades. We've managed to squander this resource much faster, and it shows that we live on a small planet—and there's nowhere left to hide our waste. Everywhere is our doorstep now.

Vitamin D

Nobody could accuse us of overusing vitamin D. To begin with, we are almost all deficient, both in northern Europe and in the northern half of the USA.[5] The final paper in this year's crop[6] shows that the higher your blood level of vitamin D, the lower your risk of catching flu, or respiratory infections in general.

The study found this to be true up to a vitamin D blood level over 100 nanomoles per liter (nmol/L), which we used to think was excessive. But nowadays we don't; the D*Action (http://www.grassrootshealth.org/daction/index.php) group located in San

Diego has shown that you need to get even higher, above 125 nmol/L, in order to minimize your risk of developing most cancers, multiple sclerosis, and other autoimmune diseases.[7] Chances are the same applies to flu and chest infections. The problem is finding people with a vitamin D level that high in order to study them; D*Action found that it takes 9,600 international units (IU) per day of vitamin D by mouth to reliably get people above 100 nmol/L (specifically, to get 97.5 percent of people there).

In a UK study, those with the highest vitamin D level—over 100 nmol/L—had about 50 percent the risk of getting respiratory infections of those with the lowest level—below 25 nmol/L, which is truly deficient. All the subjects were Caucasians living in the UK, and you might expect that fair-skinned people would have a higher level of vitamin D, but this turns out not to be so—according to a 2009 study, again in the UK,[8] Caucasian women have a slightly lower level of vitamin D than darker-skinned ones—no doubt because they heed the health warnings about skin cancer (now that's a story for another time). They didn't ask whether the subjects took any supplements, which could have made an even greater difference; a previous study in African-American women[9] found that a supplement of 800 IU per day of vitamin D reduced, and 2,000 IU effectively wiped out, the risk of winter flu.

This was partly confirmed by a randomized controlled trial in Japanese schoolchildren which showed that 1,200 IU reduced the incidence of confirmed influenza by 40 percent,[10] and a study at Yale which found that people with a serum vitamin D level over 38 ng/ml (equivalent to 95 nmol/L, very close to the 100 nmol/L used in the UK study) had half the chance of catching acute respiratory infections.[11]

Before we get bogged down in the numbers, this is how I see it: if you live north of New York or Madrid you're unlikely to have enough vitamin D in your system. You can improve that somewhat with diet, but with supplements you can probably make almost 100 percent certain (96 percent in fact) that you don't get flu. How much vitamin D? At least 5,000 IU for an adult, and 10,000 IU is completely safe (or better still, get it from sunlight—take a sunshine break now!). And if you do choose to have the vaccine, vitamin D might even make it work better.[12]

The *Orthomolecular Medicine News Service* (OMNS) is not specifically antivaccine, but we are very pro-personal choice; you can read our previous posting on this topic.[13] Get the facts, make up your own mind. Don't accept coercion or baloney from governments. As Vera Hassner Sharav said, "Public health officials on both sides of the Atlantic have lost the public trust because they have been in league with vaccine manufacturers in denying that safety problems exist."

Vaccines are a valuable asset and we shouldn't squander them the way we did antibiotics. You're not going to turn down rabies vaccine if you need it. But, equally, why ignore a gift of nature such as vitamin D?

REFERENCES FOR "FLU VACCINE"

1. Osterholm M, Kelley NS, Sommer A, et al. Efficacy and effectiveness of influenza vaccines: a systematic review and meta-analysis. *Lancet Infect Dis* 2012;12(1):36–44. doi: 10.1016/S1473–3099(11)70295-X.

2. Tomljenovic L, Shaw CA. Aluminum vaccine adjuvants: are they safe? *Curr Med Chem* 2011;18(17):2630–2637.

3. Tamiflu. Side effects and safety. Available at: http://www.tamiflu.com/hcp/tamiflu-side-effects-and-safety.

4. Järhult JD. Tamiflu: use it and lose it? Uppsala: Acta Universitatis Upsaliensis, 2011, p60. Available at: http://uu.diva-portal.org/smash/record.jsf?pid=diva2:453789.

5. Influenza. Vitamin D Council. http://www.sunarc.org and also https://www.vitamindcouncil.org/health-conditions/influenza/.

6. Berry DJ, Hesketh K, Power C, et al. Vitamin D status has a linear association with seasonal infections and lung function in British adults. *Br J Nutr* 2011;106(9):1433–1440. doi: 10.1017/S0007114511001991.

7. http://www.grassrootshealth.net/.

8. Glass D, Lens M, Swaminathan R, et al. Pigmentation and vitamin D metabolism in Caucasians: low vitamin D serum levels in fair skin types in the UK. *PLoS One* 2009;4(8):e6477. doi: 10.1371/journal.pone.0006477.

9. Cannell JJ, Vieth R, Umhau JC, et al. Epidemic influenza and vitamin D. *Epidemiol Infect* 2006;134(6):1129–1140.

10. Urashima M, Segawa T, Okazaki M, et al. Randomized trial of vitamin D supplementation to prevent seasonal influenza A in schoolchildren. *Am J Clin Nutr* 2010;91(5):1255–1260. doi: 10.3945/ajcn.2009.29094.

11. Sabetta JR, DePetrillo P, Cipriani RJ, et al. Serum 25-hydroxyvitamin d and the incidence of acute viral respiratory tract infections in healthy adults. *PLoS One* 2010;5(6):e11088. doi: 10.1371/journal.pone.0011088.

12. Cannell JJ, Zasloff M, Garland CF, et al. On the epidemiology of influenza. *Virol J* 2008;5:29. doi: 10.1186/1743–422X-5–29.

13. Downing D. The health hazards of disease prevention, *Orthomolecular Medicine News Service,* Apr 8, 2011. Available at: http://www.orthomolecular.org/resources/omns/v07n02.shtml.

WHICH SUPPLEMENTS SHOULD YOU TAKE TO PROTECT YOURSELF AGAINST COLDS AND FLUS?

by Jack Challem

From *The Nutrition Reporter* 15(12), 2004.

It has been years since I've had a flu shot—they used to leave me feeling lethargic—and it has been years since I caught the flu. With the extreme shortage of flu vaccines this year, I've decided to share my personal supplement regimen for both preventing and fighting cold and flu symptoms.

My suggestions fall into two areas, covering general prevention and the aggressive suppression and reversal of symptoms. The research suggests that these supplements work best preventively and on the first day of an apparent cold or flu infection. If you wait until the second or third day, the supplements will be of less, and possibly no, benefit. The reason is that viral concentrations increase sharply after the first day, and they become more difficult for the body to control. By using NAC and at least some of the other supplements described here, I have been able to consistently reduce a standard seven-day cold to a mild two- to three-day cold.

N-acetylcysteine

In one of the most dramatic clinical studies I've ever read, NAC supplements significantly reduced flu symptoms in a group of elderly subjects. Silvio De Flora, MD, of the University of Genoa, Italy, asked 262 subjects to take 600 milligrams (mg) of NAC twice daily or placebos for six months overlapping the cold and flu season.

First, De Flora studied general flu-like symptoms among his subjects. These symptoms included fever, headache, achiness, nasal discharge, cough, and sore throat. Each month, subjects taking NAC had one-third to one-half fewer flu-like symptoms, compared with people taking placebos.

De Flora then looked at a subgroup with laboratory-confirmed flu. Only 25 percent of them developed symptoms, compared with 79 percent of those taking placebos. In other words, NAC supplements reduced the likelihood of having flu symptoms by about two-thirds. He also found that people taking NAC spent less time in bed recovering from the flu. Of ten people who had flu-like symptoms and were not bedridden, nine were taking NAC. What to take: I take 500 mg of NAC daily throughout the year, doubling it during the cold and flu season. When I sense initial cold or flu symptoms, I immediately increase the dosage to 2,000 to 3,000 mg daily. If I end up developing a cold, I may take up to 4,000 to 6,000 mg daily. NAC's only drawback is that the capsules have a strong rotten-egg smell.

Vitamin C

More than two dozen clinical studies have found that vitamin C can reduce the symptoms and severity of the common cold (and presumably the flu). The most effective dosages range from 2,000 to 6,000 mg daily. In general, your body's optimal level of vitamin C is based on bowel tolerance—that is, the amount (divided up two or three times a day) just below what causes loose stools. When you're fighting a cold or flu, your vitamin C requirements increase sharply. If you follow the bowel-tolerance concept, you may find yourself temporarily taking 10,000 or 20,000 mg of vitamin C daily. As you recover, your vitamin C requirements will decrease.

Vitamin E

A study found that seniors who took vitamin E supplements were less likely to suffer colds and other upper respiratory infections. Take 200 international units (IU) to 400 IU of natural-source vitamin E daily.

Selenium

This mineral is a component of the body's four glutathione peroxidase compounds, potent antioxidants, and immune stimulants. Clinical and animal studies by Melinda A. Beck, PhD, of the University of North Carolina, Chapel Hill, along with Chinese researchers, have found that selenium deficiencies increase the likelihood of mutations in flu and Coxsackie viruses, leading to more severe infections. Take 200 micrograms (mcg) daily, 400 mcg if you are actually fighting cold or flu.

Lysine

This amino acid inhibits the growth of many viruses, including those that cause herpes infections. To fight a cold or flu, take 500 to 1,000 mcg daily with the other supplements recommended here.

Zinc

This mineral inhibits the replication of the virus that causes colds. Although some studies have yielded conflicting results, zinc can often reduce the severity and length of cold and flu symptoms. Take about 13 mg of zinc every couple of hours, starting at the first sign of symptoms.

Vitamin A

Several studies have found that large amounts of vitamin A can reduce the severity and risk of death in vitamin-deficient children with measles, chicken pox, and respiratory viral infections. In addition, very, very high dosages of pure vitamin A (not beta-carotene) have been used in developing nations to reduce the risk of death from pneumonia in children. These dosages are 100,000 IU daily, but for only two days over a month. Lower regular dosages should be helpful, such as 10,000 IU daily. When fighting a cold or flu, consider taking 25,000 to 50,000 IU daily—but not for more than three days. If you are pregnant, do not take more than 5,000 IU of pure vitamin A daily. *Editor's note: Up to 10,000 IU day of vitamin A is considered safe during pregnancy. More about vitamin A dosage and safety during pregnancy is discussed in* Vitamins & Pregnancy: The Real Story *(2016).*

Echinacea

While some of the research is conflicting, there's sufficient evidence to take echinacea to help prevent colds and flus. The herb boosts activity of various immune cells, in a sense putting the body on a "yellow alert," ready to quickly fight an infection. Because of the many different forms (capsules, tablets, tinctures, liquids), follow label directions.

Oscillococcinum

This is a homeopathic remedy, and the theory is that smaller dosages are more potent than larger ones, an idea that's in direct opposition to medical pharmacology. Whatever the rationale, it does seem to work (at least in this instance). A prestigious Cochrane database review cautiously acknowledged that oscillococcinum (pronounced os-sill-uh-cos-sih-num) "probably reduces the duration of illness in patients presenting with influenza symptoms." A separate review found that oscillococcinum for influenza-like illnesses was "promising." Take one dose at the onset of symptoms, with additional doses six and 12 hours later.

Washing Your Hands

The most important steps you can take to prevent a cold or flu are to avoid contact with an infected person and to avoid touching objects the infected person has used. Because it is not always possible to follow these two steps, it is essential that you regularly wash your hands in hot soapy water, especially after being in contact with an infected person and before you touch your mouth or nose.

A Reminder

Again, it is important to ramp up the dosages of the recommended supplements at the first sign of cold or flu symptoms. That ticklish nose or cough may not be from an infection, but given the potential consequences of a serious infection, it is better to err on the side of caution. If the symptoms completely disappear by the second day, you can resume your preventive dosages. If you still have any symptoms at all, continue taking the supplements for three to seven days.

SELECTED REFERENCES FOR "WHICH SUPPLEMENTS SHOULD YOU TAKE?"

De Flora S, Grassi C, Carati L. Attenuation of influenza-like symptomatology and improvement of cell-mediated immunity with long-term N-acetylcysteine treatment. *European Respiratory Journal* 1997;10:1535–1541.

Hemilä H. Does vitamin C alleviate the symptoms of the common cold? A review of current evidence. *Scandinavian Journal of Infectious Disease* 1994;26:1–6.

Mossad SB, Macknin ML, Medendorp SV, et al. Zinc gluconate lozenges for treating the common cold. A randomized, double-blind, placebo-controlled study. *Annals of Internal Medicine,* 1996;125:81–88.

Beck MA, Shi Q, Morris VC, et al. Rapid genomic evolution of a non-virulent coxsackievirus B3 in selenium-deficient mice results in selection of identical virulent isolates. *Nature Medicine* 1995;1:433–436.

Nelson HK, Shi Q, Van Dael P, et al. Host nutritional selenium status as a driving force for influenza virus mutations. *FASEB Journal* 2001;15:1481–1483.

Zakay-Rones Z, Varsano N, Zlotnik M, et al. Inhibition of several strains of influenza virus in vitro and reduction of symptoms by an elderberry extract (*Sambucus nigra L.*) during an outbreak of influenza B panama. *J Altern Complement Med* 1995;1:361–369.

Vickers AJ, Smith C. Homeopathic Oscillococcinum for preventing and treating influenza and influenza-like syndromes. *Cochrane Database Syst Rev* 2000;CD001957.

Linde K, Hondras M, Vickers A, et al. Systematic reviews of complementary therapies—an annotated bibliography. Part 3: homeopathy. *BMC Complement Altern Med* 2001;1:4.

ASCORBATE SUPPLEMENTATION REDUCES HEART FAILURE

by Andrew W. Saul, PhD, and Robert G. Smith, PhD

From the *Orthomolecular Medicine News Service,* November 22, 2011.

New research has reported that risk of heart failure decreases with increasing blood levels of vitamin C.[1] Persons with the lowest plasma levels of ascorbate had the highest risk of heart failure, and persons with the highest levels of vitamin C had the lowest risk of heart failure.

According to the US Centers for Disease Control and Prevention (CDC), there are about 600,000 deaths from heart disease each year.[2] This is an enormous number. The definition of heart failure used by the study authors was on the basis of drugs prescribed, which would include all forms of heart disease that cause death. This agrees well with the CDC definition.

Specifically, the study found that each 20 micromole/liter (μmol/L) increase in plasma vitamin C was associated with a 9 percent reduction in death from heart failure. That works out to 54,000 fewer deaths from heart failure for each increase in 20 μmol/L plasma vitamin C. If everyone took high-enough doses of vitamin C to reach the highest quartile (80 μmol/L), that would work out to approximately 216,000 fewer deaths per year. Just from taking vitamin C.

What Is Heart Failure?

The heart muscle fails for many reasons. As we get older, it weakens and may not get enough nutrients to keep it healthy. A severe heart attack that does not kill the patient but causes significant damage to the heart muscle may leave the heart in a very weakened state. Long-standing or acute high blood pressure can put a massive strain on the heart and cause it to fail. An abnormal beating of the heart—such as a very fast heart rate, an irregular beat, or a lot of missed beats—will result in less effective pumping and eventual failure. Anemia will make the heart pump harder and faster in an attempt to deliver enough oxygen to the organs. The valves in the heart which direct blood flow are made up of an important fibrous strengthening tissue called collagen. Weakness or tearing of these valves can cause the blood to flow backwards, making the heart pump very inefficiently and eventually causing it to fail. When the heart muscle begins to fail, there is a buildup of carbon dioxide and waste products, resulting in weakening of the kidneys and liver. Eventually, fluid builds up in all the organs, and the person presents with severe fatigue, shortness of breath (from fluid in the lungs), and swelling of the ankles.

Viruses and other microorganisms can attack the heart and weaken the heart muscle cells permanently by causing viral myocarditis. As the heart muscle cells get older they may require more energy to work and a greater level of protection from free-radical damage. Nutrients such as magnesium, orotic acid, coenzyme Q_{10}, acetyl L-carnitine, and others may be required. Toxins, chemotherapeutic drugs, alcohol, and deficiencies of some nutrients such as selenium may cause the heart to increase the size of its cells to compensate for the weakness. An enlargement of the heart muscle is called cardiomyopathy. These hearts are much more likely to fail.

Medical treatment of cardiac failure uses drugs that open the arteries, reduce blood pressure, and force the excessive fluid out of the body (diuretics). Drugs known as ACE inhibitors improve quality of life and survival. Diet, fluid and salt restriction, and tolerable exercise are essential. For the most severe cases, a heart transplant may be required. However, many of these treatments have significant side effects. For example, treatment with diuretics to remove excess fluid will tend to lower the plasma vitamin C level and exacerbate the causes of cardiac failure.

How Much Vitamin C Is Needed?

It takes less vitamin C than you may have thought. To achieve a plasma level of 80 µmol/L, and thereby reduce deaths by 216,000 per year, requires a daily dosage of about 500 milligrams (mg) of vitamin C. This is only one or two tablets per day, costing less than 10 cents.

Taking 3,000 to 8,000 mg per day, in continued divided doses, can achieve a plasma level twice as high (160 µmol/L). This much C could save an additional 216,000 lives as it is an additional 80 µmol/L, assuming the relationship holds.

We can go still higher, and without intravenous administration. Taking 1,000 mg of oral vitamin C per hour for 12 hours (12,000 mg per day) will result in a plasma level of about 240 µmol/L. A single 5,000 mg dose might take you to a peak of 240 µmol/L, but only for about two to four hours after the intake. That is why the dosage needs to be spread out: better absorption, gradual excretion, higher plasma levels . . . and better results.

Conclusion

Optimizing vitamin C intake optimizes the health of a person taking it. This includes persons with potentially life-threatening disorders. It is a simple, cheap, effective, and safe therapy. Vitamin C is no longer a "controversial" therapy. It is an ignored therapy. It is time for the medical profession to fully awaken to what this study confirms: higher vitamin C intakes mean less heart failure. That means that higher vitamin C intakes mean fewer deaths. 200,000 per year fewer.

With just two vitamin C tablets per day.

REFERENCES FOR "ASCORBATE SUPPLEMENTATION REDUCES HEART FAILURE"

1. Pfister R, Sharp SJ, Luben R, et al. Plasma vitamin C predicts incident heart failure in men and women in European Prospective Investigation into Cancer and Nutrition-Norfolk prospective study. *Am Heart J* 2011;162:246–253.

2. Centers for Disease Control and Prevention (CDC). Leading causes of death. Available at: http://www.cdc.gov/nchs/fastats/leading-causes-of-death.htm.

NEGATIVE NEWS MEDIA REPORTS ON VITAMIN SUPPLEMENTS

by Andrew W. Saul, PhD

Excerpted from the *Orthomolecular Medicine News Service,* November 12, 2013.

There have been a number of widely publicized negative reports about vitamins in the news media.[1] While trumpeting those select few, they just possibly may have missed these:

- *Multivitamin supplements lower your risk of cancer by 8 percent.* An 8 percent reduction in deaths means the lives of 48,000 people in the US alone could be saved each year, just by taking an inexpensive daily vitamin pill.[2]
- *72 percent of physicians personally use dietary supplements.* The multivitamin is the most popular dietary supplement taken by doctors.[3]
- *High serum levels of vitamin B_6, methionine, and folate are associated with a 50 percent reduction in lung cancer risk.* Those with higher levels of these nutrients had a significantly lower risk of lung cancer whether they smoked or not.[4]
- *Vitamin D reduces cancer risk.* Studies on breast and colorectal cancer found that an increase of serum 25(OH)D concentration of 10 nanomoles per milliliter (ng/ml) was associated with a 15 percent reduction in colorectal cancer incidence and 11 percent reduction in breast cancer incidence.[5]

- *Vitamin D increases breast cancer survival.* In women diagnosed with breast cancer, those with higher serum 25(OH)D concentrations had increased survival rates. In those with lower vitamin D concentrations, mortality increased by 8 percent.[6]
- *Risk of heart failure decreases with increasing blood levels of vitamin C.* Each 20 micromole/liter (µmol/L) increase in plasma vitamin C was associated with a 9 percent reduction in death from heart failure. If everyone took high enough doses of vitamin C to reach 80 µmol/L, it would mean 216,000 fewer deaths per year. To achieve that plasma level requires a daily dosage of about 500 milligrams (mg) of vitamin C.[7]
- *Vitamin C prevents and reverses radiation damage.*[8] To learn more, please see "Effect of vitamin C and anti-oxidative nutrition on radiation-induced gene expression in Fukushima nuclear plant workers," by Atsuo Yanagisawa, MD. A free download of the full presentation is available at http://www.doctoryourself.com/Radiation_VitC.pptx.pdf.

The Japanese College of Intravenous Therapy has produced a video for people wishing to learn more about large doses of vitamin C:

Part 1: http://www.youtube.com/watch?v=Rbm_MH3nSdM

Part 2: http://www.youtube.com/watch?v=j4cyzts3lMo

Part 3: http://www.youtube.com/watch?v=ZYiRo2Oucfo

Part 4: http://www.youtube.com/watch?v=51le8FuuYJw

All four parts of the video are available at http://firstlaw.wordpress.com/.

Vitamin C arrests and reverses cancer.[9] Oncologist Victor Marcial, MD, says, "We studied patients with advanced cancer (stage 4). Forty patients received 40,000–75,000 mg intravenously several times a week. . . In addition, they received a diet and other supplements. The initial tumor response rate was achieved in 75% of patients, defined as a 50% reduction or more in tumor size."

The news media have also reported claims that "vitamin E does no good at all in preventing cancer or heart disease." Here's more of what they failed to report:

- *Natural vitamin E factor yields a 75 percent decrease in prostate tumor formation.* Gamma-tocotrienol, a cofactor found in natural vitamin E preparations, kills prostate cancer stem cells.[10]
- *Gamma-tocotrienol also is effective against existing prostate tumors.*[11]
- *Vitamin E reduces mortality by 24 percent in persons 71 or older.*[12]
- *300 IU vitamin E per day reduces risk of lung cancer by 61 percent.*[13]

- *Vitamin E is an effective treatment for atherosclerosis.* "Subjects with supplementary vitamin E intake of 100 IU per day or greater demonstrated less coronary artery lesion progression than did subjects with supplementary vitamin E intake less than 100 IU per day."[14]
- *400 to 800 IU of vitamin E daily reduces risk of heart attack by 77 percent.*[15]

Here are additional studies showing special health benefits from vitamin E:

- *Increasing vitamin E with supplements prevents COPD [chronic obstructive pulmonary disease, emphysema, chronic bronchitis].*[16]
- *800 IU vitamin E per day is a successful treatment for fatty liver disease.*[17]
- *Alzheimer's patients who take 2,000 IU of vitamin E per day live longer.*[18]
- *400 IU of vitamin E per day reduces epileptic seizures in children by more than 60 percent.*[19]
- *Vitamin E supplements help prevent amyotrophic lateral sclerosis (ALS.)* This important finding is the result of a ten-year-plus Harvard study of over a million persons.[20]
- *Vitamin E is more effective than a prescription drug in treating chronic liver disease (nonalcoholic steatohepatitis.)* Said the authors, "The good news is that this study showed that cheap and readily available vitamin E can help many of those with this condition."[21]

REFERENCES FOR "NEGATIVE NEWS MEDIA REPORTS ON VITAMIN SUPPLEMENTS"

1. National Broadcasting Company (NBC). Available at: http://www.nbcnews.com/health/vitamins-dont-prevent-heart-disease-or-cancer-experts-find-2D11577445.

2. Gaziano JM, Sesso HD, Christen WG, et al. Multivitamins in the prevention of cancer in men: the Physicians' Health Study II randomized controlled trial. *JAMA* 2012; 308(18):1871–1880. doi:10.1001/jama.2012.14641.

3. Dickinson A, Boyon N, Shao A. Physicians and nurses use and recommend dietary supplements: report of a survey. *Nutrition Journal* 2009, 8:29 doi:10.1186/1475–2891–8-29.

4. Johansson M, Relton C, Ueland PM, et al. Serum B vitamin levels and risk of lung cancer. *JAMA* 2010;303(23):2377–2385.

5. Gandini S, Boniol M, Haukka J, et al. Meta-analysis of observational studies of serum 25-hydroxyvitamin D levels and colorectal, breast and prostate cancer and colorectal adenoma. *Int J Cancer* 2011;128(6):1414–1424.

6. Vrieling A, Hein R, Abbas S, et al. Serum 25-hydroxyvitamin D and postmenopausal breast cancer survival: a prospective patient cohort study. *Breast Cancer Res* 2011;13(4):R74.

7. Pfister R, Sharp SJ, Luben R, et al. Plasma vitamin C predicts incident heart failure in men and women in European Prospective Investigation into Cancer and Nutrition-Norfolk prospective study. *Am Heart J* 2011; 162:246–253.

8. Korkina L, et al. Antioxidant therapy in children affected by irradiation from the Chernobyl nuclear accident. *Biochem Soc Trans* 1993; 21:314S.

9. Victor M. Presentation at the Medical Sciences Campus, University of Puerto Rico, April 12, 2010. You can download the intravenous vitamin C protocol that he used free of charge at http://www.doctoryourself.com/RiordanIVC.pdf or http://www.riordanclinic.org/research/vitaminc/protocol.shtml. See also: Intravenous vitamin C therapy for cancer is presented in detail on video, available for free access at http://www.riordanclinic.org/education/symposium/s2009 (twelve lectures) and http://www.riordanclinic.org/education/symposium/s2010 (nine lectures).

10. Luk SU, Yap WN, Chiu YT, et al. Gamma-tocotrienol as an effective agent in targeting prostate cancer stem cell-like population. *Int J Cancer* 2011; 128(9):2182–2191.

11. Nesaretnam K, Teoh HK, Selvaduray KR, et al. Modulation of cell growth and apoptosis response in human prostate cancer cells supplemented with tocotrienols. *Eur J Lipid Sci Technol* 2008; 110: 23–31. See also: Conte C, Floridi A, Aisa C, et al. Gamma-tocotrienol metabolism and antiproliferative effect in prostate cancer cells. *Ann N Y Acad Sci* 2004; 1031: 391–394.

12. Hemila H, Kaprio J. Vitamin E may affect the life expectancy of men, depending on dietary vitamin C intake and smoking. *Age Ageing* 2011; 40(2): 215–220.

13. Mahabir S, Schendel K, Dong YQ, et al. Dietary alpha-, beta-, gamma- and delta-tocopherols in lung cancer risk. *Int J Cancer* 2008;123(5):1173–1180.

14. Hodis HN, Mack WJ, LaBree L, et al. Serial coronary angiographic evidence that antioxidant vitamin intake reduces progression of coronary artery atherosclerosis. *JAMA* 1995; 273:1849–1854.

15. Stephens NG, Parsons A, Schofield PM, et al. Randomized controlled trial of vitamin E in patients with coronary artery disease: Cambridge Heart Antioxidant Study (CHAOS). *Lancet* 1996; 347:781–786.

16. Agler AH, Kurth T, Gaziano JM, et al. Randomized vitamin E supplementation and risk of chronic lung disease (CLD) in the Women's Health Study. *Thorax* 2011;66(4):320–325.

17. Sanyal AJ, Chalasani N, Kowdley KV, et al. Pioglitazone, vitamin E, or placebo for nonalcoholic steatohepatitis. *N Engl J Med* 2010;362(18):1675–1685.

18. Pavlik VN, Doody RS, Rountree SD, et al. Vitamin E use is associated with improved survival in an Alzheimer's disease cohort. *Dement Geriatr Cogn Disord* 2009;28(6):536–540. See also: Grundman M. Vitamin E and Alzheimer disease: the basis for additional clinical trials. *Am J Clin Nutr* 2000 Feb;71(2):630S-636S.

19. Ogunmekan AO, Hwang PA. A randomized, double-blind, placebo-controlled, clinical trial of D-alpha-tocopheryl acetate [vitamin E], as add-on therapy, for epilepsy in children. *Epilepsia* 1989; 30(1):84–89.

20. Wang H, O'Reilly EJ, Weisskopf MG, et al. Vitamin E intake and risk of amyotrophic lateral sclerosis: a pooled analysis of data from 5 prospective cohort studies. *Am J Epidemiol* 2011; 173(6): 595–602.

21. Sanyal AJ, Chalasani N, Kowdley KV, et al. Pioglitazone, vitamin E, or placebo for nonalcoholic steatohepatitis. *N Engl J Med* 2010;362(18):1675–1685.

CHAPTER 13

A Pharmaceutical Plot Is Afoot? Of Course Not.

"It is difficult to get a man to understand something when his salary depends on his not understanding it."

—UPTON SINCLAIR

Surely it is just *coincidence* that none of this information has made it into your hands. Or is it?

We want to believe that the health care industry is inherently good. We want to believe that the makers of medicine have our best interests at heart. We want to think that doctors would do their very best to share the safest, most practical, and cost effective methods for curing sickness, that do the least possible harm and the most possible good. We want to believe that they truly seek to relieve our suffering.

Unfortunately, the health care system is incredibly flawed. We shouldn't confuse how we think things should be with how they actually are. It is in the interests of the medical industry to keep you—and your checkbook—buying into what has been sold to us lock, stock, and barrel: that pharmaceutical drugs (which kill lots of people) are the only way to cure illness, and that vitamins (which kill nobody) are, at worst, supposedly dangerous, and, at best, ineffective for treatment or prevention of real disease.

The pharmaceutical industry now more than ever drives research, study design, doctor training, media "health" reports, and publications in medical journals. Their seemingly bottomless pockets are filled by, well, us.

Well-brought-up folks tend to scoff at the word "conspiracy." (Using the word makes us sound a little crazy, right?) But we have got to realize that this is one step beyond that. The pharmaceutical industry is blatantly, persistently, and without (evident) remorse driving the way health care works and what information we get to access.

All we can do is *more.* We can spread the healing, health-giving message and try to show folks another, safer, cheaper, more effective way of maintaining and restoring health.

How to Make People Believe Any Antivitamin Scare

by Andrew W. Saul, PhD

Excerpted from the *Orthomolecular Medicine News Service,* October 20, 2011.

It just takes lots of pharmaceutical industry cash.

Cash to Study Authors

Many of the authors of a highly publicized negative vitamin E paper[1] have received substantial income from the pharmaceutical industry. The names are available in the last page of the paper (1556) in the "Conflict of Interest" section. A number of the study authors have received money from pharmaceutical companies, including Merck, Pfizer, Sanofi-Aventis, AstraZeneca, Abbott, GlaxoSmithKline, Janssen, Amgen, Firmagon, and Novartis. You will not see the conflicts in the brief summary at the *Journal of the American Association (JAMA)* website.

Advertising Revenue

Many popular magazines and almost all major medical journals receive income from the pharmaceutical industry. The only question is, how much?

Look in them all: *Readers Digest, JAMA, Newsweek, Time, AARP Today, NEJM, Archives of Pediatrics.* Even *Prevention* magazine. Practically any major periodical is full of pharmaceutical advertising.

Count the pharmaceutical ads. The more space sold, the more revenue for the publication. If you try to find a periodical's advertisement revenue, you'll likely see that they don't disclose it.

Rigged Trials

Studies of the health benefits of vitamins and essential nutrients can be easily rigged by using:[2]

- Low doses to guarantee failure
- Biased interpretation to show a statistical increase in risk

You can set up any study to fail. One way to ensure failure is to make a meaningless test. A meaningless test is assured if you make the choice to use insufficient quantities of the substance to be investigated:

- If you shoot beans at a charging rhinoceros, you are not likely to influence the outcome.
- If you give every homeless person you meet on the street 20 cents, you could easily prove that money will not help alleviate poverty.
- If you give Recommended Dietary Allowances (RDA) levels of vitamins, do not expect therapeutic results.

One reason commonly offered to justify conducting low-dose studies is that high doses of vitamins are somehow dangerous. What is dangerous is failure to supplement. The battle over vitamin supplements has been going on for nearly 70 years. You can say one thing for vitamin critics: at least they are consistent. Consistently wrong, but consistent. The oldest political trick in the book is to create doubt, then fear, and then conformity of action. The pharmaceutical industry knows this full well.

One does not waste time and money attacking something that does not work. Vitamin supplementation works well and works safely.

Bias in What Is Published, or Rejected for Publication

The largest and most popular medical journals receive very large income from pharmaceutical advertising. Peer-reviewed research indicates that this influences what they print, and even what study authors conclude from their data.[3]

Other research showed that more pharmaceutical company advertising results in a medical journal having more articles with "negative conclusions about dietary supplement safety." The authors stated, "The percentage of major articles concluding that supplements were unsafe was 4 percent in journals with fewest and 67 percent among those with the most pharmads ($P = 0.02$)." They concluded that "the impact of advertising on publications is real," and that "the ultimate impact of this bias on professional guidelines, health care, and health policy is a matter of great public concern."[4]

Censorship of What Is Indexed and Available to Doctors and the Public

There are nearly 6,000 journals indexed by the US taxpayer-funded National Library of Medicine (NLM), and over 1 billion PubMed/Medline searches each year. (PubMed/Medline is the NLM's primary online database of references and abstracts, free to Internet users.) Not one of those searches found a single paper from the peer-reviewed *Journal of Orthomolecular Medicine.*[5] PubMed/Medline does, however, index material from *Time* magazine, *Consumer Reports,* and even *Reader's Digest.* After nearly half a century of continuous peer-reviewed publication, perhaps the *Journal of Orthomolecular Medicine* should be included by the world's largest public medical library.

It is ironic that critics of vitamins preferentially cite low-dose studies in an attempt to show lack of vitamin effectiveness, yet they cannot cite any double-blind, placebo-controlled studies of high doses that show vitamin dangers. This is because vitamins are effective at high doses, and vitamins are also safe at high doses. Yet it is probable that the main, persistent roadblock to widespread examination and utilization of nutrition therapeutics is the widespread belief that there simply must be dangers with vitamin and mineral supplements. The opposite is true. There is a long and extraordinarily safe track record of high-dose nutrient therapy, dating back to the early 1940s.

Don't Believe It?

How well were these provitamin, antidrug studies covered in the mass media?

- A Harvard study showed a 27 percent reduction in AIDS deaths among patients given vitamin supplements.[6]
- There have been no deaths from vitamins in over thirty years.[7]
- Antibiotics cause 700,000 emergency room visits per year, just in the US.[8]
- Modern drug-and-cut medicine is at least the third leading cause of death in the USA. Some estimates place medicine as the number-one cause of death.[9]
- Over 1.5 million Americans are injured every year by drug errors in hospitals, doctors' offices, and nursing homes. If in a hospital, a patient can expect at least one medication error every single day.[10]
- More than 100,000 patients die every year, just in the US, from drugs properly prescribed and taken as directed.[11]

Daily Aspirin Use Linked with Pancreatic Cancer

Here's something you may have not seen. Research has shown that women who take just one aspirin a day, "which millions do to prevent heart attack and stroke as well as to treat headaches—may raise their risk of getting deadly pancreatic cancer. . . . Pancreatic cancer affects only 31,000 Americans a year, but it kills virtually all its victims within three years. The study of 88,000 nurses found that those who took two or more aspirins a week for 20 years or more had a 58 percent higher risk of pancreatic cancer."[12] *Women who took two or more aspirin tablets per day had an alarming 86 percent greater risk of pancreatic cancer.*

Study author Dr. Eva Schernhammer of Harvard Medical School was quoted as saying, "Apart from smoking, this is one of the few risk factors that have been identified for pancreatic cancer. Initially we expected that aspirin would protect against pancreatic cancer."

How about that.

Say: What if there was one, just *one* case of pancreatic cancer caused by a vitamin? What do you think the press would have said about that?

The fact is, vitamins are known to be effective and safe. They are essential nutrients, and when taken at the proper doses over a lifetime, are capable of preventing a wide variety of diseases. Because drug companies can't make big profits developing essential nutrients, they have a vested interest in agitating for the use of drugs and disparaging the use of nutritional supplements.

REFERENCES FOR "HOW TO MAKE PEOPLE BELIEVE ANY ANTIVITAMIN SCARE"

1. Klein EA, Thompson Jr, IM, Tangen CM, et al. *JAMA* 2011;306(14):1549–1556.

2. *Orthomolecular Medicine News Service.* Rigged trials: drug studies favor the manufacturer. Nov 5, 2008. Available at: http://orthomolecular.org/resources/omns/v04n20.shtml.

3. *Orthomolecular Medicine News Service.* Pharmaceutical advertising biases journals against vitamin supplements. Feb 5, 2009. Available at: http://orthomolecular.org/resources/omns/v05n02.shtml.

4. Kemper KJ, Hood KL. Does pharmaceutical advertising affect journal publication about dietary supplements? *BMC Complement Altern Med* 2008; 8:11.

5. *Orthomolecular Medicine News Service.* NLM censors nutritional research: Medline is biased, and taxpayers pay for it. Jan 15, 2010. Available at: http://orthomolecular.org/resources/omns/v06n03.shtml. See also: How to fool all of the people all of the time: US taxpayers fund library censorship. Jan 21, 2010. Available at: http://orthomolecular.org/resources/omns/v06n05.shtml.

6. Fawzi WW, Msamanga GI, Spiegelman D, et al. A randomized trial of multivitamin supplements and HIV disease progression and mortality. *N Engl J Med* 2004 Jul 1;351(1):23–32.

7. Saul AW, Vaman JN. No deaths from vitamins—none at all in 27 years. Jun 14, 2011. Available at: http://orthomolecular.org/resources/omns/v07n05.shtml See also: http://orthomolecular.org/resources/omns/v12n01.shtml.

8. The Associated Press. Bad drug reactions send 700,000 to ER yearly. Oct 17, 2006. http://www.msnbc.msn.com/id/15305033/.

9. Null G, Dean C, Feldman M, et al. Death by medicine. *J Orthomolecular Med* 2005; 20(1): 21–34.

10. The Associated Press. Drug errors injure more than 1.5 million a year. July 20, 2006. http://www.msnbc.msn.com/id/13954142.

11. Leape LL. Institute of Medicine medical error figures are not exaggerated. *JAMA* 2000;284(1):95–97. Leape LL. Error in medicine. *JAMA* 1994;272(23):1851–1857. Lazarou J, Pomeranz BH, Corey PN. Incidence of adverse drug reactions in hospitalized patients: a meta-analysis of prospective studies. *JAMA* 1998;279(15):1200–1205.

12. Fox M. Daily aspirin use linked with pancreatic cancer. *Reuters.* Oct 27, 2003. http://www.cnn.com/2003/HEALTH/10/27/cancer.aspirin.reut/index.html.

Confessions of a Frustrated Pharmacist

by Stuart Lindsey, PharmD

From the *Orthomolecular Medicine News Service*, January 30, 2012.

"When an insider breaks ranks with pharmaceutical orthodoxy, it is time to take notice. 'Whistleblower' may be an overused term, but the article that follows might be well worth readers' consideration before standing in line for their next prescription refill."

—Andrew W. Saul, Editor

I'm a registered pharmacist. I am having a difficult time with my job. I sell people drugs that are supposed to correct their various health complaints. Some medicines work like they're supposed to, but many don't. Some categories of drugs work better than others. My concern is that the outcomes of treatment I observe are so unpredictable that I would often call the entire treatment a failure in too many situations.

How It Started

In 1993, I graduated with a BS in Pharmaceutical Sciences from University of New Mexico (UNM). I became pharmacy manager for a small, independent neighborhood drugstore. Starting in the year 2000, nutrition became an integral part of our business. The anecdotal feedback from the customers who started vitamin regimens was phenomenal. That same year, my PharmD clinical rotations began with my propensity for nutritional alternatives firmly in place in my mind. On the second day of my adult-medicine rotation, my preceptor at a nearby hospital informed me that he had every intention of beating this vitamin stuff out of me. I informed him that probably wouldn't happen. Three weeks later I was terminated from my rotations. The preceptor told my supervisor at UNM that there were acute intellectual differences that couldn't be accommodated in their program. What had I done? I was pressuring my preceptor to read an article written by an MD at a hospital in Washington state that showed if a person comes into the emergency room with a yet-to-be diagnosed problem and is given a 3,000 to 4,000 milligram (mg) bolus of vitamin C, that person's chance of dying over the next ten days in ICU dropped by 57 percent![1]

One would think that someone who is an active part of the emergency room staff might find that an interesting statistic. His solution to my attempting to force him to read that article was having me removed from the program.

Pecking Order

The traditional role of the pharmacist in mainstream medicine is subordinate to that of the doctor. The doctor is responsible for most of the information that is received from and given to the patient. The pharmacist's responsibility is to reinforce the doctor's directions. The doctor and the pharmacist both want to have a positive treatment outcome, but there is a legally defined "standard of care" looking over their shoulder.

The training that I received to become a PharmD motivated me to become more interested in these treatment outcomes. After refilling a patient's prescriptions a few times, it becomes obvious that the expected positive outcomes often simply don't happen. It's easy to take the low road and blame it on "poor compliance by the patient." I'm sure this can explain some treatment-failure outcomes, but not all. Many (indeed most) drugs such as blood pressure regulators can require several adjustments of dose or combination with alternative medicines before a positive outcome is obtained.

Wrong Drug; Wrong Disease

One drug misadventure is turning drugs that were originally designed for a rare (0.3 percent of the population) condition called Zollinger-Ellison syndrome into big pharma's treatment for occasional indigestion. These drugs are called proton-pump inhibitors (PPI).[2] After prolonged exposure to PPIs, the body's true issues of achlorhydria start to surface.[3]

These drugs are likely to cause magnesium deficiency, among other problems. Even the Food and Drug Administration (FDA) thinks their long-term use is unwise.[4]

The original instructions for these drugs were for a maximum use of six weeks . . . until somebody in marketing figured out that people could be on the drugs for years. Drug usage gets even more complicated when you understand that excessive use of antibiotics could be the cause of the initial indigestion complaints. What you get from inserting proton-pump inhibitors into this situation is a gastrointestinal nightmare. A better course of medicine in this type of case might well be a bottle of probiotic supplements (or yogurt) and a few quarts of aloe vera juice.

Many doctors are recognizing there are problems with overusing PPIs, but many still don't get it. An example of this occured in my school in NM, where a lot of students went into a nearby impoverished area for rotations. They have blue laws in this area with no alcohol sales on Sunday. The students saw the pattern of the patients going into the clinics on Monday after abusing solvents, even gasoline vapors, and having the doctors put them on omeprazole (e.g., Prilosec) long term, because their stomachs are upset. This is medicine in the real world.

Reliability or Bias?

Mainstream medicine and pharmacy instill into their practitioners from the beginning to be careful about where you get your information. Medical journals boast of their peer review process. When you discuss with other health professionals, invariably they will ask from which medical journal did you get your information. I actually took an elective course in pharmacy on how to evaluate a particular article for its truthfulness. The class was structured on a backbone of caution about making sure, as one read an article, that we understand that real truthfulness only comes from a few approved sources.

I was never comfortable with this concept. Once you realized that many of these "truthfulness bastions" actually have a hidden agenda, the whole premise of this course became suspect. One of my preceptors for my doctoral program insisted that I become familiar with a particular medical journal. If I did, she said, I would be on my way to understanding the "big picture." When I expressed being a little skeptical of this journal, the teacher told me I could trust it as the journal was nonprofit, and there were no editorial strings attached.

Weirdly enough, what had started our exchange over credibility was a warm can of a diet soft drink on the teacher's desk. She drank the stuff all day. I was kidding around with her, and asked her if she had seen some controversial articles about the dangers of consuming quantities of aspartame. She scoffed at my conspiracy theory–laden point of view and I thought the subject was closed. The beginning of the next day, the teacher gave me an assignment: to hustle over to the medical library and make sure I read a paper she assured me would set me straight about my aspartame suspicions, while simultaneously demonstrating the value of getting my information from a nonprofit medical journal. It turned out that the article she wanted me to read, in the "nonprofit medical journal" was funded in its entirety by the Drug Manufacturers Association.

Flashy Pharma Ads

As I read the literature, I discovered that there is very decidedly a barrier between two blocks of information: substances that can be patented vs. substances that can't be. The can-be-patented group gets a professional discussion in eye-pleasing, four-color-print, art-like magazines. This attention to aesthetics tricks some people into interpreting, from the flashy presentation method, that the information is intrinsically truthful.

The world's drug manufacturers do an incredibly good job using all kinds of media penetration to get the word out about their products. The drug industry's audience used to be confined to readers of medical journals and trade publications. Then, in 1997, direct-to-consumer marketing was made legal.[5]

Personally, I don't think this kind of presentation should be allowed. I have doctor friends that say they frequently have patients that self-diagnose from TV commercials and demand the doctor write them a prescription for the advertised product. The patients then threaten the doctor, if he or she refuses their request, that they will change doctors to get the medication. One of my doctor friends says he feels like a trained seal.

Negative Reporting on Vitamins

A vitamin article usually doesn't get the same glossy presentation. Frequently, questionable vitamin research will be published and get blown out of proportion. A prime example of this was the clamor in the press in 2008 that vitamin E somehow caused lung cancer.

I studied this 2008 experiment[6] and found glaring errors in its execution. These errors were so obvious that the experiment shouldn't have gotten any attention, yet this article ended up virtually everywhere. Antivitamin spin requires this kind of research to be widely disseminated to show how "ineffectual" and even "dangerous" vitamins are. I tracked down one of the article's original authors and questioned him about the failure to define what kind of vitamin E had been studied. A simple literature hunt shows considerable difference between natural and synthetic vitamin E. This is an important distinction because most of the negative articles and subsequent treatment failures have used the synthetic form for the experiment, often because it is cheap. Natural vitamin E with mixed tocopherols and tocotrienols costs two or three times more than the synthetic form.

Before I even got the question out of my mouth, the researcher started up, "I know, I know what you're going to say." He ended up admitting that they hadn't even considered the vitamin E type when they did the experiment. This failure to define the vitamin E type made it impossible to draw a meaningful conclusion. I asked the researcher if he realized how much damage this highly quoted article had done to vitamin credibility. If there has been anything like a retraction, I have yet to see it.

Illness Is Not Caused by Drug Deficiency

If you've made it this far in reading this article you have discerned that I'm sympathetic to vitamin arguments. I think most diseases are some form of malnutrition. Taking the position that nutrition is the foundation of disease doesn't make medicine any simpler. You still have to figure out who has what and why. There are many disease states that are difficult to pin down using the "pharmaceutical solution to disease." A drug solution is a nice idea, in theory. It makes the assumption that the cause of a disease is so well understood that a man-made chemical commonly called "medicine" is administered, very efficiently solving the health problem. The reality, though, is medicine doesn't understand most health problems very well. A person with a heart rhythm disturbance is not low on digoxin. A child who is diagnosed with attention-deficit hyperactivity disorder (ADHD) does not act that way because the child is low on Ritalin. By the same logic, a person with type 2 diabetes doesn't have a deficit of metformin. The flaw of medicine is the concept of managing (but not curing) a particular disease state. I'm hard pressed to name any disease state that mainstream medicine is in control of.

Voltaire allegedly said, "Doctors are men who pour drugs of which they know little, to cure diseases of which they know less, into human beings of whom they know nothing." Maybe he overstated the problem. Maybe he didn't.

REFERENCES FOR "CONFESSIONS OF A FRUSTRATED PHARMACIST"

1. Nathens AB, Neff MJ, Jurkovich, et al. Randomized, prospective trial of antioxidant supplementation in critically ill surgical patients. *Ann Surg* 2002; 236(6): 814–822. Free full text paper at: http://www.ncbi.nlm.nih.gov/pmc/articles/PMC1422648/?tool=pubmed.

2. Maton PN, Vinayek R, Frucht H, et al. Long-term efficacy and safety of omeprazole in patients with Zollinger-Ellison syndrome: a prospective study. *Gastroenterology* 1989;97(4):827–836.

Maton PN, Lack EE, Collen MJ, et al. The effect of Zollinger-Ellison syndrome and omeprazole therapy on gastric oxyntic endocrine cells. *Gastroenterology* 1990;99(4):943–950.

3. Laria A, Zoli A, Gremese E, et al. Proton pump inhibitors in rheumatic diseases: clinical practice, drug interactions, bone fractures and risk of infections. *Reumatismo* 2011;63(1):5–10. Fohl AL, Regal RE. Proton pump inhibitor-associated pneumonia: Not a breath of fresh air after all? *World J Gastrointest Pharmacol Ther* 2011;2(3):17–26. doi: 10.4292/wjgpt.v2.i3.17.

4. U. S. Department of Health and Human Services. Food and Drug Administration. Proton pump inhibitor drugs (PPIs): drug safety communication—low magnesium levels can be associated with long-term use. Mar 2, 2011. http://www.fda.gov/Safety/MedWatch/SafetyInformation/SafetyAlertsforHumanMedicalProducts/ucm245275.htm.

5. Donohue JM, Cevasco M, Rosenthal MB. A decade of direct-to-consumer advertising of prescription drugs. *N Engl J Med* 2007; 357:673–681. doi: 10.1056/NEJMsa070502.

6. Slatore CG, Littman AJ, Au DH, et al. Long-term use of supplemental multivitamins, vitamin C, vitamin E, and folate does not reduce the risk of lung cancer. *Am J Respir Crit Care Med* 2008; 177(5): 524–530. doi: 10.1164/rccm.200709–1398OC.

BIG NAMES, BIG MISTAKES: CONSUMERS MISLED BY SUPPLEMENT BASHING

by Gert Schuitemaker, PhD, and Bo Jonsson, MD, PhD

From the *Orthomolecular Medicine News Service,* October 20, 2015.

Big names: the *New England Journal of Medicine* (NEJM), arguably the most prestigious medical journal in the world. Plus, the *New York Times.* On October 14th, the latter mentioned, "Dietary Supplements Lead to 20,000 E.R. Visits Yearly, Study Finds." It was a report of a study published in the NEJM with the headline "Emergency Department Visits for Adverse Events Related to Dietary Supplements."

Whoa! What is that again? Is there *really* something new and terrible about vitamin C or magnesium?

Naturally, it was time to investigate. First, a look at the original paper from NEJM, and a direct examination as to how the study was designed.[1] This was a revelation in itself, which can best be explained as follows: Let's say someone is exercising on a Sunday morning and suddenly gets palpitations. Oh, he thinks, what's going on here? A little bit frightened, and just to be sure, he decides to go to the ER. He says, "Doctor, something is going wrong. I have palpitations." The doctor examines him and asked about the circumstances. Then he learned that the visitor had used that morning a dietary supplement. Aha! That's it! Dietary supplements! Suspicious!

There is not even one death caused by any dietary supplement, according to the most recent information collected by the U.S. National Poison Data System.[2]

This observational report is done by just the one doctor serving at that time. The data collection in this investigation can be considered poor as well as subjective. It falls scientifically short. Moreover, as we already know, too many physicians 1) have little affinity for dietary supplements, and 2) are virtually untrained as to nutrition and supplements.

But Wait: There's More

We continued by looking over the results section. We had already noticed that the researchers drew the conclusion that problems with dietary supplements were underestimated. Duffy Mackay, a spokesman for the Council for Responsible Nutrition, a supplement industry trade group, argued that the results showed that only 0.01 percent of all Americans demonstrated an adverse effect from dietary supplements. So he came to an opposite conclusion: the study highlighted how relatively safe supplements are given how many people took them.[3]

In the study, it was striking that the biggest segment of that 0.01 percent was 20- to 34-year-olds who took energy products and weight loss products. They showed symptoms like chest pain, heart palpitations, and irregular heart rhythms. What kind of supplements could these be? We are not aware that vitamin C, vitamin B_3, or any of the essential nutrients show these types of adverse effects.

> *"The most misleading part of the* NY Times *article's headline is 'lead.' It is important to distinguish causation from correlation, and guilt from association."*
>
> —W. TODD PENBERTHY, PHD

Where, then, is the problem? Mainly it's with the so-called "supplements" containing alkaloid substances, in most cases caffeine, but also ephedra, already banned in 2004 by the Food and Drug Administration as a supplement, but still offered for sale via the internet. Therefore, a comparison with "energy drinks" is more apt than to label these products as dietary supplements. However, caffeine-laden drinks were for some reason not included in the study. Aside from being available as both tablets and capsules, caffeine and nutrients have very little in common. Caffeine is a (medicinal) stimulant; nutrients are part of the human metabolism which are necessary for maintaining proper health.

It is significant that neither the *New York Times* nor the original *NEJM* paper mentioned caffeine or coffee-extract. The researchers only mentioned energy products and weight loss products, not specifying the substances involved. In order to find out that the study mainly concerned caffeine, we had to get into a separate annex which was somewhat difficult to for the public to find, and only available via the website of the *NEJM*.

And what is in the future for unsuspecting consumers? The headline "Dietary Supplements Finally Banned"?

It could happen. You can be sure the media will let you know when it does.

REFERENCES FOR "BIG NAMES, BIG MISTAKES"

1. Geller AI, Shehab N, Weidle NJ, et al. Emergency Department Visits for Adverse Events Related to Dietary Supplements. *N Engl J Med* 2015;373(16):1531–1540. doi: 10.1056/NEJMsa1504267.

2. Saul AW. No deaths from vitamins. Absolutely none. Jan 14, 2015. Available at: http://orthomolecular.org/resources/omns/v11n01.shtml. See also: Saul AW. No deaths from ANY dietary supplement. Jan 16, 2015. Available at: http://orthomolecular.org/resources/omns/v11n02.shtml.

3. O'Connor A. Dietary supplements lead to 20,000 E.R. visits yearly, study finds. *The New York Times*. Well. Oct 14, 2015.

PHARMACEUTICAL DRUG MARKETING TO OUR CHILDREN: BORDERING ON CRIMINAL

by Helen Saul Case

From the *Orthomolecular Medicine News Service,* June 11, 2013.

I can't be the only one noticing. In fact I'm pretty sure I'm not. Drugs are being marketed directly to our children. If you don't believe me, just take a closer look at the commercials plastered about our TV shows at an estimated and alarming 80 an hour,[1] many targeting our little ones with images of animals and cartoons. Everywhere in the world, except the United States and New Zealand, direct-to-consumer pharmaceutical drug advertising is prohibited.[2] Perhaps it's time to think about why it should be banned here, too.

TV ads are designed to make an impact. They are meant to foster brand familiarity and loyalty. They appeal to our emotions. They often emphasize our shortcomings as fathers, mothers, friends, and spouses. Commercials influence us into thinking that using a particular product is a normal, ordinary, good idea: an everyday thing to do that everybody is doing.

I remember being shocked the first time I saw a pharmaceutical drug ad on TV. I couldn't believe that anyone would take a medication with a list of side effects that seemed so much worse than the disease it supposedly helped treat. Now, it is easy to become numb to them. The sheer volume of drug advertisements we are inundated with on a regular basis practically ensures we accept them as a natural part of life. Now that their presence isn't as shocking, it is easy to pay more attention to the beautiful imagery on the screen rather than the described dangers of the drug. I can rattle off brand name after brand name, and I'm not even paying attention, nor do I have any interest in them.

Until recently. When my baby girl starting pointing at cartoons and animals in pharmaceutical ads, I had had enough.

Profits and Preschoolers

There is no money in selling something nobody believes in. Drug companies want their commercials to be appealing. When I was little, I once asked my dad why they called a certain candy a "Thin Mint." He said because no one would buy them if they called them "Fat Mints."

Drug ads are alluring, especially to young eyes. The commercial for the drug Abilify, a buddy for your antidepressant, has a friendly little cartoon "A" coming to the rescue of a happy little Rx pill and a lovely cartoon woman. Variants of their commercial showcase a childish depression cloud and a rainy cartoon umbrella. A quick glance would have you believing you are watching children's programming meant to teach about the alphabet or the weather.

The antidepressant Zoloft's bouncing cartoon ball can't be described as anything but cute (who doesn't love a cowlick?), and even more "adult" commercials like those for the inhaler Spiriva have real-live elephants capturing the attention of my toddler.

How about those positively mesmerizing Lunesta commercials with the peaceful glowing butterflies? (My daughter loves those.) An entire nation appears to be on drugs as the butterflies, indicated with thousands of illuminated specks, glow across a map of the United States. They capture your attention as a voice softly coos, "Join us." This particular ad doesn't even tell you the name of the drug, and therefore doesn't have to tell you what is wrong with the drug, either. The commercial advises you to seek out their website, ProjectLuna.com, which dons a name rather similar to their "unnamed" product. Of course, they've already made you familiar with their drug in numerous other broadcasts, so they don't even *need* to tell you what it's for. It's kind of like the Nike swoosh. We all know what it means.

Do adults really need cartoons to understand what a drug can do? Or is there a more sinister plot afoot?

Drugs for the Whole Family

Some of you are telling me to turn my TV off. What business has a toddler watching *Let's Make a Deal* anyway. And while I hear you, I can tell you that unless I leave the TV off all the time, she's going to see a drug ad sooner or later. She does love books and magazines, especially ones with animals. Maybe we will just stick to those. Of course, the most recent publication we received wasn't any better.

My cat receives a magazine in the mail from her veterinarian. It encourages her to come in for her checkups. She can't read very well, but if she could, she'd see that the pages are dotted with drug ads appealing to the emotions of her owner.

Drugging pets is big business. For example, Pfizer Animal Health is now Zoetis, a multi-billion dollar company, just one in a multi-billion dollar industry. There is real money to be made medicating our "companion animals." And unless you have some sort of animal prescription drug coverage, which is highly unlikely, you will be paying for those meds out of pocket. And we are. A *New York Times* article about our "Pill-Popping Pets" indicated that "surveys by the American Pet Products Manufacturers Association found that 77 percent of dog owners and 52 percent of cat owners gave their animals some sort of medication in 2006."[3] That means half to three-quarters of our furry friends are being drugged. By us. (Apparently, there is even a pill for all that puking my cat has been doing.[4] Who knew?)

A Lesson to Be Learned, Again

Have we forgotten about Joe? Perhaps we should take a step back in time and consider the R. J. Reynolds Tobacco Company. Joe Camel, the cartoon character promoting Camel cigarettes, "which the Federal Trade Commission (FTC) alleges was successful in appealing to many children and adolescents under 18, induced many young people to begin smoking or to continue smoking cigarettes and as a result caused significant injury to their health and safety." R .J. Reynolds was accused of promoting a "dangerous" product through "a campaign that was attractive to those too young to purchase cigarettes legally." Joe Camel was "as recognizable to kids as Mickey Mouse." After the campaign started, the FTC claimed "the percentage of kids who smoked Camels became larger than the percentage of adults who smoked Camels."[5] Were kids starting to smoke, and continuing to smoke, because of good ol' Joe? Were they too young to know what hit 'em?

"As to 'medicine,' I used to use very little of this stuff for infants. Now, I categorically state: just say no to drugs."

—PEDIATRICIAN RALPH K. CAMPBELL, MD

We're Asking for It

Maybe kids can't get their own prescription, but they know someone who can get it for them. We lead by example. We are going to our doctors and *asking* for drugs for ourselves and for our children. Our doctors are all too happy to dole them out. They'll even throw in some free samples to get you started. There are billions of dollars spent every year advertising drugs directly to us, and it is working. The most heavily advertised pharmaceuticals see the largest increase in prescriptions and purchases.[6]

A Slippery Slope

I believe advertising drugs in a child-friendly way is dangerous. For example, what kid doesn't have a bad day? Or a ton of them? Being moody is part of being human, and it is certainly part of being an adolescent. Putting the idea in a young mind that being upset is an emotion that should be medicated is tricky territory. Critics of the pharmaceutical industry agree that "a lot of money can be made from healthy people who believe they are sick."[7]

Kids want to be happy. Parents want to help their children feel better. They may see minimized risk due to the positive associations drawn from drug commercials. We may be overconfident in drugs and in the doctors that prescribe them. We may think, "Well, if my physician gave it to me, it must be okay."

Making drugs a common and everyday part of life: it appears that's what pharmaceutical companies are trying to do. I think back to school trips I took with my middle school students. We are required to carry their medications when we travel, and each year, over the course of many, the hefty Ziploc bags I lugged around filled with medications grew and grew until I practically had my backpack overflowing with them. Eight to twelve kids, and a backpack full of meds. What was happening? I was surprised, but perhaps I shouldn't have been: one out of every two people in America is taking prescription medications.[8] And so too is their cat.

It took 23 years before Joe Camel was taken out. How long before we pop the Zoloft bubble and squash the Nasonex bumblebee?

Safety of Supplements vs. the Dangers of Drugs

I believe drug treatment for disease should be last on the list, and nutrition should be first. Are there folks that need medicines? Yes. But what about natural, effective, and safe ways we can combat allergies, depression, and trouble sleeping? I haven't seen any commercials about niacin (B_3) for mental disorders. Or about the importance of high-dose vitamin C. Or about the health benefits of optimal doses of vitamin D. We often turn away from nutrition and toward medication. This, ladies, gentlemen, and children, is wrong.

Just Say No

Drugs are dangerous.[9] The front page of Zoloft's own website states, "Antidepressant medicines may increase suicidal thoughts or actions in some children, teenagers, and young adults especially within the first few months of treatment."[10] *With over a hundred thousand deaths every year due to pharmaceuticals taken as directed,*[11] I really don't want my kid to be among them.

The old adage is true: just say no to drugs. And if the results of the "Say No to Drugs" campaign[12] are any indication of how well it works to do so, it will be a sorry success indeed.

REFERENCES FOR "PHARMACEUTICAL DRUG MARKETING TO OUR CHILDREN"

1. Spiegel A. Selling sickness: how drug ads changed health care. Oct 13, 2009. National Public Radio. Available at: http://www.npr.org/templates/story/story.php?storyId=113675737.

2. Woodward LD. Pharmaceutical ads: good or bad for consumers? ABC News, February 24, 2010. Available at: http://abcnews.go.com/Business/Wellness/pharmaceutical-ads-good-bad-consumers/story?id=9925198.

3. Vlahos J. Pill-popping pets. *The New York Times Magazine,* July 13, 2008. Available at: http://www.nytimes.com/2008/07/13/magazine/13pets-t.html?pagewanted=all&_r=0.

4. Cerenia. Cerenia.com.

5. Federal Trade Commission. Joe Camel advertising campaign violates federal law, FTC says. Agency charges R.J. Reynolds with causing substantial injury to the health and safety of children and adolescents under 18. May 28, 1997. Available at: http://www.ftc.gov/opa/1997/05/joecamel.shtm.

6. Findlay S. Research brief: prescription drugs and mass media advertising. National Institute for Health Care Management Foundation (NIHCM Foundation), Sept 2000. Available at: http://www.nihcm.org/pdf/DTCbrief.pdf.

7. Ibid.

8. Carroll J. Half of Americans currently taking prescription medication. Gallup News Service, Dec 9, 2005. Available at: http://www.gallup.com/poll/20365/halfamericans-currently-taking-prescription-medication.aspx.

9. Mercola J. Pharmaceutical drugs are 62,000 times more likely to kill you than supplements. Jul 24, 2012. Available at: http://articles.mercola.com/sites/articles/archive/2012/07/24/pharmaceutical-drugs-vs-nutritional-supplements.aspx.

10. Zoloft. Zoloft.com.

11. Starfield B. Is US health really the best in the world?" *JAMA* 2000; 284(4):483–485.

12. Reaves J. Just say no to DARE. Feb 15, 2001. Available at: http://www.time.com/time/nation/article/0,8599,99564,00.html#ixzz2Va6a9TK7.

ANTIVITAMIN PUBLICATIONS: MISINFORMATION PRESENTED AS TRUTH

by Rolf Hefti

From the *Orthomolecular Medicine News Service,* July 18, 2013.

Some anti-supplement publications[1–4] by a prominent spokesman for the medical industry, Paul A. Offit, MD, received broad mainstream media coverage.

Let's take a closer look at some of the studies that Dr. Offit proffers to substantiate his generalized antivitamin charges.

CLAIM: Offit claimed that a study[5] from 1942 had already refuted the proposition made by dual Nobel Prize winner Linus Pauling, PhD (1901–1994), during the 1970s that high-dose vitamin C supplements can ameliorate the unpleasant experience of the common cold.[3]

FACT: The cited study[5] actually showed a significant decrease in the severity and duration of symptoms of the common cold with the use of moderate-high dose vitamin C supplements.[6]

CLAIM: Offit dismissed Pauling's claim that high-dose vitamin therapy is useful in the treatment of cancer, calling Pauling "arguably the world's greatest quack."[3] Offit referred to two Mayo clinic studies[7,8] that asserted to have replicated, and refuted, Pauling's (and a colleague's) studies,[9,10] which demonstrated impressive supplement benefits against cancer.

FACT: Pauling described in detail that the two Mayo clinic papers were not following his (and his colleague's) study procedures; thus those studies were meaningless and irrelevant in debunking his vitamin claims.[11] Offit fails to mention this crucial point, thus presenting an established scientific falsehood as a scientific fact. Research has confirmed that vitamin C therapy is beneficial in the fight against cancer if the proper protocols are followed.[12]

CLAIM: Offit claimed that only four types of supplements (calcium, folic acid, omega-3 fatty acid, and vitamin D) "might be of value for otherwise healthy people."[1–3]

FACT: Many dietary supplements are of value for our ever-increasingly unhealthy population, validated by sound scientific data, including randomized controlled studies.[13,14,24–27]

CLAIM: Offit claims that taking megavitamins (doses above RDA amounts) could increase the risk of cancer, heart disease, and mortality in "otherwise healthy" consumers. He advises the public to "stop taking vitamins."[1–4]

FACT: Several of the studies that Offit cited are either misleading or flawed. For example, some findings only applied to chain-smokers who also consumed alcohol, elderly people, or gravely ill people [20–23] rather than "otherwise healthy" people. Contrary to Offit's claim, many meaningful studies have documented that nutritional supplements, especially in large doses, significantly reduce the risk of heart disease, cancer, and mortality in both "otherwise healthy" and sick people.[13–19,24–29]

Looking at any annual report of the American Association of Poison Control Centers[30] shows very few deaths from supplement consumption. Far more people die from the intake of aspirin, commonly perceived as a rather safe substance. Most disturbing, scientific data from medical journals and government health statistics reveal that the proper consumption of pharmaceutical medications kills over 100,000 people every year in the US alone.[31,32]

Conclusion

Dr. Offit's vitamin-bashing accusations have little to do with accuracy. Politics, or profit, provides the most plausible explanation for such unfounded attacks.

The field of alternative medicine has grown dramatically since the 1990s, particularly the supplement industry. Alternative medicine's products and services have increasingly become a significant competitor to the big business of orthodox medicine, which is aimed instead at the treatment of long-term disease. Alternative medicine cuts into the bottom line of the medical industry's profit-generating model of disease care.

Dr. Offit's sweeping, nonscientific generalizations against the use of dietary supplements appear to be an attempt to diminish the influence of a steadily growing competitor. Above all, Offit's incorrect and biased antisupplement accusations reaffirm the importance of following first principles to arrive at the whole truth: take a look at the facts yourself, and do not put your trust in authorities.

REFERENCES FOR "ANTIVITAMIN PUBLICATIONS"

1. Offit PA. *Do You Believe in Magic? The Sense and Nonsense of Alternative Medicine.* New York: HarperCollins, 2013.

2. Offit PA. *Killing You Softly: The Sense and Nonsense of Alternative Medicine.* Fourth Estate, 2013.

3. Offit PA. Vitamins: stop taking the pills: Vitamin supplements are good for you, right? Wrong, says a new book—they're a multibillion-pound con and in high doses can increase your risk of heart disease and cancer. *The Guardian,* Jun 7, 2013.

4. Offit PA. Don't take your vitamins. *The New York Times,* Jun 8, 2013.

5. Cowan DW, Diehl HS, Baker AB. Vitamins for the prevention of colds. *J Am Med Assoc* 1942;120: 1267–1271.

6. Pauling L. Early evidence about vitamin C and the common cold. *Orthomolecular Psychiatry* 1974;3(3):139–151.

7. Creagan ET, Moertel CG, O'Fallon JR, et al. Failure of high-dose vitamin C (ascorbic acid) therapy to benefit patients with advanced cancer. A controlled trial. *N Engl J Med* 1979;301(13):687–690.

8. Moertel CG, Fleming TR, Creagan ET, et al. High- dose vitamin C versus placebo in the treatment of patients with advanced cancer who have had no prior chemotherapy. A randomized double-blind comparison. *N Engl J Med* 1985;312(3):137–141.

9. Cameron E, Pauling L. Supplemental ascorbate in the supportive treatment of cancer: Prolongation of survival times in terminal human cancer. *Proc Natl Acad Sci U S A* 1976;73(10):3685–3689.

10. Ibid.

11. Pauling L. *How to Live Longer and Feel Better.* Oregon State University Press, 2006.

12. Ohno S, Ohno Y, Suzuki N, et al. High-dose vitamin C (ascorbic acid) therapy in the treatment of patients with advanced cancer. *Anticancer Res* 2009;29(3):809–815.

13. Canner PL, Berge KG, Wenger NK, et al. Fifteen year mortality in Coronary Drug Project patients: long- term benefit with niacin. *J Am Coll Cardiol* 1986;8(6):1245–1255.

14. Berge KG, Canner PL. Coronary drug project: experience with niacin. Coronary Drug Project Research Group. *Eur J Clin Pharmacol* 1991;40 Suppl 1:S49–51.

15. Lee IM, Cook NR, Gaziano JM, et al. Vitamin E in the primary prevention of cardiovascular disease and cancer: the Women's Health Study: a randomized controlled trial. *JAMA* 2005;294(1):56–65.

16. Gaziano JM, Sesso HD, Christen WG, et al. Multivitamins in the prevention of cancer in men: the Physicians' Health Study II randomized controlled trial. *JAMA* 2012;308(18):1871–1880.

17. Clark LC, Combs GF Jr, Turnbull BW, et al. Effects of selenium supplementation for cancer prevention in patients with carcinoma of the skin. A randomized controlled trial. Nutritional Prevention of Cancer Study Group. *JAMA* 1996;276(24):1957–1963.

18. Fawzi WW, Msamanga GI, Spiegelman D, et al. A randomized trial of multivitamin supplements and HIV disease progression and mortality. *N Engl J Med* 2004;351(1):23–32.

19. Shimizu M, Fukutomi Y, Ninomiya M, et al. Green tea extracts for the prevention of metachronous colorectal adenomas: a pilot study. *Cancer Epidemiol Biomarkers Prev* 2008;17(11):3020–3025.

20. The effect of vitamin E and beta carotene on the incidence of lung cancer and other cancers in male smokers. The Alpha- Tocopherol, Beta Carotene Cancer Prevention Study Group. *N Engl J Med* 1994;330(15):1029–1035.

21. Omenn GS, Goodman GE, Thornquist MD, et al. Effects of a combination of beta carotene and vitamin A on lung cancer and cardiovascular disease. *N Engl J Med* 1996;334(18):1150–1155.

22. Miller ER 3rd, Pastor-Barriuso R, Dalal D, et al. Meta-analysis: high-dosage vitamin E supplementation may increase all-cause mortality. *Ann Intern Med* 2005;142(1):37–46.

23. Lonn E, Bosch J, Yusuf S, et al. Effects of long-term vitamin E supplementation on cardiovascular events and cancer: a randomized controlled trial. *JAMA* 2005;293(11):1338–1347.

24. White E, Shannon JS, Patterson RE. Relationship between vitamin and calcium supplement use and colon cancer. *Cancer Epidemiol Biomarkers Prev* 1997;6(10):769–774.

25. Watkins ML, Erickson JD, Thun MJ, et al. Multivitamin use and mortality in a large prospective study. *Am J Epidemiol* 2000;152(2):149–162.

26. Harris HR, Bergkvist L, Wolk A. Vitamin C intake and breast cancer mortality in a cohort of Swedish women. *Br J Cancer* 2013. doi: 10.1038/bjc.2013.269.

27. Enstrom JE, Kanim LE, Klein MA. Vitamin C intake and mortality among a sample of the United States population. *Epidemiology* 1992;3(3):194–202.

28. Tovar J, Nilsson A, Johansson M, et al. A diet based on multiple functional concepts improves cardiometabolic risk parameters in healthy subjects. *Nutr Metab (Lond)* 2012;9:29. doi: 10.1186/1743–7075–9-29.

29. Gaziano JM, Sesso HD, Christen WG, et al. Multivitamins in the prevention of cancer in men: the Physicians' Health Study II randomized controlled trial. *JAMA* 2012;308(18):1871–1880.

30. American Association of Poison Control Centers. Annual Report from 1983- 2008. http://www.aapcc.org.

31. Starfield B. Is US health really the best in the world? *JAMA* 2000;284(4):483–485.

32. Dean C, Feldman M, Rasio D, et al. Death by Medicine. Independent review commissioned by the Nutrition Institute of America, 2003.

TRASHING VITAMINS WITH GARBAGE ARTICLES

by Travis V. Meyer

From the *Orthomolecular Medicine News Service,* September 3, 2013.

Recently, while browsing the news, I found yet another article trashing vitamins: "Stop swallowing vitamins and the claims about their effects, doctors urge."[1]

I found this article interesting due to some of the outrageous statements made in the article by a Dr. Paul Offit and Dr. Donald Hensrud. I'll be the first to tell you that I'm not in the health industry, nor do I have any advanced degrees in health sciences (my master's degree is in business administration, not health care). Still, some of these claims are so outrageous you wonder how they can print this stuff with a good conscience.

Here are some quotes from the article that had me shaking my head, along with my own layman's opinion regarding such statements:

"Vitamin pills are not merely of uncertain benefit. In some cases, and especially in large doses, they are downright dangerous."

This is a very charged statement, as it is asserting that you are potentially risking your life by talking supplements in large doses. However, where is the evidence supporting claims that vitamins in large doses are "downright dangerous"? I have read articles that exalt the values of megadose vitamin therapy, and all of them have had one thing in common: references to the scientific research backing up their position. If the article is to be believed, it should specify which vitamins are so "dangerous" and precisely what that means, with abundant supporting citations.

Analysis of US Poison Control Center annual report data indicates that there have been no confirmed deaths from vitamins in the 28 years that such data has been available.[2]

How about this statement:

"Megavitamins contain many times greater than the recommended daily allowance. Five times, 10 times, sometimes 20 times more. And I think therein danger lies. There are a number of studies showing that you can actually get too much of a good thing, that this can actually increase your risk of cancer and heart disease. I think most people don't know that."

I have to admit that this was surprising to me. In fact, I've never seen even one reliable study showing that taking vitamins in any dose can increase my risk of cancer and heart disease. Again, I'd love to see this great number of studies. Logic dictates if vitamins were that dangerous, and had a number of studies supporting this claim, that this news would have been put out long ago, especially since big pharma would be popping champagne and sending their propaganda officers into overtime if such news came out. Not to mention the safety alerts and probable market withdrawals of said vitamins. And that brings me to another point. Many prescription drugs can be hazardous to health, and several big money makers have had to be withdrawn because of dangerous side effects. Compared to drugs, vitamins look pretty safe to me.

Continuing:

"Even a multivitamin might be a little bit too much. . . If you're taking just one nutrient, it may be throwing off the balance of the overall milieu."

Really? I'll tell you what has thrown *my* milieu out of balance: taking just one antibiotic. My milieu was so out of balance that I was stuck in the bathroom every 30 minutes. If taking one vitamin, say extra vitamin C, may be throwing off nutritional balance, I want proof, not assumptions or speculation.

Antibiotics put over 142,000 into emergency rooms every year, just in the USA. Common antibiotics, the ones most frequently prescribed and regarded as safest, cause nearly half of these emergencies.[3]

That supposedly reliable news sources publish such throw-away articles just blows my mind. How can you make such speculative claims without any facts to back up such statements? These are supposed to be scientists who base their statements on facts and research, not charlatans who speculate on what may or may not shift your "milieu" out of sorts.

Which brings us to the statements that rankle me the most about this article:

"Offit argued in a recent opinion article in the *New York Times* that 'people need only the recommended daily allowance— the amount of vitamins found in a routine diet.'"

That depends on both how you quantify need, and how you quantify what makes up a routine diet. I suppose if you don't want to develop scurvy, all you need is the Recommended Dietary Allowance (RDA). But is that really the point? I don't want to get sick, I don't want to get cancer, and I don't want to need antibiotics, so perhaps I need a bit more than the RDA. How do we know that the processed foods we've been purchasing for the last 50 years are all that nutritious? In fact, hasn't there been much ado about how our routine diet of processed foods is making us obese and ill?

You don't need a medical degree to cock your head and say, "Wait a minute, something smells fishy here, and it's not my omega-3 pills." I'd like to close with this: my wife and son have significantly reduced their terrible allergies by taking large doses of vitamin C daily. Also, my son seems to have increased his focus after starting on niacin supplements. All this, and no sign of cancer or heart disease.

REFERENCES FOR "TRASHING VITAMINS"

1. MPR News. Stop swallowing vitamins and the claims about their effects, doctors urge. Aug 13, 2013. Available at: http://minnesota.publicradio.org/display/web/2013/08/13/daily-circuit-vitamins-health.

2. Saul AW, Vaman JN. No deaths from vitamins—none at all in 27 years. Jun 14, 2011. Available at: http://orthomolecular.org/resources/omns/v07n05.shtml.

3. Shehab N, Patel PR, Srinivasan A, et al. Emergency department visits for antibiotic-associated adverse events. *Clin Infect Dis* 2008;47(6):735–743. doi: 10.1086/591126.

FDA CLAIMS "FOOD SUPPLEMENT" DEATHS; HIDES DETAILS FROM THE PUBLIC

From the *Orthomolecular Medicine News Service,* October 9, 2008 (updated June 20, 2011).

"There is a principle which is a bar against all information, which is proof against all argument, and which cannot fail to keep man in everlasting ignorance. That principle is condemnation without investigation."

—HERBERT SPENCER

"Dietary supplements cause 600 'adverse events,'" reported *USA Today*. In an article that looks much like an official US Food and Drug Administration (FDA) press release, it said that "[s]erious side effects from the use of food supplements resulted in 604 'adverse-event' reports—a list that includes at least five deaths—through the first six months that such accounts have been required by law."[1]

Good grief! Looks like all those supplement-popping health nuts really are nuts after all. Food supplements simply must be dangerous!

Or are they?

Later on in the article, far from the headline, *USA Today* conceded that "[a]n adverse event can be anything from a concern that a supplement isn't working to a serious illness that follows consumption." And, FDA spokesman Michael Herndon admitted that of the five deaths and 85 hospitalizations reported, "Some of these deaths were likely due to underlying medical conditions."

FDA's method of gaining data is suspect at best and biased at worst. Their "Dietary Supplement Adverse Event Reporting" webpage states, "FDA would like to know when a product causes a problem even if you are unsure the product caused the problem or even if you do not visit a doctor or clinic."[2] The measure of uncertainty involved in publicly soliciting adverse reports "even if you are unsure that the product caused the problem" is noteworthy.

But most significant of all is that FDA refused to disclose exactly which supplements allegedly were causing problems. Doesn't the public have a right to know? In the absence of FDA disclosure to the contrary, it is likely that the five or fewer deaths attributed to "food supplements" were in fact due to medicinal substances marketed as dietary supplements. FDA acknowledges this in a roundabout way at their website.[3] There you will find an "Important Message," which asks health professionals to "Report Serious Adverse Events Associated with Dietary Supplements Containing GBL, GHB, or BD . . . a group of products sold as dietary supplements for bodybuilding, weight loss and sleep inducement which have been determined to pose a significant public health hazard. These products are chemically related to gamma butyrolactone (GBL), gamma hydroxybutyric acid (GHB), and 1,4 butanediol (BD), and can cause dangerously low respiratory rates (intubation may be required), unconsciousness/coma, vomiting, seizures, bradycardia and death. GBL, GHB and BD have been linked to at least 122 serious illnesses reported to FDA, including three deaths."

But these substances are not foods. They are not vitamins, and they are not minerals, and they are not amino acids. They should not be considered with or as food supplements. Over half of all Americans safely take nutritional supplements every day. If each of those persons took only one tablet per day, that would be some 145,000,000 individual doses daily, for a total of over 53 billion doses annually. Many healthy people take more. And yet, according to national statistics compiled by the authoritative American Association of Poison Control Centers, there is not even one death per year from vitamins.[4] Look at the reports, which detail each individual vitamin, mineral, amino acid, and herb, and see for yourself at: http://www.aapcc.org/dnn/NPDS/AnnualReports/tabid/125/Default.aspx.

By comparison, FDA acknowledges that prescription drugs resulted in 482,154 adverse-event reports in the year 2007. That is nearly 400 times as many adverse events from prescription drugs per six-month period. And this much higher number does not include over-the-counter drugs, a striking omission. Many nonprescription drugs, such as Tylenol (acetaminophen), are a long way from safe. Liver toxicity from acetaminophen poisoning is by far the most common cause of acute liver failure in the United States. Acetaminophen accounted for 51 percent of all acute liver failure cases in 2003.[5] Indeed, the Associated Press previously reported that common drug dangers are so bad that "[h]armful reactions to some of the most widely used medicines—from insulin to a common antibiotic—sent more than 700,000 Americans to emergency rooms each year."[6]

Vitamin supplements compete with FDA-sponsored drugs. FDA has been trying to eliminate availability of vitamin supplements for over 45 years. As early as 1962, writes constitutional attorney Jonathan W. Emord, "FDA perceived a competitive threat emerging to drug regulation from the sale of dietary ingredients at above RDA doses." In 1966, "FDA published a rule that any dietary supplement exceeding 150% of the RDA for a vitamin or mineral would automatically be regulated as a drug." In 1976, after a "public outcry," the Proxmire Amendment prohibited FDA from deeming a vitamin or mineral a drug solely because of potency. "Undaunted," continues Emord, "FDA tried yet again to rid the market of vitamins in the 1970s by claiming on a case by case basis that they were adulterated based on their potency." FDA also tried to have supplements declared to be unapproved food additives. "FDA's position was a logical absurdity: Single ingredient dietary supplements were food additives because the ingredients were added to a gelatin capsule which was, FDA said with a wink and a smirk, a food. . . The United States Court of Appeals for the Seventh Circuit described FDA's position as an 'Alice in Wonderland' approach." In 1980, FDA tried to get vitamins classified as over-the-counter drugs. . . "FDA has repeatedly exceeded the limits of its statutory authority to bring about changes designed to protect drug companies from competition."[7]

Additional evidence comes directly from FDA, whose own Dietary Task Force Report, released June 15, 1993, said, "The task force considered many issues in its deliberations including to ensure that the existence of dietary supplements on the market does not act as a disincentive for drug development." There is also this statement that was made by the FDA Deputy Commissioner for Policy, David Adams, at the Drug Information Association Annual Meeting, July 12, 1993: "Pay careful attention to what is happening with dietary supplements in the legislative arena . . . If these efforts are successful, there could be created a class of products to compete with approved drugs. The establishment of a separate regulatory category for supplements could undercut exclusivity rights enjoyed by the holders of approved drug applications."

FDA wants control of vitamins. Their latest ploy is to frighten the public into thinking vitamin supplements are dangerous, without proof, and without even naming the supplements they accuse. Don't fall for what Abram Hoffer, MD, calls "the FDA's grand lie that, if told over and over again, is accepted as somehow true."

Vitamin supplements are not the problem. Poor eating habits, and too many medicines, are the problem. Food supplements are a solution. They are effective, and vastly safer than drugs. The US Food and Drug Administration knows this full well.

REFERENCES FOR "FDA CLAIMS 'FOOD SUPPLEMENT' DEATHS"

1. Perez AJ. Dietary supplements cause 600 'adverse events'. *USA Today,* Sept 22, 2008. Available at: http://www.usatoday.com/news/health/2008–09–22-supplements-adverse-events_N.htm.

2. U.S. Department of Health and Human Services. U.S. Food and Drug Administration. Dietary supplements adverse event reporting. Available at: http://www.fda.gov/food/dietarysupplements/reportadverseevent/ucm111110.htm.

3. http://vm.cfsan.fda.gov/~dms/mwgblghb.html (no longer available). See instead: Henney JE. Warning on dietary supplements. *JAMA*. 1999;282(13):1218. doi:10.1001/jama.282.13.1218.

4. Annual Reports of the American Association of Poison Control Centers' National Poisoning and Exposure Database. Download any report from 1983–2014 at http://www.aapcc.org/annual-reports/ free of charge. The "Vitamin" category is usually near the end of the report. Summary and commentary at: http://www.doctoryourself.com/vitsafety.html. See also: http://orthomolecular.org/resources/omns/v12n01.shtml and http://orthomolecular.org/resources/omns/v12n02.shtml.

5. Larson AM et al. Acetaminophen-induced acute liver failure: results from a United States multicenter, prospective study. *Hepatology* 2005;42:1364–1372.

6. Associated Press. Bad drug reactions send 700,000 to ER yearly. Oct 17, 2006. Available at: http://www.msnbc.msn.com/id/15305033/.

7. Emord JW. FDA violation of the rule of law. Speech from the Health Freedom Exposition in Richmond, Virginia September 23, 2006. Available at: http://www.emord.com/Read-FDA-Violation-of-the-Rule-of-Law.html.

Truth in Pharmaceutical Advertising: Now There Is an Oxymoron for You

by Ralph K. Campbell, MD

From the *Orthomolecular Medicine News Service,* June 27, 2013.

Advertising is a powerful and effective tool for promoting the sale of products, especially from the drug and food industries, due to their huge profits. Awareness of a need for government to keep advertisers in line goes back to the end of the 19th century. The very first US Pure Food and Drug Act was passed in 1906, when Theodore Roosevelt was president. Currently, the Federal Trade Commission requires that advertising must be "truthful and non-deceptive." Advertisers must have evidence to back up their claims. Advertisements cannot be "unfair," and must inform about anything that may "materially affect" the consumer's decision. However, those terms are not easily defined. And corporations redefine them for their own benefit.

There has been a culture shift. We still like to stick it to the big corporations, but there is little concern for the nuances of false advertising. Many people today don't have the background to discern what they read, and may be inclined to trust a well-constructed ad. Even lawyers can barely determine what is "legal," let alone what is "right." More often, the aim is simply to construct effective advertising that boosts sales irrespective of morality.

Historically, the American Medical Association (AMA) was the official "ethics police" for advertising of drugs, hospitals, clinics, individual physicians, and medical devices. Initially, most advertising was forbidden. Members of the AMA were fined for violations. Since social standing in the community is important to a practicing physician, this embarrassment was enough to effectively chastise most offenders. Claims of the superiority of one clinic, hospital, or specialist over another were rarely made. Advertising of drugs was minimal for many decades, but recently has been growing exponentially. I attribute this to two factors: the pharmaceutical industry's great power and influence on medical practice, and the private insurance industry that provides accessibility of drugs to its clients by covering the cost—whatever it is. The uninformed patient is usually not aware of the actual cost covered by the insurer. This enables a for-profit insurance company to have full say of what expenses are covered, because it does not have to face challenges from those covered.

Use as Directed. . . by the Advertiser

One look at an evening TV news broadcast illustrates this influence. Drug ads, through the efforts of marketing specialists, are presented to specifically targeted audiences. Who watches the five o'clock news? Lots of people, including a whole lot of retirement-aged folks. Many are taking numerous prescriptions and over-the-counter (OTC) medications of their choosing. These include everything from an OTC product that helps keep a dental plate where it belongs to potent immune-system modifiers that can have life-threatening side effects. The retired viewer will likely have interest in a drug upon being convinced that it will alleviate a medical condition.

In the world of drug advertising, signs and symptoms and their treatment are organized into specific motifs. After clearly describing how a drug can help you, without a clear description of its drawbacks, the final admonition is: "Ask your doctor about . . . " Of course, since only a doctor can prescribe, this statement becomes a veiled suggestion that the doctor will agree. The problem here is that it is usually better for a patient to get medical information from the doctor, with whom a trusting relationship has been formed, than from an advertisement designed for maximum profit. In many cases, to fully inform a patient about a disease and its treatment takes hours or even days.

An advertisement from early TV is still prominent in my mind because of its impropriety. A drug that is generally prescribed only by a specialist such as an oncologist should not be advertised. After chemotherapy, many patients are found to be anemic, due to the treatment having interfered with the bone marrow's ability to form new red blood cells (erythrocytes). The process is called erythropoiesis; the stimulating hormone is erythropoietin. Pharmaceutical companies developed a drug that, chemically, is a look-alike of the hormone; it is prescribed only when absolutely necessary. Certainly, this is not the kind of drug that is freely dispensed. With all the safeguards from agencies such as the US Food and Drug Administration (FDA), how could this be allowed? A win-at-all-costs culture seems to be the driving force that can affect doctors, athletic-event participants, and all in between. Unfortunately the FDA is not the watchdog it is cracked up to be.

The Risk Is Yours

We joke about ads that loudly proclaim the attributes of the sponsor's specific drug for a disorder, or actual disease, that the viewer is convinced he has, while softly listing the side effects. For example, the ad for the only recognized "stop smoking" drug has such dire warnings that to continue smoking might seem a better choice. Listen carefully for soft enunciation of such words as "occasional fatalities," which might well provide cause for reflection. Because of the savvy marketing from the business end of the drug company, the lawyers, and the PR specialists, the "Fair" Trade Commission never seems to be concerned about such advertising, evidently because it is considered inconsequential.

New drugs are being advertised at an astonishing rate. When a successful drug's patent runs out, and it becomes a generic drug, immediately another company will market their own look-alike with a catchy name. Some of the conditions and drug names may even sound humorous. But I see no humor in advertising an immune-system suppressor—a type of drug that is only prescribed after all safer pharmaceuticals have failed. This drug is designed to inhibit tumor necrosis factor (TNF), an active component of a well-functioning immune system. The FDA approves its use for rheumatoid arthritis, ankylosing spondylitis (crippling arthritis of the spine), and psoritic arthritis—a few of the severe auto-immune diseases. Since it disrupts immune-system function, only specialists should prescribe it, and only when they have exhausted all the other possibilities. The warnings about side effects should include the risk that a drug will contribute to the development of new infections or to severe flareups of present infections, and to more serious problems such as inflammation of the optic nerve and heart failure. This type of drug can also cause autoimmune diseases, and even a fast-growing type of lymphoma (cancer). The ads gloss over the severity of the side effects, so that the viewer gets the impression that the drug is simply a new and improved super aspirin.

Food Ads

Half-truths are a big part of food advertising as well. The words "natural" and "organic" are freely used, much to the dismay of a real organic farmer who has gone through the certification process. "Free range" chickens—that are free of depression from living in an overcrowded space—are now happy birds that are able to run around, even if they are fenced in an area without vegetation to provide insects to eat. The size of the "range" is not defined—measured in square feet or inches? Is the range free of chemicals? Powerful companies such as Monsanto and DuPont are doing their best to prevent labeling of GMOs (genetically modified foods), blocking a step that would give consumers the ability to know what they are eating. Monsanto is succeeding on a national level but cannot completely overcome the actions of private organic food producers whose patrons are demanding labeling. What is Monsanto concerned about? Probably this: the European Union has already adopted required labeling of GMO foods.

Everyone knows that making money is the driving force for advertising. Let the consumer beware.

A CONSTANT STREAM OF EXPENSIVE DRUGS

by Helen Saul Case

From the *Orthomolecular Medicine News Service,* November 16, 2015.

It would be novel indeed to see a news media report entitled "Life-Saving Vitamins." That's a headline about vitamins that would be true for once.

Instead, I see folks on TV speaking about those drugs they so desperately "need" while they plead with drug companies to just make them more affordable. "It's tough when it comes to medical stuff costing so much because you *can't* say no to medication," says one patient who seeks an expensive drug to help lower his high cholesterol.[1]

"[It's] a kind of blackmail: if you want drug companies to keep turning out life-saving drugs, you will gratefully pay whatever they charge."

—MARCIA ANGELL, MD

Take comfort, consumer. NBC News is on it. On Wednesday, November 4, 2015, they presented a news bit ominously titled "Your Money or Your Life." NBC asked Leonard Schleifer, MD, CEO of Regeneron, "Why do the same medications cost so much more here than in other countries?"

After all, NBC pointed out that drugs cost twice as much in the United States than they do in Canada, the United Kingdom, or Australia. And they noted that Regeneron's new drug Praluent is particularly costly.

Dr. Schleifer justified the price tag on his company's expensive new drug because of the high cost of the product's development. "Do we want cheap drugs now, and no drugs in the future?" he asks. "Or more expensive drugs now, and a constant stream of drugs?"[2]

Ah, yes.

This pharmaceutical CEO would have us enjoy an endless stream of expensive drugs. *Of course* he would. For many people who take cholesterol-lowering drugs every day, a constant supply is exactly what they end up paying for.

The Drug Marketing Machine

The pharmaceutical industry is "primarily a marketing machine to sell drugs of dubious benefit," says Marcia Angell, MD, a senior lecturer at Harvard Medical School and former editor-in-chief of the *New England Journal of Medicine.*[3] In her bestselling book, *The Truth about the Drug Companies,*[4] she says that the supposedly high cost of research and development has very little to do with how high they price their products. Basically, drug companies charge what they think they can get. And while you will hear it claimed otherwise, far more is spent on marketing than on research and development. She even points out that "news" about drugs is just another way to promote drugs. "Contrary to the industry's public relations," says Dr. Angell, "you don't get what you pay for."

"New drug" does not automatically mean "improved," "better," or "safe." It means that at least in a couple of trials, it beat a placebo. "Clearly drug companies are more concerned with profits than with patients," says Andrew W. Saul, PhD.[5]

Get Out Your Checkbook

Praluent costs $40 *a day.*[6] That's $14,600 a year. NBC reported that this is significantly more costly than it should be. They referred to a watchdog study that suggested a more reasonable price would be $2,200 to $7,700 a year, or just $6 to $21 a day. Golly, thanks so much, NBC! That's much more reasonable.

Believe it or not, there is an even cheaper, more effective option to reduce "bad" LDL cholesterol, and we've known about it for over 60 years.[7]

Niacin Is Better than Any Cholesterol Drug

Back in the 1950s, William Parsons, MD, and colleagues reported that niacin lowers bad cholesterol, increases good cholesterol, and lowers triglycerides, among other benefits, such as living longer.[8] Abram Hoffer, MD, who pioneered the use of niacin to cure schizophrenia, says Dr. Parsons provides the evidence that niacin is the "only practical, effective, safe, and cost effective method for restoring lipid levels to normal."[9]

"Niacin should probably be the first-line medication for people who want to lower their cholesterol levels," say Drs. Hilary Roberts and Steve Hickey, authors of *The Vitamin Cure for Heart Disease.* Additionally, the health advantages of niacin extend well beyond its ability to reduce cholesterol. "[N]iacin inhibits inflammation and protects the delicate linings of the arteries," say Dr. Roberts and Dr. Hickey, and "helps maintain the arterial wall and prevents atherosclerosis."[10]

"A vitamin can act as a drug,
but a drug can never act as a vitamin."
—ANDREW W. SAUL, PHD

The dose is the key. "[T]he data on patients with problem cholesterol/LDL levels still support 3,000 to 5,000 milligrams (mg) of immediate-release niacin as the best clinically-proven approach to maintaining a healthy lipid profile," says researcher, professor, and niacin expert W. Todd Penberthy, PhD. And, despite what you may have heard, niacin is "far safer than the safest drug."[11]

And Niacin Is Cheaper Too

The cost of a bottle of regular, flush niacin comes in under eight bucks. Taking six to ten 500 mg niacin tablets per day ($0.03 a tablet) would cost $0.19 to $0.30. The yearly investment to take the best cholesterol-lowering substance out there, would be $70 to $110. That's 20 to 100 times cheaper than statins. That's up to 200 times cheaper than Praluent. And niacin is safer then all of them.

"We've all been carefully taught that drugs cure illness, not vitamins," says Dr. Saul. "The system is remarkably well-entrenched."[5] Instead of being hailed as the safe, effective, affordable, lifesaving vitamin it is, niacin is bashed in the media, and dangerous drugs are practically revered. Is the only fault we can find with them is that they cost too much?

We can do better. We *can* say no to medication. We can do something about high cholesterol, and it doesn't have to cost a pile. We don't have to buy into or believe what we see on TV. And until a headline reads, "Lifesaving Vitamins," I sure won't.

Editor's Note: Niacin is likely to cause a flush. Niacinamide and inositol hexaniacinate do not. There is much more to know than this, however. If you intend to take therapeutic, high doses of niacin, please read Niacin: The Real Story, *by the world's leading niacin, expert Abram Hoffer, MD, PhD.*

REFERENCES FOR "A CONSTANT STREAM OF EXPENSIVE DRUGS"

1. NBC News. Regeneron CEO explains the high cost of cholesterol drug Praluent. Available at: http://www.nbcnews.com/video/regeneron-ceo-explains-the-high-cost-of-cholesterol-drug-praluent-559474243915.

2. Ibid.

3. Angell, M. *The Truth About the Drug Companies.* New York: Random House, Inc., 2004.

4. Review at http://orthomolecular.org/library/jom/2005/pdf/2005-v20n02-p120.pdf.

5. Saul AW. Rigged Trials: Drug Studies Favor the Manufacturer. *Orthomolecular Medicine News Service,* Nov 5, 2008. Available at: http://orthomolecular.org/resources/omns/v04n20.shtml.

6. CBS News. New cholesterol lowering drug Praluent far more expensive than statins. Available at: http://www.cbsnews.com/news/praluent-cholesterol-lowering-drug-high-cost-statin-alternative/.

7. Hoffer A. Niacin, coronary disease and longevity. Available at: http://www.doctoryourself.com/hoffer_cardio.html.

8. Parsons WB. *Cholesterol Control Without Diet!* Lilac Press, 2000.

9. Hoffer A, Saul AW, Foster H. *Niacin: The Real Story*. Laguna Beach, CA: Basic Health Publications, Inc., 2012.

10. Roberts H, Hickey S. *The Vitamin Cure for Heart Disease*. Laguna Beach, CA: Basic Health Publications, Inc., 2011.

11. Penberthy WT. Laropiprant is the bad one; niacin is/was/will always be the good one. *Orthomolecular Medicine News Service*, July 25, 2014. Available at: http://orthomolecular.org/resources/omns/v10n12.shtml.

"It comes down to this: living healthfully is prevention AND cure for most ailments of humanity. That is indeed simple. It is also true, it works, and you can prove it."

—ANDREW W. SAUL, PHD

Are There No Hospitals? Are There No Nursing Homes?

by Andrew W. Saul

From the *Orthomolecular Medicine News Service*, December 23, 2013.

Might be fun, but I have never shopped at Neiman Marcus, Hammacher Schlemmer, or Saks Fifth Avenue. Years ago, as a Big Apple tourist, I did have a long look in the window of the Waldorf Astoria restaurant and read the lunch menu. A small green side salad cost more than I would have wanted to spend for an entire dinner anywhere else. When luxuries are predictably expensive, we can scoff, wish, or drool.

But what really grabbed my ever-miserly attention was a recent visit to a supermarket. Not an upscale munchie boutique, just a run-of-the-mill chain store in a working-class community. Over to the produce department, and there they were, oranges, one dollar. Each. Grapefruits were even more.

Later, I was at a well-known big-box department store. Ascorbic acid vitamin C, 500 milligrams (mg), was under ten bucks for 500 tablets. That's two cents a tablet, four cents per 1,000 mg.

One store-bought medium-sized orange might contain 60 mg of vitamin C. I think that figure would be substantially lower for most tired-looking, out-of-state oranges you are likely to purchase mid-winter. Even if we allow a generous 62 mg, it takes eight oranges to equal the ascorbic acid in one single 500 mg tablet. Eight oranges can cost eight bucks. The vitamin C tablet can cost two cents. That means, milligram for milligram, *vitamin C from tablets is four hundred times cheaper* than vitamin C from oranges. Even if those oranges were an incredible 75 percent-off special, they'd still cost 100 times more than the supplement.

I am fully aware that there are many side benefits of eating oranges. Among other things, oranges contain bioflavonoids, fiber, and are delicious. But their price remains an obstacle.

A few daily oranges are Waldorf salads seen through the window; virtually unaffordable luxury for millions of people. On the other hand, anyone, and I mean anyone, can find $7.30 per year for a vitamin C tablet each day.

Many people eat really lousy, utterly unbalanced diets. Some do so by choice, some by circumstances. If you have money, you can still eat wrong. Look around and see. But if you are truly poor, you cannot afford the quantity and variety of fresh produce needed to eat right.

It is far cheaper to get vitamins and other micronutrients from supplementation than it is to get those nutrients from foods. I wish that were not the case, but it is. That is why the multivitamin is the biggest health bargain on the planet.

This especially matters to the poor.

With apologies to Charles Dickens, and with a deep bow to *Forbes*,[1] NBC,[2] CBS,[3] *Annals of Internal Medicine*,[4] the *New York Times*,[5] *The Week*,[6] and other pharmaphilic (drug-loving) media, I offer holiday greetings:

"At this festive season of the year, Mr. Scrooge," said the gentleman, "it is more than usually desirable that we should make some slight provision for the poor and destitute, who suffer greatly at the present time. Hundreds of thousands are in want of adequate nutrition, sir."

"Are there no hospitals?" asked Scrooge.

"Plenty of hospitals," said the gentleman.

"And the nursing homes," demanded Scrooge. "Are they still in operation?"

"They are. Still," returned the gentleman, "I wish I could say they were not."

"Oh. I was afraid, from what you said at first, that something had occurred to stop them in their useful course," said Scrooge.

"Under the impression that they scarcely furnish adequate health of mind or body to the multitude," returned the gentleman, "a few of us are endeavoring to change matters."

"Those establishments are sufficient," said Scrooge. "Those who are badly off must go there."

"Many can't go there; and many would rather die."

"If they would rather die," said Scrooge, "they had better do it, and decrease the surplus population."

Later that night, when Scrooge was with the Spirit of Christmas Present:

From the foldings of its robe, the Spirit brought two children. They knelt down at its feet, and clung upon the outside of its garment. They were a boy and a girl, meager and ragged. Scrooge started back, appalled.

The Spirit said: "This boy is Ignorance. This girl is Want. Beware them both, but most of all beware this boy."

Ignorance is indeed the greater threat. The news media by their own words are the very personification of ignorance. They warn people off supplements when supplementation is the very thing people need to be healthier, or at the very least, less sick. Of course, if people were less sick, they'd use fewer drugs. Pharmaceutical advertising income lines the media's pockets. That would explain those hatchet jobs on vitamins.

But we can fix it. Improving essential vitamin and mineral intake through inexpensive multivitamins and vitamin C tablets will improve health nationwide, worldwide. Until we can get everyone eating healthfully, supplementation is an immediately available, affordable answer.

REFERENCES FOR "ARE THERE NO HOSPITALS?"

1. Husten L. Case closed: multivitamins should not be used. *Forbes*, Dec 16, 2013. Available at: http://www.forbes.com/sites/larryhusten/2013/12/16/case-closed-multivitamins-should-not-be-used/.

2. *NBC Nightly News*. New studies dispel multivitamin myths. Dec 16, 2013. Available at: http://www.nbcnews.com/video/nightly-news/53848559/#53848559.

3. Jaslow R. Multivitamin researchers say "case is closed" after studies find no health benefits. CBS, Dec 16, 2013. Available at: http://www.cbsnews.com/news/multivitamin-researchers-say-case-is-closed-supplements-dont-boost-health/.

4. Guallar E, Stranges S, Mulrow C, et al. Enough is enough: stop wasting money on vitamin and mineral supplements. *Ann Intern Med* 2013; 159(12):850–851.

5. Offit P, Erush S. Skip the supplements. *The New York Times*, Dec 14, 2013. Available at: http://www.nytimes.com/2013/12/15/opinion/sunday/skip-the-supplements.html?_r=0.

6. Weber P. How the vitamin industrial complex swindled America. *The Week*, Dec 18, 2013. Available at: http://theweek.com/article/index/254290/how-the-vitamin-industrial-complex-swindled-america.

CHAPTER 14

Do I Need *All* Those Vitamins?

"It's amazing how you can live so well without modern medicine."

—The Great Human Odyssey, The Adaptable Ape.

Yes, you need all those vitamins. Vitamins are *vital.* That's how they got their name. We need all of them every day. We must take in essential nutrients as we cannot manufacture them on our own. The only question, then, is quantity.

Ideally, we wouldn't have to think about supplementation. Vitamins would be abundant in all of our foods, and all of our foods would be fresh, nutritious, varied, whole, and predominantly plant-based.

But even the most carefully selected diet will still lack optimal levels of certain nutrients. And no diet could ever provide the therapeutic levels of vitamin C or vitamin E or B complex. It simply cannot be done. We can choose to accept this inadequacy and accept the consequences of that choice, or we can choose to take safe, inexpensive supplements to, yes, *supplement* that good diet we should already be eating.

We can survive on inadequate levels of nutrients for some time. People do it every day. The question is, how sick do you want to be? How often do you want to feel unwell? Do you want to "learn to live with" chronic illness? You can play out that hand of cards, but you are playing a losing game. Taking supplements stacks the deck in our favor. There is no substitute for great nutrition. There is no quick fix. There is no one-pill solution.

We don't want to be sick, and sick people want to get well. There is an available answer for those who choose to hear it: orthomolecular nutrition works. It is not speculation or make-believe. Orthomolecular physicians have proven that in optimal doses vitamins can do what so many pharmaceutical drugs fail to do, fail to do well, or fail to do without the risk of dangerous side effects, even death. Year after year, there is not one confirmed death from any vitamin. Not one.

The pharmaceutical industry has "nearly limitless influence over medical research, education, and how doctors do their jobs" through control of clinical trials, media advertising, politics, and what doctors are taught in medical school and continuing education.[1] Your doctor may not know about orthomolecular treatment. Medical students are certainly not hearing about it in school.

We can only ignore ignorance for so long. Today, we would not excuse doctors who did not wash their hands between deliveries. I believe we can no longer excuse physicians for not knowing about nutritional therapy. If your doctor isn't recommending vitamins, it is time to find another doctor.

I am not against using drugs when necessary, but not when there is a safer, healthier, more effective alternative. And there is. Let's look in another physician's tool bag. Let's learn from doctors who have moved away from commercial medicine and toward what works: inexpensive, safe, nutritional solutions.

It's hard to prove "prevention." Proof is simply good health. It seems that every day you hear about folks fighting this or that health problem. When I take a look at my husband and kids, I think, "Well, we don't have that." Or, "We got that, but not as badly." Our family jumps on sickness with high-dose nutrient therapy *before* it becomes a clearly diagnosable illness. If an illness only develops into a stuffy nose or a slight cough, isn't that almost as good as not getting sick at all? We only have little problems, because we address the little problems before they become big ones. When teaching classes full of middle schoolers, if you fail to address the little issues, all you have are big ones. A lack of prevention practically ensures a problem.

Many of us see vitamins as optional. They aren't. People may fuss about having too many pills to swallow. They say there is no time to take them, or they won't remember. No one would say that about water or food. If our need for vitamins were as apparent as thirst, we could not ignore it. All too many people discover that if they do not prioritize health, they get sick. Then health becomes the priority whether they like it or not.

What are we willing to do to achieve better health? I ate a salad for lunch. Have I had "enough" vegetables? When it comes to vitamins, our government's idea of what is "enough" has been proven time and time again to be inadequate if you want to prevent, arrest, and reverse chronic disease. We must get rid of old-fashioned notions of "enough" when it comes to vitamins. Instead, let our bodies do the talking, and take time to listen. Illness is the body's cry for better nutrition.

You cannot argue with your body. You can certainly try, but it will win every time. In one way or another, it is taking into account all it is exposed to. It cannot be fooled. Your body works and functions independently of your desire to have it do so.

Biology is rather involuntary. Our heart beats without our advance permission. Our body operates as it does because that is was it was designed to do. Our "control" of our body is the extent to which we choose to participate in its successful, healthy functioning. We can offer it good food, clean water, exercise, and vitamins. We can provide it with the right tools for wellness.

My grandfather taught me, as he taught my father, that health is the most important area of focus in life. Health deserves attention *first.* Everything else is second. In the event of a problem on an airplane, you are required to put your oxygen mask on before your children's. You take care of yourself first so you can take care of others.

CHAPTER 14 REFERENCE

1. Angell, M. *The Truth about the Drug Companies: How They Deceive Us and What to Do about It.* New York, NY: Random House LLC, 2004.

Appendix 1

"Health in America is the fastest growing failing business in the Western civilization."

—EMANUEL CHERASKIN, MD

Our system of health care is really one of disease care. The focus at the doctor's office is far more about treatment than it has ever been about prevention. The facts remain: drugs and surgery are expensive and do not address the underlying causes of illness. This next article discusses this broken "health" care system, and how orthomolecular medicine may very well be the answer we are looking for.

Orthomolecular Medicine: The Best Cost-Effective, Rational, and Scientific Choice for Disease Treatment

by Michael J. Gonzalez, DSc, NMD, PhD, FACN, and Jorge R. Miranda-Massari, PharmD

From *J Orthomolecular Med* 2013; 28 (1): 5–8.

The current health care system doesn't work. For the past several decades medical practice in the United States of America has become excessively dependent on drugs and technology. Medical science and health care policy are influenced by a myriad of powerful private interest groups. This is the main reason why medical care in the USA is by far the most expensive in the world but, sadly, by no means the best. Many countries have higher longevity and lower mortality rates in many diseases. The "USA way" of practicing medicine is just profit-oriented and not consistent with public health priorities.

In 2009, the National Health Expenditure Accounts estimated that the US expenditure in healthcare was $2.5 trillion, although an independent study claimed that the amount reached was $2.8 trillion.[1] This represents 17.3 percent of our gross national product, more than double the percentage of the gross national product spent by any other nation on health care.[2] Seventy-eight percent of our health care costs are aimed at treating the 133 million Americans who have chronic diseases. Despite this, we rank 12th out of 13 industrialized nations in 16 major indicators of the health status of a population, such as life expectancy for different groups, neonatal and age-adjusted mortality.[3] We wait for illness to develop and then we spend huge sums on heroic measures. We practice "Rescue Medicine." We have a large population of vertically ill people: they are not sick enough to lie down (horizontally ill) but are sufficiently unhealthy to pose a substantial risk of needing major therapeutic investments. When we talk about health insurance what we really mean is disease-care reimbursement. We spend more but feel worse. This is a very expensive and ineffective system of health care (or rather disease-care).

Moreover, we should have in mind that acute and emergency care cannot effectively treat chronic disease. This kind of medicine focuses only on getting rid of the immediate symptoms, not the disease. Not only does our current approach fail to effectively diagnose and treat the underlying causes of chronic disease, it does great harm at a high economic cost. Since the Renaissance, science, especially medicine, has taken a particular path in its analytical evaluation of the world. It is rooted in the assumption that complex problems are solvable by dividing them into smaller, simpler units. By reducing it into smaller units, this approach has been termed "reductionist" and has been the predominant paradigm of science over the past four centuries. Reductionism pervades the medical sciences and affects the way we diagnose, treat, and prevent disease. Is reductionist medicine part of our overall health care problem? Probably!

Reductionist medicine is a direct product of Cartesian ideas about the body, specifically, the long-held view that the mind is separate from the body. The philosopher René Descartes (1596–1650) argued that the mind and body are made of totally different substances: mind is spiritual matter and body is material matter. Within conventional scientific thinking, there was no way to link the activities of the mind with the functions of the body. In general, reductionism is the process of learning more and more about less and less until eventually one knows everything about nothing. Such symptom-driven treatment lacks a curative effect since it fails to identify and eradicate underlying causes of disease. At some point the late Dr. Emanuel Cheraskin stated, "Health in America is the fastest growing failing business in the Western civilization."

Is our health care status a product of capitalism? Should we add to our constitution the right to be healthy? That would be the right thing to do, but unfortunately this ideal is not part of our current health care system.

> *"Nutritional supplementation is not the answer to every health problem, but it does not have to be. Nutrient therapy, properly dosed and administered, is the answer to many chronic medical problems."*
>
> —ANDREW W. SAUL, PhD

Orthomolecular Medicine to the Rescue

A better approach that leads to health and wellness is to focus on optimizing the biological functioning in our bodies' core biochemical/physiological systems. This approach is called orthomolecular medicine (OM). OM utilizes nutrition and supplementation as important corrective metabolic tools, tools that are effective and inexpensive. Nutritional science has always been neglected in medicine. It is seen as a secondary, less relevant factor in health. Physicians have abdicated the science and practice of nutrition. This is why we do not have concise nutritional guidelines or consensus related to nutrition and disease, despite abundant evidence. It is also why there is so much professional and public confusion around nutrition and supplementation in general.

The standard American diet is lacking in necessary nutrients. This state of nutritional insufficiency is a possible reason why millions are walking around with headaches, body aches, digestive upset, skin problems, sinus problems, frequent colds, and many other diseases that may quickly disappear when they start taking the necessary vitamins and minerals. Nutrition is enhanced through supplementation.

The current dietary reference intakes (DRIs) recommends only a minimum amount of nutrients, enough to prevent deficiency diseases, not the varying amounts needed by a polymorphic population for optimal health that may be hundreds of times the DRIs. Most physicians and consumers do not realize that DRIs are the minimum necessary to prevent deficiency diseases. Medicine has failed to recognize that nutrients are multifunctional metabolic substances with multiple biochemical/physiological roles. For example, vitamin D not only prevents rickets, but may have a role in treating or preventing heart disease, multiple sclerosis, polycystic ovarian syndrome, depression, epilepsy, type 1 diabetes, and cancer.[4–6] Folate not only prevents megaloblastic anemia, but also prevents neural tube defects, cardiovascular disease, dementia, depression, and colon and breast cancer.[7,8]

Conventional medical thinking has been biased against the therapeutic use of vitamins/minerals in disease and has largely ignored the fact that vitamins/minerals have a role in optimizing health. Here are just a few of the diseases common in our population, along with the nutritional deficiencies or insufficiencies associated with them:

- Cardiovascular disease: Significant deficiencies in vitamin D have been linked to peripheral artery disease,[9,10] which usually precedes cardiovascular disease. Also, vitamins C, D, E, folate, pyridoxine, and cobalamin promote healthy endothelial function,[11–13] which reduces the risk of heart disease. Coenzyme Q_{10} deficiencies also cause cardiac problems.[14–15]
- Osteoporosis: Long-term calcium deficiencies usually bring about problems in bone structure and strength.[16] Vitamin D and magnesium are necessary for calcium absorption.
- Prostate disease: Zinc is essential for a healthy prostate and for male reproductive and urinary health in general.[17] Zinc supplementation in some cases helps overcome erectile dysfunction.
- Hypothyroidism: We need at least 200 micrograms daily of iodine for general health. That dose is the bare minimum. Lack of iodine translates to millions of people feeling tired or cold, and has also been linked to breast cancer.[18] Long-term iodine deficiencies often turn into hypothyroidism.

These common deficiencies/insufficiencies are just the tip of the disease iceberg. Every chronic disease or illness can be traced to a nutritional deficiency or insufficiency. We are actually treating nutritional deficiencies/insufficiencies with drugs.

The Hidden Hunger Concept

Since we are not eating enough of the proper nutrient-dense foods, what we end up eating is lacking in vital nutrients and too high in calories. Hidden Hunger or the "Occult Hunger Concept" refers to subclinical deficiencies or nutrient insufficiencies that our population suffers due to excessive consumption of calorie-rich, nutrient-poor, refined food. This is likely the basis of metabolic disruptions that underlie many pathological/disease states.

Nutrients restore normal function, and they do so by optimizing normal biological functions, mostly by their action as coenzymes/cofactors in thousands of biochemical reactions. They function within the genetic and cellular environment of the cell to enhance and facilitate the optimal functioning of our physiology. Failure to utilize nutritional interventions when such interventions are clinically indicated is inconsistent with the delivery of quality health care and should be considered malpractice.[19] To get the most benefit from supplements, they should be taken every day, long-term, and not as drugs that are only taken when a person is sick or diseased. The goal of nutritional supplementation is to create optimal physiologic nutrient levels capable of producing what is known as "Metabolic Correction."[20]

Are Supplements Toxic?

Over the years, there have only been two or three times when a dietary supplement was deemed unsafe and pulled off the market. One of the banned supplements was ephedra, which was used to help with weight loss/energy. Ephedra is a stimulant and, if abused, it can cause problems. The other case was tryptophan, an amino acid substance present in turkey, milk, and many other foods. One manufacturer (from Japan) shipped contaminated tryptophan, so the FDA banned the supplement completely for many years. Tryptophan itself is completely safe; the problem was the contaminant.

On the other hand, there is a long list of disasters with prescription drugs causing deaths and severe, permanent adverse effects. Hundreds of thousands of people are rushed to an emergency room every year with an adverse reaction to a prescription drug. Moreover, the incidence of serious and fatal ADRs from prescription medication in US hospitals has been reported to be extremely high, reaching 2,216,000 serious adverse reactions and 106,000 deaths.[21] ADRs also significantly increase length of hospital stay and total hospitalization costs.[22] Overall, the cost of drug-related morbidity and mortality exceeded $177.4 billion in 2000. Given the economic and medical burdens associated with medication-related morbidity and mortality, new models and strategies for preventing this problem are urgently needed.[23]

Orthomolecular Medicine Is a Viable Scientific Strategy to Prevent and Treat Disease

An essential aspect of OM is that it seeks to provide a molecular understanding for how our nutrient intake affects health by altering the expression and/or structure of the genes. The progression from a healthy phenotype to a chronic disease phenotype must occur by changes in gene expression or by differences in activities of proteins and enzymes and those dietary components that directly or indirectly regulate the expression of genomic information. In this sense, dietary intervention and nutritional supplementation based on knowledge of nutritional requirements, nutritional status, and particular genotype (i.e., individualized OM) can be used to prevent, mitigate, or cure chronic disease. Genes are selectively activated or suppressed when molecules such as neurotransmitters, hormones, growth factors, or other signal molecules bind to and activate cell-surface receptors, initiating a cascade of biochemical reactions in which enzymes play a central role. These enzymes require cofactors to enable their catalytic activity. These cofactors are vitamins and minerals.

OM can also compensate for short-term nutrient deficiencies or insufficiencies that, if uncorrected, lead to infirmity and chronic diseases. Dr. Bruce N. Ames' "Triage

Theory" of optimal nutrition describes how the human body prioritizes the use of vitamins and minerals when receiving an insufficient amount of them in order to sustain functionality.[24] Under such a limited nutritional environment, the body will always direct nutrients toward short-term health and survival and away from the regulation and repair of cellular DNA and proteins that optimize health and increase longevity. OM affords all individuals the opportunity for robust health, so that short-term nutrient deficiencies or insufficiencies are adequately dealt with, and thus do not result in increased morbidity and early mortality.

The term "metabolic correction," introduced by Drs. Michael J. Gonzalez and Jorge R. Miranda-Massari in 2011, is a functional term that explains how nutrients are capable of correcting biochemical disruptions that promote disease and infirmity.[25] Thus, another scientific rationale for OM is derived in part from the recognition that altered enzymatic function due to distorted enzyme structures can be metabolically corrected by the administration of supraphysiologic doses of nutrients.

Conclusion

The focus of medicine should be on repairing and correcting the imbalances which allow illness to develop in the first place. It requires a change in thinking, which is thinking "outside the box." OM is preventive, protective, and corrective. The principles and practices of OM are now sufficiently established to change medicine forever, from a pathology-based system to a health-based practice.

REFERENCES FOR APPENDIX 1

1. Deloitte Center for Health Solutions. The hidden costs of U.S. health care: consumer discretionary health care spending. 2012. Available at: http://content.hcpro.com/pdf/content/287442.pdf (accessed May 2016).

2. Truffer CJ, Keehan S, Smith S, et al. Health spending projections through 2019: the recession's impact continues. *Health Aff March* 2010;29:522–529.

3. Starfield B. *Primary Care: Balancing Health Needs, Services and Technology*. New York, NY. Oxford University Press, 1998.

4. Holick MF. The vitamin D deficiency pandemic and consequences for nonskeletal health: mechanisms of action. *Mol Aspects Med* 2008; 29: 361–368.

5. Holick MF. Vitamin D: evolutionary, physiological and health perspectives. *Curr Drug Targets* 2011;12:4–18.

6. Cannell JJ, Hollis BW. Use of vitamin D in clinical practice. *Altern Med Rev* 2008;13:6–20.

7. Stanger O, Fowler B, Piertzik K, et al. Homocysteine, folate and vitamin B12 in neuropsychiatric diseases: review and treatment recommendations. *Expert Rev Neurother,* 2009;9:1393–1412.

8. Duthie SJ. Epigenetic modifications and human pathologies: cancer and CVD. *Proc Nutr Soc* 2011;70 47–56.

9. Gaddipati VC, Bailey BA, Kuriacose R, et al. The relationship of vitamin D status to cardiovascular risk factors and amputation risk in veterans with peripheral arterial disease. *J Am Med Dir Assoc* 2011;12:58–61.

10. Chua GT, Chan YC, Cheng SW. Vitamin D status and peripheral arterial disease: evidence so far. *Vasc Health Risk Manag* 2011;7:671–675.

11. Traber MG, Stevens JF. Vitamins C and E: beneficial effects from a mechanistic perspective. *Free Rad Biol Med* 2011;51:1000–1013.

12. Wang X, Qin X, Demirtas H, et al. Efficacy of folic acid supplementation in stroke prevention: a meta-analysis. *Lancet* 2007; 369: 1876–1882.

13. Brewer LC, Michos ED, Reis JP. Vitamin D in atherosclerosis, vascular disease, and endothelial function. *Curr Drug Targets* 2011;12:54–60.

14. Gao L, Mao Q, Cao J, et al. Effects of coenzyme Q10 on vascular endothelial function in humans: a meta-analysis of randomized controlled trials. *Atherosclerosis* 2012;22:311–316.

15. Fotino AD, Thompson-Paul AM, Bazzano LA. Effect of coenzyme Q10 supplementation on heart failure: a meta-analysis. *Am J Clin Nutr* 2013;97:268–275.

16. Joo NS, Dawson-Hughes B, Kim YS, et al. Impact of calcium and vitamin D insufficiencies on serum parathyroid hormone and bone mineral density: Analysis of the fourth and fifth Korea National Health and Nutrition Examination Survey (KNHAENS IV-3, 2009 and V-1, 2010). J *Bone Miner Res* 2012.

17. Franklin RB, Costello LC. Zinc as an anti-tumor agent in prostate cancer and in other cancers. *Arch Biochem Biophys* 2007;463:211–217.

18. Eskin BA: Iodine Metabolism and Breast Cancer. *Transac NY Acad Sci,* 1970; 32:911–947.

19. Fletcher RH, Fairfield KM. Vitamins for chronic disease prevention in adults: clinical applications. *JAMA* 2002; 287: 3127–3129.

20. Gonzalez MJ, Miranda-Massari JR. Metabolic correction: a functional explanation of orthomolecular medicine. *J Orthomolecular Med* 2012; 27:13–20.

21. Lazarou J, Pomeranz BH, Corey PN. Incidence of adverse drug reactions in hospitalized patients: a meta-analysis of prospective studies. *JAMA* 1998; 279:1200–1205.

22. Suh DC, Woodall BS, Shin SK, et al. Clinical and economic impact of adverse drug reactions in hospitalized patients. *Ann Pharmacother* 2000;34:1373–1379.

23. Ernst FR, Grizzle AJ. Drug-related morbidity and mortality: updating the cost-of-illness model. *J Am Pharm Assoc* (Wash) 2001;41:192–199.

24. Ames BN. Low micronutrient intake may accelerate the degenerative diseases of aging through allocation of scarce micronutrients by triage. *Proc Natl Acad Sci USA,* 2006; 103:17589–17594.

25. Miranda-Massari JR, Gonzalez MJ, Jimenez FJ, et al. Metabolic correction in the management of diabetic peripheral neuropathy: improving clinical results beyond symptom control. *Curr Clin Pharmacol* 2011;6:260–273.

Appendix 2

Probiotics—Good Bacteria—Help Maintain Our Health in Many Ways

by Jack Challem

From *The Nutrition Reporter,* January 2013: 24(1).

Our digestive tract contains a teeming city of beneficial bacteria—with a population that's ten times larger than the number of cells in our body. It is a true symbiotic relationship, one that can positively influence our health while we provide a supportive environment to these microorganisms. Doctors have known for years that these "probiotics" make tiny amounts of some vitamins and can help prevent diarrhea. But the latest research shows that their positive effects on our health may be far greater—influencing how we fare as we age, preventing potentially deadly bacterial infections, and maybe even affecting our weight.

In a recent article Patrizia Brigidi, PhD, and her colleagues at the University of Bologna, Italy, reviewed some of the benefits of maintaining a healthy population of gut bacteria.[1] After all, as Brigidi, wrote, "Microbes are our life-long companions." But as we age, the dominant species of gut bacteria often shift. For example, Firmicutes species, which have anti-inflammatory benefits, tend to decrease, while Bacteroidetes species increase. Indeed, some of the beneficial bacteria produce butyrate, a substance that has anti-inflammatory and anticancer benefits. Citing an animal study, Brigidi noted that *Bifidobacterium lactis* supplements increased longevity in mice, apparently by reducing the age-promoting effects of inflammation.

Animal and some human studies have found that the predominant species of gut bacteria are very different between overweight and normal-weight individuals. It has not been clear whether the differences contribute to obesity or are a consequence, although eating habits do seem to influence the types of bacteria present in the gut.

Peter J. H. Jones, PhD, of the University of Manitoba, Canada, and his colleagues tested two types of "novel probiotics" on 28 overweight men and women.[2] The subjects ate the same diet, and the probiotics were consumed in yogurt. People in the study consumed each of the two probiotics—*Lactobacillus amylovorus* and *L. fermentum*—for 43 days, as well as a "control" yogurt for the same period of time. The three study phases was separated by a six-week period in which none of the subjects were given yogurt. Men and women getting *L. amylovorus* lost an average 4 percent of their body weight over a 43-day period, while *L. fermentum* led to a 3 percent decrease in body weight. When the subjects ate the standard yogurt in the crossover study, they lost only 1 percent of their body weight.

Another group of Canadian researchers analyzed data from 20 human studies, including 3,818 people, in which probiotics were given to prevent *Clostridium difficile* infection after using antibiotics. Oral antibiotics disrupt the bacterial environment of the gut, leading to diarrhea, colitis, and sometimes death. *C. difficile* is a toxic species of bacteria that often fills the probiotic void created by antibiotics. Bradley C. Johnston, PhD, of the Hospital for Sick Children Research Institute, Toronto, found that consuming probiotics reduced the risk of *C. difficile*-related diarrhea by 66 percent.[3]

In a separate analysis, Marina L. Ritchie, PhD, of Dalhousie University, Nova Scotia, Canada, looked at the benefits of probiotics in a variety of gastrointestinal diseases, include antibiotic-associated diarrhea, infectious diarrhea, irritable bowel syndrome, *C. difficile* infection, among others.[4] According to Ritchie, probiotics were helpful in resolving most of the gastrointestinal problems, except for "traveler's diarrhea."

Finally, Lyudmila Boyanova, MD, and Ivan Mitov, MD, of the University of Sofia, Bulgaria, discussed the specific use of probiotics in the journal *Expert Review of Anti-Infective Therapy*.[5] They wrote that probiotics can prevent or reduce antibiotic- and *C. difficile*-associated diarrhea. "For this purpose, *L. rhamnosus GG* and *Saccharomyces bloulardii* [a beneficial yeast] are used, the latter inhibiting *C. difficile* toxic effects."

Boyanova and Mitov added, "Probiotics are often prescribed for one to three weeks longer than the duration of antibiotic treatment. They should be taken with food because the increased gastric pH is more favorable for the probiotics."

REFERENCES FOR APPENDIX 2

1. Biagi E, Candela M, Turroni S, et al. Ageing and gut microbes: perspectives for health maintenance and longevity. *Pharmacol Res* 2013;69(1):11–20.

2. Omar JM, Chan YM, Jones ML, et al. *Lactobacillus fermentum* and *Lactobacillus amylovorus* as probiotics alter body adiposity and gut microflora in healthy persons. *Journal of Functional Foods* 2013; 5(1): 116–123 [Epub ahead of print].

3. Johnston BC, Ma SS, Goldenberg JZ, et al. Probiotics for the prevention of *Clostridium difficile*-associated diarrhea: a systematic review and meta-analysis. *Ann Intern Med* 2012; 157(12):878–888 [Epub ahead of print].

4. Ritchie ML, Romanuk TN. A meta-analysis of probiotic efficacy for gastrointestinal diseases. *PLoS One* 2012: doi 10.1371/journal.pone. 0034938.

5. Boyanova L, Mitov I. Coadministration of probiotics with antibiotics: why, when and for how long? *Expert Rev Anti Infect Ther* 2012;10(4):407–409.

Appendix 3

Nutritional Therapy at the Crossroads

by Jack Challem

From *J Orthomolecular Med* 1994; 9(3). Presented at the 23rd Annual Nutritional Medicine Today Conference, April 30,1994, Vancouver, Canada.

Nutritional therapy is at a crossroads.

Many of us have for years recognized the value of vitamins, minerals, and other nutritional factors in the prevention and treatment of disease. For years, however, we were the heretics and the quacks in the mind of the medical establishment.

We are now witnessing a revolution in medicine. Almost overnight, nutritional research and therapy have become acceptable—or at least are on the fast track toward acceptability.

But there are still dangers facing people, like us, who want to use vitamins and other supplements.

Nutritional therapy is at a crossroads. But it's only one of many crossroads that have existed in this field.

The Early Days

Let's step back briefly in history.

You all know the story of Dr. James Lind, the British naval physician. In the 15th and 16th centuries, the crews of one ship after another were decimated by scurvy, the extreme deficiency of vitamin C. More British sailors were lost to scurvy than to war. In 1754, in *A Treatise on Scurvy,* Lind documented the association between sailors eating citrus fruit—high in vitamin C—and *not* dying of scurvy.

Of course, Dr. Lind did not know that sailors were dying because of an extreme vitamin C deficiency. But he did recognize that citrus contained something that kept them alive and healthy.

Now, let's fast forward to the 19th and early 20th centuries. Many vitamin-deficiency diseases were originally thought to be caused by bacteria, fungi, and other "mysterious" substances—outside forces and agents, rather than something internally wrong or missing.

In March, in an antique store on the Oregon coast, I came across a medical textbook on diet and disease, published in 1905 in England. According to the book, beriberi was obviously caused by a microbe, not by a lack of vitamin B_1 (thiamine). Of course, no one knew what a vitamin was at that time.

Then, in 1912, Casimir Funk, a Polish biochemist working in London, theorized that foods contained "vita amines," substances vital to life.

Nutrition had reached an important crossroads.

Quickly, other vitamin discoveries were made. In 1913, researchers discovered vitamin A. In 1922, vitamin D and vitamin E. Vitamin B_2 was discovered in 1933, vitamin K in 1935, B_6 in 1936, pantothenic acid in 1938, biotin in 1940, folic acid in 1944, and vitamin B_{12} in 1948.

To understand the significance of these discoveries, in particular in the teens and 1920s, you have to understand that diseases like scurvy, pellagra, beri-beri, and pernicious anemia were as serious and commonplace as heart disease, cancer, Alzheimer's, and AIDS are today.

But the discovery of these vitamins, and the context of their discovery, also led to the creation of a "nutritional paradigm" we've had to suffer with for some 80 years. The paradigm held that vitamins cured vitamin-deficiency diseases like scurvy and pernicious anemia. But beyond that, they were of little use in the body.

If vitamin discoverers had crystal balls, they could have realized that diseases like heart disease, cancer, and Alzheimer's are, in large part, caused by nutritional deficiencies. Not entirely, of course, because subtle genetic defects and environmental toxins also contribute to the cause of disease.

Another thing happened that retarded the recognition of vitamins. Vitamins weren't medicines. They were foods. Because most doctors were male, and dieticians were predominantly female, vitamins were relegated downward to the realm of home economics and dietetics. Meanwhile, doctors concentrated on the "serious stuff"—surgery, medicines, and radiation.

In the 1930s, though, nutrition almost reached another crossroads. It was then that Albert Szent-Gyorgyi, PhD, isolated crystalline vitamin C. This meant researchers could do experiments with it, and they they found that it could do more than just cure scurvy.

In 1934, doctors realized how dependent the heart valves and muscles were on vitamin C. In 1935, they found that vitamin C could combat polio and provide resistance to diphtheria. In 1936, doctors realized that vitamin C influenced glucose tolerance. In 1937, they found that vitamin C could control tuberculosis, and that vitamin C and the amino acid glutathione could inactivate viruses. In 1938, they recognized that vitamin C could alleviate allergies and allergy-like sensitivities.

It's amazing what we knew back then.

A similar story unfolded for vitamin E. In the 1930s, based on the findings of a Danish veterinarian, Evan Shute, MD, found it useful for preventing spontaneous abortion in his obstetrical patients. Within a few years, he realized that it could have value in treating heart disease.

Nutrition Interruptus

But then, World War II interceded.

The good news: there's nothing like a war to advance surgical techniques and to develop new medicines. The bad news: vitamins and nutritional therapies moved to the back burner. After the war, vitamin research never regained the momentum it had in the 1930s—at least not for another 50 years.

Still, there were glimmers of hope, hints of crossroads that might have been.

The June 10, 1946, issue of *Time* magazine reported, "Out of Canada last week came news of a startling discovery: a treatment for heart disease (the nation's No. 1 killer) which so far has succeeded against all common forms of the ailment . . . Large concentrated doses of vitamin E . . . benefited four types of heart ailment (95 percent of the total): arteriosclerotic, hypertensive, rheumatic, old and new coronary heart disease. The vitamin helps a failing heart. It eliminates anginal pain."

And then the attacks came. For decades, vitamin E was mocked as a "sex vitamin" because its deficiency resulted in sterility in rats. It was eschewed by the medical establishment as a "cure in search of a disease." Dr. Evan Shute and his brother Dr. Wilfrid Shute, both cardiologists, continued to treat patients with vitamin E. They documented their clinical findings, but finding no journal willing to publish them, Dr. Evan Shute began publishing his own medical journal, *The Summary*.

In the 1950s, Abram Hoffer, MD, PhD, and Humphry Osmond, MD, demonstrated that niacin—vitamin B_3—and vitamin C could control some types of schizophrenia. They conducted the first double-blind study in psychiatry, which was published in the *Menninger Bulletin,* to demonstrate the effectiveness of niacin and vitamin C.

They have been largely ignored by the psychological and psychiatric establishment.

Still, niacin has been recognized for its ability to lower cholesterol—another discovery by Dr. Hoffer — although most conventional physicians still prefer to prescribe cholesterol-lowering drugs, such as lovastatin.

Orthomolecular Medicine

It's time to fast-forward to 1968—a major crossroads for nutrition.

In the April 19, 1968, issue of *Science,* Linus Pauling described his concept of orthomolecular psychiatry—a concept that has become the underpinning for all of orthomolecular, or nutritional, medicine.

We sometimes take the greatness of Linus Pauling, PhD, for granted. But let me remind you that he was awarded two Nobel prizes—and would probably have gotten a third, had the political terrorism of Joseph McCarthy, in the 1950s, not delayed Dr. Pauling from traveling to England. He had figured out the double-helix before Watson and Crick. But this time, political politics, not medical politics, stepped in the way.

Anyway, in the *Science* article, Dr. Pauling said essentially this: to achieve *optimal* health, a person must obtain optimal concentrations of the beneficial nutrients normally present in the body's cells. In a sense, these nutrients help prime the cell to its maximum efficiency—and maximum lifespan.

Pauling formalized a new nutrition paradigm, one based not on deficiency states but one based on optimal intakes. In defining orthomolecular medicine, Pauling was at least 25 years ahead of the medical community.

And it's my prediction that advances in genetic research will soon recognize that Dr. Pauling has been right all along, because researchers will realize that nutritional deficiencies are one of the factors that express the genes that cause cancer, Alzheimer's, and other diseases.

But I'm getting a little ahead of myself.

Of course, we all know that the medical establishment did not respond by saying, "Gee thanks, Linus." Instead, it attacked—even more so when Dr. Pauling published his book on vitamin C and the common cold two years later.

In the 1970s, medical journals were replete with articles attacking vitamin C and vitamin E. For example, in the fourth edition of *Human Nutrition and Dietetics,* published in 1970, Stanley Davidson and R. Passmore wrote, "Vitamin E is one of those embarrassing vitamins that have been identified, isolated and synthesized by physiologists and biochemists and then handed to the medical profession with the suggestion that a use should be found for it, without any satisfactory evidence to show that human beings are ever deficient of it or even that it is a necessary nutrient for man."

But Dr. Pauling had gotten people thinking about nutrition as something more than what people shovel into their stomachs. Research on vitamins and minerals began to quietly accumulate in the 1970s.

Nineteen eighty-two was another crossroads. It was in that year that the US National Academy of Sciences published *Diet, Nutrition and Cancer,* a report that conceded that diets high in beta-carotene and low in fat could protect against cancer, heart disease, and other degenerative diseases. Suddenly, nutrients could prevent something besides a deficiency disease.

The 1980s were a time of change, one small crossroad after another. More and more researchers focused on vitamins, minerals, and other food factors. More and more research on vitamins and minerals was funded by government agencies.

In the 1980s, momentum also grew for the free-radical theory of aging and disease, a theory originally proposed back in 1955. Free radicals are missing an electron, and nature abhors a vacuum. So as free radicals try to replace the missing electron, they steal one from healthy molecules. The effect is like a nuclear chain reaction, with free radicals spreading out like neutrons, damaging and aging cells.

But here's the catch. When you buy into the free-radical theory, you have to then buy into the "antioxidant vitamin" theory, because vitamins A, and C, and E, and selenium donate electrons to quench the free-radical cascade. So the growing evidence supporting the free-radical theory directly supports orthomolecular medicine.

The Impact of the Personal Computer

Something else happened in the 1980s. The personal computer changed the way people used computers, and this changed the way people disseminated and learned about medical research.

The vast Medline database, developed by the National Library of Medicine, which is part of the US National Institutes of Health, became directly accessible by end-users in the late 1980s.

Let me tell you what this means. Medical libraries have traditionally been oppressive places—really, obstacles to knowledge. In the "old days" thousands of medical journals crowded the shelves, discouraging a lot of people from using them by their sheer volume.

With Medline, I can access abstracts from more than 3,000 medical journals over the last 20 or so years. By typing a few keystrokes, I can discover in seconds that almost 700 articles on vitamin E were published in 1992. By cross-referencing vitamin E with Parkinson's disease, I can quickly see all the abstracts for articles on this subject. At the same time, I find out who the author was, the journal, the date of publication . . . and then all I have to do is walk over, pick up the specific journal, and read it to find out the details.

The Medline computer database has made information about nutritional medicine much easier to access than ever before. Medline has made my job as a medical reporter easier, and it has made library research easier for physicians. You still have to ask the computer to search for something specific, but it has turned a discouraging, laborious process into something that's about at the level of a computer game.

These days, if someone pooh-poohs vitamin E, or vitamin C, or coenzyme Q_{10}, you'll probably hear me say, "Why don't you read the literature." With Medline so easy to use, the only thing that keeps conventional doctors from learning about nutritional therapy is overbooking their patients—or laziness.

Let me tell you just a little bit about what has been in the medical journals over the past year.

- In light of the Shutes' experiences, at the top of the list are the well-designed epidemiological studies on vitamin E by Meir Stampfer, MD, and Eric Rimm, ScD. They were published in the May 20, 1993, *New England Journal of Medicine.* Stampfer set out to disprove an association between vitamin E and heart disease. As it turned out, he confirmed that supplements—not ordinary dietary levels—of vitamin E dramatically reduced the incidence of heart disease. While Stampfer stopped short of recommending that the average person take vitamin E supplements, he did acknowledge to a *New York Times* reporter that he takes the vitamin himself.
- If you read the medical literature, you'll find that vitamin E also increases the success rate of both balloon angioplasty and bypass surgery. See the article on vitamin E and bypass surgery by Coghlan in the *Journal of Thoracic and Cardiovascular Surgery* (Aug. 1993;106:268–74).
- We all know about the wonders of beta-carotene. The *American Journal of Clinical Nutrition* (Feb. 1994;59:409–12) reported a experiment in which beta-carotene protected against genetic damage caused by radiation. Other research is showing that less well-known carotenoids, such as alpha-carotene and lycopene, may be even more potent.
- The flavonoids, or bioflavonoids, once considered part of the vitamin C complex, are also emerging as nutrients in their own right. A study of 805 Dutch men found that diets high in the flavonoids protect against heart disease and heart attacks, according to an article in *Lancet* (Oct. 23, 1993; 342:1007–11).
- The flavonoids, which function as antioxidants, are high in vegetables, soybeans, and tofu. Finnish and Japanese researchers reported in *Lancet* (Nov. 13, 1993;342:1209–10) that a high intake of flavonoids found in soy products probably reduces the risk of death from prostate cancer.
- Garlic, too, is recognized in the medical literature for its therapeutic potential. One study published in the *American Journal of Medicine* (June 1993;94:632–5) reported that people taking garlic capsules benefited from an 11 percent reduction in their serum low-density lipoprotein levels.
- In *Biochemical and Biophysical Research Communications* (April 15, 1993;192:241–5), Karl Folkers, PhD, MD, of the University of Texas at Austin, reported using coenzyme Q_{10}, a nutrient that Folkers regrets not calling a vitamin, to treat ten cancer patients. Some of the patients have lived for three, nine, ten, and 15 years—recovering from heart failure and showing no signs of recurring cancer.

- Here's one more piece of research on propolis, the stuff bees use to seal their hives. People either swear by propolis—or swear about it. In *Cancer Research* (Sept. 15, 1993;53:1482–88), researchers reported that several naturally occurring caffeic acid esters found in honey and propolis significantly inhibited colon cancer in a dose-dependent manner.

Insurance Companies

Nutrition research reached another crossroads last year, when Blue Cross/Blue Shield Insurance decided it would pay for heart patients to enroll in Dean Ornish's heart-disease-reversal program, based on diet instead of drugs and surgery. The $3,000 program is 10 percent of the cost of coronary artery bypass surgery.

Insurance companies have traditionally been the bane of nutritional therapies. They don't like paying for "experimental" treatments. But with today's health care crisis—a crisis triggered by the greed and marketing of hospitals, drug companies, and medical instrument companies—vitamins are the inexpensive alternative. Even more important, nutritional therapies focus on prevention as well as treatment—instead of high-priced, high-tech, late-stage medical care.

I predict that, once they realize how much money they can save, insurance companies may become one of our strongest allies in nutritional medicine.

But even the insurance companies are up against some tough opposition.

Coenzyme Q_{10}

This is where things get a little sinister. For years, most of us believed that the drug companies ignored vitamins because they couldn't be patented and, thus, they cannot make a lot of money off them. In most respects, they can't be patented. But people can acquire "use-patents" for specific nutrients.

For example, Richard Wurtman, PhD, of Massachusetts Institute of Technology, who has done some excellent research on tryptophan and serotonin and brain chemistry, has use-patent #4,377,595 for tryptophan in the treatment of depression. He also has use-patent #4,737,489 for choline in the treatment of neurological diseases and aging. The pharmaceutical giant Sigma Tau has been marketing a prescription version of carnitine—acetyl-L-carnitine—in Italy for several years, and the company has just completed a double-blind, crossover study of 430 Alzheimer's patients at 27 US medical centers.

While I'm not sure there's a grand conspiracy at work—there may be, or there may not be—there are powerful, greedy forces at work. These use-patents are virtually worthless as long as these substances are available over the counter as nutritional supplements.

I'd like to talk a little more about coenzyme Q_{10} in this context. CoQ_{10} is a nutrient found almost universally in food, but is exceptionally high in organ meats and tuna.

The body makes it, also, in a 17-step enzymatic process dependently largely on the B-complex vitamins. CoQ_{10}'s primary function is in producing adenosine triphosphate (ATP) and stimulating the mitochondria, the energy factories of our cells. Secondary to that, it functions as an antioxidant.

Much of what we know about CoQ_{10} goes back to Karl Folkers at the University of Texas, Austin. In 20 years of reporting nutritional medicine, I don't think I've seen anything quite like it.

CoQ_{10} is an effective treatment for cardiomyopathy and other forms of heart failure. Cardiologists typically treat cardiomyopathy with ACE (angiotensin-converting enzyme) inhibitors, digitalis, diuretics, or beta-blockers. Cardiothoracic surgeons consider a heart transplant the ideal treatment—at $150,000 for the surgery, and $2,000 a month for lifelong medication. CoQ_{10} will cure cardiomyopathy for $30–$40 a month. It's all superbly documented in the medical literature.

James Ryan, an investment banker, was one of the patients in Karl Folker's first trial of CoQ_{10} in the early 1980s. Ryan had been diagnosed with congestive heart failure and told he had 18 months to live. Fourteen years later, he is still very much alive. The only people who live that long with cardiomyopathy are people who take CoQ_{10}, and Ryan had been taking it since that study over ten years ago.

In 1988, Karl Folkers and the late Per Langsjoen, MD, a cardiologist, become the "inventors" of the CoQ_{10} treatment of AIDS. They published a paper in *Biochemical and Biophysical Research Communications* (June 16, 1988;153:888–96) describing the treatment of seven AIDS patients. The results were dramatic.

The University of Texas, where they did the research, applied for a use-patent on September 21, 1987, and was granted it—#5,011,858 on April 30, 1991. In 1992, Ryan created Ryan Pharmaceuticals Inc., and bought the use-patent from the University of Texas. He, in turn, sold Ryan Pharmaceuticals and the CoQ_{10} use-patent for the treatment of AIDS to Receptagen, a joint US/Canadian biotechnology company, in 1993, for about $2 million.

What's the use-patent worth? Not much, as long as CoQ_{10} is still available as a dietary supplement. But take CoQ_{10} off the market, and it's probably worth hundreds of millions of dollars.

Problems with Medical Journalists

Now, let me turn my attention to medical reporters. The question I've asked about CoQ_{10} and other nutrients for years—and I'm sure the question you've asked—is why you don't read all this in the daily newspapers or news magazines.

I'll give you my opinion, an opinion based on my experience as a medical reporter and as someone who has also worked in advertising and public relations. In most of journalism, reporters are taught to get a statement from the "other side." This ensures some semblance of balanced reporting. In politics, it may be calling a Democrat when a Republican makes an announcement, or getting a comment from a consumer group when a company makes some pronouncement.

If the average political reporter related what a senator or president said—without seeking a contrasting opinion—he'd be viewed as little more than a public relations hack posing as a journalist. Of course, no political reporter in his right mind would accept statements at face value from a politician.

Yet this lack of critical perspective permeates medical reporting. Most medical reporters report only what's described by "the experts" and by the public relations people who work for hospitals, pharmaceutical manufacturers, and other companies that make their profits from health care. They think medicine is a single-party system in which decisions are arrived at rationally.

Most medical reporters ignore the fact that "nonprofit" hospitals compete as fiercely for market share as profit-making businesses. They report high-tech advances as if they are miraculous benefits for humankind, rather than as new profit centers. Reporters dutifully describe the value of carpal tunnel surgery, but ignore an effective, low-cost nonsurgical treatment, like vitamin B_6. And they faithfully repeat the need for more donor hearts for transplants, but remain oblivious to the medical literature on the use of CoQ_{10}.

Medical reporting has largely been devoid of the checks and balances found in political reporting. The reason is that most medical reporters have been convinced by the establishment's experts and by their public relations people that they simply cannot understand medicine. They can, of course, understand the Byzantine politics of Washington and Ottawa. They can understand nuclear power—or at least think they can. But reporters are convinced they're too dumb to understand medicine.

I don't believe that (although I know my limitations and absorb medicine a bite at a time). But that's what they've been told in very, very subtle ways. And when they believe it, they can be spoon-fed anything. That vitamin E is a cure in search of a disease. That vitamin C has no value in heart disease or cancer. That Prozac or Zoloft are the drugs of choice in depression, instead of vitamin B_6 or tryptophan. And that beta-carotene won't protect you against smoking—without asking why anything should protect you against a really disgusting, dangerous habit.

In conclusion, it's clear: nutrition is not at just one crossroads. Nutrition has crossed many roads, and it continues to. We have reached a time when the scientific evidence supporting the preventive and therapeutic use of vitamins, minerals, and other food factors is literally overwhelming. It's all in the medical literature.

In the next few years, we will finally see the acceptability of what has for years been unacceptable: nutritional therapy.

Additional Reading

This book can't possibly cover it all, nor does it intend to. To learn more about nutritional (orthomolecular) medicine and healthful living, here is a short list of some additional titles you may want to look into.

Brighthope, I.E., A.W. Saul. *The Vitamin Cure for Diabetes: Prevent and Treat Diabetes Using Nutrition and Vitamin Supplementation.* Laguna Beach, CA: Basic Health Publications, 2012.

Written by Australian physician Ian Brighthope, MD, who has tremendous experience in the area of nutrition, this book will help women (or men) who struggle with diabetes and want to know more about natural treatment approaches.

Calton, J., M. Calton. *Rich Food Poor Food: The Ultimate Grocery Purchasing System (GPS).* Malibu, CA: Primal Nutrition, 2013.

A guide for navigating the grocery store and helping work your way up the food continuum to the best food possible, this is a useful resource for anyone looking to improve their diet.

Campbell, R., A.W. Saul. *The Vitamin Cure for Children's Health Problems: Prevent and Treat Children's Health Problems Using Nutrition and Vitamin C Supplementation.* Laguna Beach, CA: Basic Health Publications, 2011.

Campbell, R., A.W. Saul. *The Vitamin Cure for Infant and Toddler Health Problems: Prevent and Treat Young Children's Health Problems Using Nutrition and Vitamin C Supplementation.* Laguna Beach, CA: Basic Health Publications, 2013.

Board-certified pediatrician Ralph Campbell, MD, and my father, Andrew W. Saul, PhD, wrote these books to help parents conquer health issues common to many children, and to do so safely and effectively with nutrition. My husband and I don't go to our pediatrician without checking these books first.

Case, H.S. *Vitamins & Pregnancy: The Real Story. Your Orthomolecular Guide for Healthy Babies and Happy Moms.* Nashville, TN: Turner Publishing, 2016.

My third book written especially for expectant parents interested in applying orthomolecular medicine to achieve a happy, healthy pregnancy and baby.

Case, H.S. *The Vitamin Cure for Women's Health Problems.* Laguna Beach, CA: Basic Health Publications, 2012.

My first book, aimed at helping women successfully treat common health problems like premenstrual syndrome, yeast infections, stress, anxiety, depression, urinary tract infections, and menopause, and more with vitamins and without pharmaceuticals.

Cass, H., K. Barnes. *8 Weeks to Vibrant Health: A Take-Charge Plan for Women to Correct Imbalances, Reclaim Energy and Restore Well-Being.* New York, NY: McGraw Hill, 2011.

Written by Hyla Cass, MD, this book takes a balanced approach, looking at both prescription drugs and nutrients for the treatment of disease with a focus on doing the least invasive, safest option first. It is easy to read and packed with valuable information by a nationally recognized expert in the field of integrative medicine.

Challem, J. *The Food Mood Solution: All-Natural Ways to Banish Anxiety, Depression, Anger, Stress, Overeating, and Alcohol and Drug Problems—and Feel Good Again.* Hoboken, NJ: Wiley, 2008.

Nutrition expert Jack Challem has written numerous books and articles. Known as "The Nutrition Reporter," he demystifies research by clearly explaining scientific studies. Here he shows you how food can work for you.

Crook, W.G., C. Dean, E. Crook. *The Yeast Connection and Women's Health.* 2nd edition. Jackson, TN: Professional Books, 2005.

Here is a book that should be on every woman's bookshelf. Yeast overgrowth is more common than most people think, and we aren't just talking about localized yeast infections.

Dean, C. *The Magnesium Miracle.* Revised and updated. New York: Ballantine Books, 2007.

That title is not a typo. You may be amazed at just how much this mineral plays a role in your health and the prevention of illness. Carolyn Dean is both a medical doctor and a naturopath and has written over two dozen books on natural health. This is a very important book worth reading.

Downing, D. *The Vitamin Cure for Allergies.* Laguna Beach, CA: Basic Health Publications, 2010.

This one is often borrowed off my bookshelf. Damien Downing, MD, has written a very real and engaging book about how to manage (and prevent) allergies naturally.

Gaby, A.R. *Nutritional Medicine.* Concord, NH: Fritz Perlberg Publishing, 2011.

If you are looking for a textbook of nutritional medicine, here you go. While Alan Gaby, MD, has intended this substantial book for health care practitioners, it is a valuable addition to anyone's alternative-medicine library.

González, M. J., Miranda, J. R., Saul, A. W. *I Have Cancer: What Should I Do? Your Orthomolecular Guide for Cancer Management.* Laguna Beach, CA: Basic Health Publications, 2009.

If you or someone you love has been diagnosed with cancer and seek to integrate orthomolecular therapy, this book shows how optimum nutrition and dietary supplements can both prevent and treat cancer.

Hickey, S. *The Vitamin Cure for Migraines: How to Prevent and Treat Migraine Headaches Using Nutrition and Vitamin Supplementation.* Laguna Beach, CA: Basic Health Publications, 2010.

If you suffer from migraines, you know you need all the help you can get. Written by Steven Hickey, who has a doctorate in medical biophysics, this book shows you why nutrition should be your first choice when it comes to the treatment of migraine headaches.

Hickey, S., A.W. Saul. *Vitamin C: The Real Story, the Remarkable and Controversial Healing Factor.* Laguna Beach, CA: Basic Health Publications, 2008.

If you want to know more about vitamin C, this is the book to read. I've been taking C my whole life, but for those getting started, or those who want to know more, this book is a wonderful resource.

Hoffer, A., A.W. Saul. *Orthomolecular Medicine for Everyone: Megavitamin Therapeutics for Families and Physicians.* Laguna Beach, CA: Basic Health Publications, 2008.

My go-to guide. Those interested in orthomolecular medicine may want to read this first. Written in part by Abram Hoffer, MD, PhD, a pioneer of orthomolecular medicine, this book is truly for everyone.

Hoffer A., A.W. Saul, H. D. Foster. *Niacin: The Real Story.* Laguna Beach, CA: Basic Health Publications, 2012.

This is an excellent resource for those who want to learn more about the value and safety of niacin for the treatment of mood disorders.

Hoffer, A., A.W. Saul, S. Hickey. *Hospitals and Health: Your Orthomolecular Guide to a Shorter, Safer Hospital Stay.* Laguna Beach, CA: Basic Health Publications, 2011.

This one is essential for anyone expecting (or not expecting) to have a hospital stay, or for those who must care for others who must.

Hoffer, A., J. Prousky. *Anxiety: Orthomolecular Diagnosis and Treatment.* Toronto, ON: CCNM Press, 2007.

A natural approach to anxiety written by experts in their field.

Hoffer, A., J. Prousky. *Naturopathic Nutrition.* Toronto, ON: CCNM Press, 2006.

Abram Hoffer, MD, PhD, and Jonathan Prousky, ND, have written a practical and easy to read book for anyone interested in adopting orthomolecular principles into their diets for better health.

Hoffer, A., A.W. Saul. *The Vitamin Cure for Alcoholism.* Laguna Beach, CA: Basic Health Publications, 2009.

Yes, even Bill W., cofounder of Alcoholics Anonymous, promoted the use of megavitamin therapy to treat alcohol addiction. Written by Abram Hoffer, MD, PhD, and Andrew W. Saul, PhD, this book shows that alcoholism is primarily a metabolic disease that can (and should) be successfully and safely treated with optimal nutrition.

Holford, P. *Optimum Nutrition for the Mind.* London: Piatkus, 2003.

Author of the popular book The Optimum Nutrition Bible *(and over thirty others), Patrick Holford writes material that is always worth reading. This one is no exception. Both a nutrition expert and psychologist, he shows how nutrition can increase IQ and concentration, improve memory, mood, and sleep, beat depression, conquer stress and anxiety, and much more.*

Jonsson, B.H., A.W. Saul. *The Vitamin Cure for Depression: How to Prevent and Treat Depression Using Nutrition and Vitamin Supplementation.* Laguna Beach, CA: Basic Health Publications, 2012.

This book gives you what you are likely not getting from your doctor: the clear value of vitamins and other nutrients to combat depression.

Levy, T.E. *Curing the Incurable: Vitamin C, Infectious Diseases, and Toxins.* Philadelphia, PA: Xlibris Corporation, 2002.

Levy, T.E. *Primal Panacea.* Henderson, NV: MedFox Publishing, 2011.

Both a medical doctor and a lawyer, Thomas Levy knows exactly what he is talking about. Readers will find great comfort in understanding the critical role that optimal vitamin C intake has for the reduction of toxins, the prevention of vaccine side effects, its antiviral and antibiotic properties, and much more, as well as its proven safety in both adults and children.

Pauling, L. *How to Live Longer and Feel Better.* Corvallis, OR: Oregon State University Press, 2006.

The classic must-read for anyone interested in orthomolecular medicine written by the guy who gave it its name, and how it can do exactly what the title claims.

Prousky, J. *The Vitamin Cure for Chronic Fatigue Syndrome: How to Prevent and Treat Chronic Fatigue Syndrome Using Safe and Effective Natural Therapies.* Laguna, Beach, CA: Basic Health Publications, 2010.

If you suffer from fatigue, muscle and joint pain, memory or concentration issues, feeling poorly after you exercise, and not feeling rested after you sleep, you may want to investigate the possibility of chronic fatigue. Written by a naturopath, Johnathan Prousky, coauthor of Anxiety: Orthomolecular Diagnosis and Treatment, *this book may be just what you are looking for.*

Roberts, H., and S. Hickey. *The Vitamin Cure for Heart Disease.* Laguna Beach, CA: Basic Health Publications, 2011.

If you want to learn what really causes heart disease, how not to get it, and how it can be treated, even reversed, with proper supplementation, you'll want to read this important and well-written book by Hilary Roberts, PhD, and Steve Hickey, PhD.

Saul, A.W. *Doctor Yourself: Natural Healing That Works.* 2nd edition. Laguna Beach, CA: Basic Health Publications, 2012.

Saul, A.W. *Fire Your Doctor: How to Be Independently Healthy.* Laguna Beach, CA: Basic Health Publications, 2005.

If you'd like to learn more about your health while actually enjoying reading about it, these books are a great place to start. Both are written by my father, who is always a great inspiration to me.

Saul, A.W., editor. *The Orthomolecular Treatment of Chronic Disease.* Laguna Beach, CA: Basic Health Publications, 2014.

This is a reference book, but it reads as enjoyably as a good novel. It's enormous, it's interesting, and it's packed with articles from over 65 experts in nutritional healing.

Saul, A.W., H.S. Case. *Vegetable Juicing for Everyone. How to Get Your Family Healthier and Happier, Faster!* Laguna Beach, CA: Basic Health Publications, 2013.

I wrote this one along with my father. It is not a juicing recipe book. (There are lots of those out there already.) If you want to get motivated and excited about juicing vegetables, while being entertained at the same time with stories about our off-kilter family, it might be just the thing.

Smith, R. G., and T. Penberthy. *The Vitamin Cure for Arthritis.* Laguna Beach, CA: Basic Health Publications, 2015.

Written by research scientist Robert G. Smith, PhD, author of The Vitamin Cure for Eye Disease, *and biochemist Todd Penberthy, PhD, this book shows that damage to our joints can be reversed through nutrition. A valuable resource for anyone seeking to prevent, treat, or reverse arthritis.*

About the Author

Helen Saul Case is the author of *The Vitamin Cure for Women's Health Problems* and *Vitamins & Pregnancy: The Real Story* and coauthor of *Vegetable Juicing for Everyone.* She appears in the film *That Vitamin Movie* (2016). Mrs. Case is Assistant Editor for the peer-reviewed *Orthomolecular Medicine News Service* and she has published in the *Journal of Orthomolecular Medicine.* She is the daughter of Andrew W. Saul, star of the movie *Food Matters* and author of many popular books, including *Doctor Yourself.* Mrs. Case currently lives with her husband and children in western New York. She can be found on Facebook and at her website helensaulcase.com.

Index

CPSIA information can be obtained
at www.ICGtesting.com
Printed in the USA
BVOW06s0926170517
484264BV00018B/86/P